# Evaluation of Health Promotion and Disease Prevention Programs

FIFTH EDITION | # Evaluation of Health Promotion and Disease Prevention Programs

## IMPROVING POPULATION HEALTH THROUGH EVIDENCE-BASED PRACTICE

**RICHARD A. WINDSOR, MS, PHD, MPH**

OXFORD
UNIVERSITY PRESS

# OXFORD
UNIVERSITY PRESS

Oxford University Press is a department of the University of
Oxford. It furthers the University's objective of excellence in research,
scholarship, and education by publishing worldwide.

Oxford   New York
Auckland   Cape Town   Dar es Salaam   Hong Kong   Karachi
Kuala Lumpur   Madrid   Melbourne   Mexico City   Nairobi
New Delhi   Shanghai   Taipei   Toronto

With offices in
Argentina   Austria   Brazil   Chile   Czech Republic   France   Greece
Guatemala   Hungary   Italy   Japan   Poland   Portugal   Singapore
South Korea   Switzerland   Thailand   Turkey   Ukraine   Vietnam

Oxford is a registered trademark of Oxford University Press
in the UK and certain other countries.

Published in the United States of America by
Oxford University Press
198 Madison Avenue, New York, NY 10016

Library of Congress Cataloging-in-Publication Data
Windsor, Richard A., author.
[Evaluation of health promotion, health education, and disease prevention programs]
Evaluation of health promotion and disease prevention programs : improving population health
through evidenced-based practice / Richard Windsor. — 5th edition.
     p. ; cm.
Preceded by Evaluation of health promotion, health education, and disease prevention programs /
Richard Windsor... [et al.]. 3rd ed. c2004.
The 4th ed. was self-published in 2010 under the title: Evaluation of health promotion and disease
prevention and management programs.
Includes bibliographical references.
ISBN 978–0–19–023507–9
I. Title.
[DNLM: 1.  Health Education—organization & administration.   2.  Evaluation Studies as Topic.
3.  Evidence-Based Practice.   4.  Health Promotion—methods.   WA 590]
RA440.5
613—dc23
2014042592

9 8 7 6 5 4 3 2 1
Printed in the United States of America
on acid-free paper

# CONTENTS

# ACKNOWLEDGMENTS

A SPECIAL NOTE OF RECOGNITION AND appreciation is extended to my colleagues, all professors of Public Health, who served as contributing authors of the first, second, and third editions: Tom Baranowski of Baylor University, Noreen Clark of the University of Michigan, and Gary Cutter of the University of Alabama at Birmingham.

Special thanks are extended to reviewers of the previous editions.

First edition reviewers (1984): Charles Baffi, Virginia Polytechnic University; Lorraine Davis, University of Oregon; Robert S. Gold, Southern Illinois University; Jennie K. Kronenfeld, University of South Carolina; and James Price, University of Toledo.

Second edition reviewers (1994): Catherine Crooks, Middle Tennessee State University; Richard Petosa, Ohio State University; and Yuzuru J. Takeshita, University of Michigan.

Third edition reviewers (2004): Rick Boyd, University of Medicine and Dentistry of New Jersey; Bob Goodman, University of Indiana; Randy Black, Purdue University; Robert E. Fullilove, Columbia University; Kimberly M. Harper, Florida A & M University; John Sciacca, Northern Arizona University; and Robert Valois, University of South Carolina.

Fourth edition reviewers (2010): Richard Boyd, Rutgers University; Sean Cleary, George Washington University; David Driscoll, University of Alaska-Anchorage; and Dwight Harshbarger, West Virginia University.

# ABOUT THE AUTHOR

**Richard Windsor, MS, PhD, MPH,** received a BS (Honors, 1969) at Morgan State College (an HBUC), and MS (1970) and PhD (1972) in Community Health Education from the University of Illinois with an emphasis in Educational-Social Psychology and Survey-Evaluation Research Methods. He was an Assistant Professor, School of Education, at Ohio State University (1972–1975). He completed a Post-Doctoral Fellowship and an MPH in Maternal and Child Health (MCH) Services Research at The Johns Hopkins University (JHU) School of Public Health (1975–1976). He was an Assistant Professor at JHU (1976–1977) and Coordinator of "COPD Evaluation Trial for Primary Care Physicians" of coal miners and families in Western Pennsylvania, funded by the National Institutes of Health (NIH) and the United Mine Workers Health & Retirement Funds, Washington, D.C.

He was recruited in 1977 to help create the University of Alabama (UAB) School of Public Health (SPH) and Department of Health Behavior (DHB). He was a participant and contributor to the first, second, and third CEPH-SPH Accreditation Self-Studies. He was Associate Professor-Tenured (1978–1983) and Professor-Chair-DHB (1984–1991), and created with his Faculty the MPH, MSPH, DrPH, PhD, and Post-Doctoral Programs in Health Promotion–Disease Prevention. He was a Senior Scientist (1978–1991) and Associate Director for Cancer Prevention and Control of the National Cancer Institute (NCI) designated Comprehensive Cancer Center of Alabama at the UAB Medical Center (1987–1991).

He was Associate Director (AD) for Prevention of the National Heart, Lung, and BIood Institute (NHLBI), Director, Office of Prevention,

Education, and Control (OPEC, 1991–1993) and was appointed to the US Government Senior Executive Service (SES 4) by the Department of Health and Human Services (DHHS) Secretary. As AD, he was a member of the NHLBI Executive Committee and supervised PhD/MD trained staff who coordinated the OPEC-based National Asthma, Blood Resources, Cholesterol, Heart Attack Alert, and High Blood Pressure Programs. Following his federal appointment at NIH, he was a Research Professor (1994–2000) and Lead Science Advisor, Robert Wood Johnson Foundation, Smoke Free Families–National Program Office, Department of Obstetrics/Gynecology, UAB School of Medicine (1994–2002). He was Primary Investigator (PI) of the NCI-funded (1997–2002) SCRIPT Trial III, a collaborative project with the Alabama Health Department.

He has been PI or Co-PI of 15 peer-reviewed evaluations funded by the NIH, NCI, NHLBI, the National Institute of Child Health and Human Development (NICHD), the National Institute on Drug Abuse (NIDA), National Center for Health Services Research (NCHSR), and the Centers for Disease Control and Prevention (CDC) (> $24 Million/Direct + Indirect). He has been PI or Co-PI of 10 "Smoking Cessation and Reduction In Pregnancy Treatment (SCRIPT) Trials" (1982–2012). He directed five projects as the Co-PI with colleagues at UAB, JHU, Mayo Clinic, Brown University, and George Washington University (GWU) Medical Centers and the leadership and clinical staff of local and state Departments of Public Health. He was the PI of the NCI-funded "WV RFTS-SCRIPT Dissemination Program" (2007–2012). It was the first evaluation to document the adoption and behavioral impact for a state-wide Perinatal Division and home-based Medicaid population of the AHRQ (2000 and 2008) recommended SCRIPT Program.

The SCRIPT Program was recommended by the Agency for Healthcare Research and Quality (AHRQ, 2000 and 2008) Tobacco Treatment Clinical Practice Guidelines, and the American Congress of Obstetricians and Gynecologists (ACOG) as an effective intervention for use in prenatal care. He has published more than 100 reports, including 50 SCRIPT Trial process, impact, and CEA-CBA evaluation reports. He received the 1997 C. Everett Koop National Health Award for his direction of the SCRIPT evaluations (1982–1997). He was elected to Delta Omega, JHU-SPH (1999), for his contributions to the fields of MCH and Program Evaluation.

He has been a Consultant to the US Agency for International Development (USAID), the World Health Organization (WHO), multiple NIH Institutes, the CDC, the Robert Wood Johnson Foundation (RWJF), and the Ministries of Health of China, Canada, Ireland,

Singapore, and the United Kingdom (NICE). He has been a Visiting Professor at 10 universities in Australia, China, England, Scotland, and Singapore. He was a past Vice President, President (1980–1982) and was elected a Distinguished Fellow of the Society of Public Health Education (1999). He is the author of *Evaluation of HP-DP Programs* (1st ed., 1984; 2nd ed., 1994; 3rd ed., 2004; McGraw-Hill). It was published in Chinese (1990) and Korean (2005). In the fall of 2009 on sabbatical as a Visiting Professor, University of London School of Hygiene and Tropical Medicine, he completing the fourth edition: *Evaluation of Health Promotion–Disease Prevention and Management Programs* (2010). This volume, published by Oxford University Press, is the fifth edition of this textbook.

The author was a tenured Professor (> 2000–2014) at George Washington University School of Public Health and was jointly appointed Presidential Professor of Public Health, University of Alaska Anchorage (2007–2013). Since 1972 he has taught "Evaluation of HP-DP Programs" courses and has mentored MS-MPH-MSPH-DrPH-PhD and Post-Doctoral students in multiple Schools of Public Health in the United States and abroad. He was elected Professor Emeritus on July 1, 2014, by the Faculty of George Washington University.

## Fifth Edition Contributing Author

**Neal Richard Boyd, MS, EdD, MSPH,** received a BA in History from Carson-Newman College (1971), a MS in Safety Education (1978), and EdD in Health Education (1981) from the University of Tennessee. He was an Assistant-Associate Professor-Chair in the Department of Health and Safety Education, University of Southern Mississippi (1981–1989). He was a Post-Doctoral Fellow in Cancer Prevention and Control, Comprehensive Cancer Center of Alabama and UAB-SPH (1989–91) and received an MSPH in Behavioral Science (1991) from the UAB-SPH. He was an NCI Cancer Prevention Fellow (1991–1993) and Senior Scientist of the Faculty of the Fox Chase Comprehensive Cancer Center (1993–1999). He was a Professor-Director, DrPH Program in the Department of Prevention and Community Health in the School of Public Health at George Washington University (2001–2006). He is Professor and was Associate Dean for Academic Programs at the School of Public Health, University of Medicine and Dentistry of New Jersey (2006–2010). He prepared Chapter 2 for the fourth and fifth editions.

## Fifth Edition Contributing Editor

**Regina Crawford Windsor, BA, MPH,** graduated from Middlebury College (2002) majoring in International Studies and Spanish Literature, and minored in the History of Art and Architecture. She worked at National Geographic in Development and Translations, Washington, DC (2002–2003), after graduation. She received an MPH (2007) in Epidemiology and Global Health from the UAB-School of Public Health (SPH). After a field experience in Sub-Saharan Africa, she was a member of the staff at the John J. Sparkman Center for Global Health, UAB-SPH (2008–2009). She served as a Science Editor at the Natural Standard Research Collaboration, a company designed to systematically review, publish, and disseminate the evidence base for Integrative and Alternative Medical Treatment Methods (Boston, 2009–2013). She is a science editor, writer, and researcher in Cambridge, Massachusetts. She served as a Contributing Editor of the fifth edition.

# 1 | Introduction to Health Promotion and Disease Prevention Program Evaluation

Chance favors the prepared.

*—Louis Pasteur*

## Introduction

Public health and population health professionals must know how to produce valid evidence; to succeed, they must know what is effective and, equally important, what does not work for whom and in what settings. Although guidelines to conduct systematic reviews and ratings of evaluations of Health Promotion and Disease Prevention and Management (HP-DP) programs have existed for decades, most published "evaluations" do not meet well-established meta-evaluation (ME) and meta-analysis (MA) criteria. Many do not meet the core standards of professional practice. Thus, one the most salient challenges to HP-DP program, policy, and evaluation leadership is to dramatically increase the percentage of the next generation of evaluations that meet established (global) standards of planning and evaluation practice. The following is an introduction to the scope of the challenge to future HP-DP program evaluations.

According to the US Census Bureau International Data Base, the world population was 3 billion in 1960, 6 billion in 2000, and is over 7 billion in 2015. The US population increased from 180 million in 1960 to over 320 million in 2015. Many factors, including large population, production, migration, and development transitions in each decade, modified the environment within and between countries, especially in the last 30 years. While large variations exist in the distribution and trends of communicable and non-communicable diseases (NCD) between and within all countries, a global consensus exists. The next generation will experience a dramatic shift in the distribution of morbidity and mortality, a shift from younger to older population, and a shift from acute to chronic conditions.

Current estimates, for example of the "Global Burden of Disease" in *Lancet* (2012), confirm that about 60%–70% of the causes of these trends are primarily, but far from exclusively, attributable to modifiable behavioral risk factors. Thus, while individual and population behavior change will always be difficult to produce, regardless of the country, problem, population, or program setting, human behavior will continue to be a primary focus of future health HP-DP programs. The equally complex, concurrent issue to be addressed is, how do we significantly improve the methodological quality of evaluations and the internal and external validity of solutions to the problems noted?

During the last three decades of population transitions, agencies in the United States (e.g., the National Institutes of Health [NIH] and the Centers for Disease Control and Prevention [CDC]) and in the European Union (e.g., the National Institute for Health and Clinical Excellence [NICE, UK]), as well as multiple nongovernmental organizations (NGO) in countries throughout the world, have examined the role that behavioral, social, and environmental determinants play in the promotion of health and prevention, and the management of disease. There is general agreement among multiple sources of insight in the public-population health science community. Typically, no single risk factor, method, model, or solution to improving health exists for future chronic or acute disease trends.

While an emphasis by programs and evaluations on individual behaviors or risk factors (*downstream indicators*) will yield results for specific problems and populations, future HP-DP initiatives will enhance their success by concurrently focusing on behavior and a combination of other salient factors and determinants, for example, family, community, and physical and social environments (*upstream indicators*). In making future decisions about solutions, planning a program and its evaluation, key stakeholders must have a clearer picture of and make adjustments to the "contextual issues" of the problem, population, and setting. Future HP-DP solutions will need to have a broader perspective: a Population Health Model (PHM). The application of a PHM and the PRECEDE-PROCEED Planning Framework, discussed in detail in Chapter 2, should increase the probability of producing more "practice-based evidence" and "evidenced-based practice."

## Chapter Overview

This chapter discusses the common purposes of evaluation and the role of evaluation in achieving an organization or a program mission. Planning and evaluation are presented as inseparable concepts and processes. Because members of an evaluation team need to know and need to be able to routinely use a common language with clarity and consistency, common evaluation terms and definitions are presented. The issues of competence and credentialing in evaluation planning as core functions of HP-DP professional practice are reviewed. Because behavior is always a determinant of a population's health, competencies in evaluation for MPH-MSPH-MS programs for health education-promotion specialists are described. We discuss the critical importance of conducting systematic reviews and syntheses of bodies of evidence—meta-evaluation (ME) and meta-analysis (MA)—as one of the first steps (1) to determine "best practice" intervention methods for a specific health problem, (2) to define valid qualitative, process, impact, and outcome measures, and (3) to describe the current types and levels of intervention efficacy or effectiveness, and program costs.

With these foundation discussions, a framework and ME methods to define the Evaluation PHASE are presented. ME is defined as an assessment of the degree of validity and maturation of the HP-DP measurement and intervention science and practice base for a specific risk factor, a problem, a defined population at risk, and a program delivery setting. Contemporary evaluations demand that planning and evaluation stakeholders develop productive and collaborative relationships to successfully implement programs and evaluations. The purpose of an Evaluability Assessment is to gather information and insight from key stakeholders about the readiness of a program to conduct an evaluation. Accordingly, we examine a basic organizational-consensus development concept in evaluation: "Science-Policy-Practice Partnerships."

We present a brief synopsis, "Evaluation Progress Reviews," ranging from 1960 to 2020, of the development of HP-DP program evaluation as a specialty field, and provide an update and brief commentary on the World Health Organization (WHO) Millennium Development Goals (MDG, 2013). The enduring "science-policy-practice gap" in HP-DP planning and evaluation is discussed, reflecting the failure of many programs in high-, middle-, and low-income countries to meet basic standards of practice. Because poorly designed evaluations of interventions cannot produce valid evidence and benefit current or future participants, discussions of the inherent ethical concerns and significant inefficiencies, and the need for a stronger, independent peer review system of new HP-DP evaluation initiatives, are presented. While no simple solution exists to resolve all issues cited in the literature, contemporary evaluation leadership and teams need to embrace and apply a trans-disciplinary philosophy to overcome the barriers to implementing a best practices approach. The chapter concludes with comments about future challenges to HP-DP program evaluation.

It is an illusion to think of evaluation as primarily a scientific and analytical endeavor. If an evaluation team is multidisciplinary, and its director and team have the necessary graduate level credentials and experience, drafting a scientifically valid plan will be the easier task in the evaluation development process. *The true test of the technical-professional competency of an evaluation team demands a much broader skill set. A successful leader and team need to have the emotional intelligence, organizational leadership, and communication skills to balance internal and external political demands while concurrently making programmatic and methodological adjustments to address professional practice and client concerns. All of these adjustments need to be made without compromising core scientific principles to produce valid evidence of implementation and effectiveness.* Topics introduced in this chapter are discussed in detail throughout the book.

## Target Audiences

This book introduces the evaluation student, members of an evaluation team, and organizational and political leadership to the multiple, enduring, and complex issues that must be addressed before a local agency, national program, or federal agency (e.g., Ministry of Health) can report, with a high degree of validity and confidence, that it has achieved its process and impact objectives. The book has three primary audiences: (1) graduate and post-graduate students in public and population health programs, especially health education–health promotion specialists, (2) HP-DP staff in planning and evaluation training courses, and (3) public-population health program leadership who plan, manage, and evaluate local, state, provincial, and national programs. A case-study approach applied in each chapter provides specific examples and data for each target audience. A variety of health problems, populations at risk, and settings are presented.

The book will also serve as a methodological guide and general reference text for HP-DP program leadership in agencies and organizations responsible for planning, reviewing, and funding evaluations. Although the content can be learned without the prerequisite courses, most individuals who will use this text, MS-MPH-DrPH-PhD students, will have had at least the following introductory courses as part of their graduate program: "Planning and Management of HP-DP Programs," "Introduction to the Application of Social-Behavioral Science Theory and Methods for Public Health," "Introduction to Biostatistics," and "Introduction to Epidemiology." The value of these courses to plan and implement an HP-DP program evaluation should be self-evident.

## Program Evaluation: A Trans-Disciplinary Process

Program evaluation is a core competency of graduate-level public and population health program planning, management, and practice. Evaluations incorporate principles, theories, and methods from multiple population science disciplines, including behavioral science–health education–health promotion, biostatistics, environmental and occupational health sciences, epidemiology, and health services policy-management-research. State-of-the-art and science HP-DP evaluations will systematically select and apply scientific theories and methods from an eclectic range of academic disciplines, including anthropology, basic biological-health sciences, communication, economics, education, engineering, information-system sciences, law, political science, psychology, and sociology. The challenge to an evaluation is to select the most salient insight.

The disciplines noted, and related scientific literatures, provide an evolving and maturing knowledge base for HP-DP professional practice. They define how to validly measure the acceptability, feasibility of delivery, efficacy or effectiveness, and cost of interventions for specific problems, target populations, and program settings. These disciplines collectively define the minimum proximal, intermediate, and distal psycho-social constructs, behaviors, and environmental and health status indicators that HP-DP programs must measure at periodic intervals. These disciplines define the "gold standard" of measurement science and analysis methods to produce valid data and rates representative of a problem and a defined population for a specific period of time.

Because of the complexity of causes and solutions, a *trans-disciplinary leadership philosophy and team* are needed to plan and evaluate HP-DP programs. Evaluation leadership needs to reflect this philosophy as it assesses and defines local, state/province, and country-level health problems and creates targeted programs for salient problems. *Regardless of the problem, however, a comprehensive HP-DP program evaluation would have at least four core objectives:*

1. To produce valid evidence to document that a tailored, replicable HP-DP program was acceptable to and was delivered with fidelity by providers and regular practice sites, and was acceptable to a representative sample of a target population at risk (*process + qualitative evaluation*);
2. To document that the HP-DP program delivered was the most plausible explanation for statistically significant (if observed) and clinically and programmatically relevant changes in cognitive, skill, psychosocial, behavioral, health, and environmental impact and health outcome rates among a target population for a defined setting during a specific time period (*behavioral impact + health outcome evaluation*);
3. To document the cost, efficiency, and cost-effectiveness or cost-benefit of an HP-DP program for a specific population, or subgroup, and practice setting (*cost-economic evaluation*); and
4. To produce evidence-insight from Objectives 1, 2, and 3 with sufficiently high internal and external validity to formulate population health policies, and to plan translational-dissemination and effectiveness evaluations of system-wide, population-focused HP-DP programs to achieve specific behavioral impact and health outcome objectives for an extended time period (*program translational-dissemination-adoption evaluation*).

## Program Evaluation Terms

Program evaluation, like all professional specialties, has a technical language. Good communications among members of a planning and evaluation team and the use of an accurate and consistent technical language are essential. Although there is some variation in the definitions of each term in the literature, a set of common terms are used throughout this text. Knowing the definition of each term is necessary to review, comprehend, and discuss evaluation methods and literature, to participate in planning an evaluation and training activities, and to prepare an evaluation written report and oral presentation. *In defining an evaluation term, each should be perceived as being applicable to a specific problem, population, or subgroup, location, or practice setting, for example, clinic-school-community, time period, (e.g., 2015–2018), and defined geographic area.*

**Meta-evaluation (ME)**: A systematic methodological review and rating of the validity of HP-DP program evaluations, using specific criteria in eight categories: (1) experimental and quasi-experimental designs; (2) measurement validity, reliability, and completeness; (3) sample size, effect size, and statistical power; (4) sample eligibility and representativeness; (5) definition, tailoring, and replicability of measurement and intervention procedures; (6) performance measurement and process evaluation; (7) level of behavioral impact and health outcome rates; and (8) cost-economic analyses and cost effectiveness–cost benefit analyses.

**Meta-analysis (MA)**: A quantitative analysis of experimental research from a meta-evaluation, using standardized methodological criteria and procedures, to assess the level of internal and external validity of the intervention, and to produce an aggregate estimate of impact and effect size for an HP-DP program.

**HP-DP program-intervention**: A planned, targeted combination of defined, replicable treatment procedures $(X_1 + X_2 + X_n)$ and observational procedures $(O_1 + O_2 + O_n)$, derived from an ME and MA and professional judgment and selected for a population, to be implemented to produce significant changes in knowledge, psychosocial constructs, behavioral impact, environmental quality, and/or health outcome rates.

**Evaluation research**: An evaluation category, including **PHASE 1** Formative Evaluations or **PHASE 2** Efficacy Evaluations, designed to establish the quality, feasibility, efficacy, and cost and cost-effectiveness or cost-benefit of a new, theory-based program delivered by specialist staff under optimal practice conditions.

**Formative evaluation**: A **PHASE 1** Evaluation of an existing or new (untested) intervention, conducted under optimal program-practice conditions, delivered by specialized staff designed to produce data and insight during the early intervention development period to document (1) the feasibility of program implementation, (2) the acceptability of program methods and materials, and (3) the efficacy to produce significant immediate (1 hour–1 week), short-term (1–6 months), or intermediate (6–12 months) changes in impact rates.

**Efficacy evaluation**: A **PHASE 2** Evaluation designed to document the extent to which a relatively new program, with an adequate **PHASE 1** Formative Evaluation evidence base documenting the feasibility of delivery of an HP-DP program by specialized staff under optimal practice conditions, produced statistically significant and programmatically important changes in an impact or outcome rate < 1 year period.

**Internal validity**: The degree to which a statistically significant change in an impact and/or outcome rate can be attributed to an HP-DP program ($Xn$): Is $Xn$ the most plausible explanation for observed significant changes ($On$) for a sample of a defined population at risk in a defined practice setting and system of care?

**Program (Impact or Outcome) evaluation**: An evaluation category of **PHASE 3** Effectiveness and **PHASE 4** Translation-Dissemination Evaluations designed to assess the degree of both internal and external validity and to document the feasibility, effectiveness, and cost-effectiveness of an HP-DP program delivered by trained, regular staff under normal practice conditions to produce significant intermediate (e.g., 1–2 years) or long-term (e.g., ≥ 3 years) changes in behavioral impact or health-environmental outcome rates.

**Effectiveness evaluation**: A **PHASE 3** Evaluation designed to document if an efficacious (tested) **PHASE 2** intervention ($Xn$) can be delivered by trained regular staff under normal practice conditions, and has produced a statistically significant change in an impact or outcome rate among a representative sample of clients and sites.

**Dissemination-translation evaluation**: A **PHASE 4** Evaluation designed to document the feasibility, acceptability, degree of delivery, and level of adoption by providers of a **PHASE 3** "evidenced-based" HP-DP program for a target population in a system-wide services program, and to document its effectiveness, cost, and cost-effectiveness and/or cost-benefit to produce significant changes in behavioral and environmental-health outcome rates.

**External validity**: The degree to which a statistically significant change in a behavioral impact or health status outcome rate from a representative sample from **PHASE 3** and **4** Evaluations can be attributable to an intervention and can be generalized to a large, defined population in a system of care and practice settings.

**Process evaluation:** A type of evaluation used in **PHASE 1, 2, 3**, and **4** Evaluations to document the degree to which standardized, replicable intervention ($Xn$) and observational ($On$) procedures were performed and measured for all trained staff to document the feasibility and fidelity of routine delivery: How much of the $Xn$ and $On$ procedures ($Pn$) were provided with fidelity to whom, where, when, how, and by whom?

**Qualitative evaluation**: A type of evaluation used in **PHASE 1, 2, 3**, and **4** Evaluations that applies indirect and direct observational and interview methods, to assess program acceptability and perceived value by managers, staff, and participants, and to describe why the HP-DP program succeeded or did not succeed?

**Cost-effectiveness analysis (CEA)**: A cost-economic analysis used by **PHASE 1, 2, 3**, and **4** Evaluations to document the relationship between intervention ($Xn$) program costs INPUT and an impact-outcome rate OUTPUT: a ratio of cost per unit and percent of behavioral impact and/or environmental-health outcome.

**Cost utility analysis**: A type of cost-effectiveness analysis designed to document outcomes in Quality Adjusted Life Years (QALY) or Disability Adjusted Life Years (DALY): a cost-utility ratio expressed as a dollar value per QALY saved or one lost year of healthy life (DALY).

**Cost-benefit analysis (CBA)**: A cost and economic analysis used primarily by **PHASE 2, 3**, and **4** Evaluations designed to document the relationship between intervention ($Xn$) costs (INPUT) and a program behavioral health outcome rates (OUTPUT), expressed as a monetary benefit/consequence: a return on investment (ROI) or a ratio of costs/unit of economic benefit and net economic benefit (savings).

## Purposes of Program Evaluation

Among the many decisions to be made by an evaluation director and an organization, two of the most important are the following: to reach a clear agreement on the purposes of an evaluation (*why*) and to define what specific types of evaluations can be conducted for this problem and the HP-DP program at this time (*what-how*). After an evaluation team has established productive science-policy-practice partnerships, has conducted a meta-evaluation of the related literature, and has prepared an Evaluability Assessment Report of a program for their organization, it should be able to draft an initial, complete evaluation plan for internal review, discussion, and revision.

All plans require many drafts, reviews, and revisions. After staff have reviewed drafts of a plan, having one or two independent, external experts review it is recommended. Conducting an annual project internal and external peer review (*Progress Review*) will provide useful insight about implementation problems and solutions. The following are 10 common evaluation purposes:

1. To determine the degree of achievement of program objectives;
2. To establish quality control methods to monitor staff performance;
3. To document strengths and weaknesses for ongoing decision-making;
4. To meet the demand for public or fiscal accountability;
5. To determine the generalizability of a program to other populations;
6. To identify hypotheses about behavior changes for future evaluations;
7. To contribute to the science-evidence base of population health programs;
8. To improve staff skills required to plan, implement, and evaluate programs;
9. To promote positive public relations and community awareness; and
10. To fulfill grant or contract requirements.

All 10 purposes need to be considered when an evaluation director and team are preparing their plans and reports. Although each evaluation may not achieve all 10 goals, an experienced, reality-based team needs to consider the relevance of each purpose for its program plan. The ability of a program to achieve these purposes is directly related to the competency and experience of the evaluation team, the capacity of program staff, the purposes of an evaluation, and the complexity and characteristics of the health problem and target population. While all of these are important issues to consider, the time frame and availability of resources to conduct the program and evaluation are critical parameters that predict success or failure for almost all evaluations.

Most organizations that fund or manage HP-DP services or programs require an evaluation to determine the effectiveness of services provided, measured as behavioral or health outcome rates. The identification of methods to document reasons for achievement or non-achievement of salient program objectives will be expected. A valid evaluation report should routinely provide data insight about program development and modification. This information may (or may not) be used in current and future decisions about resource allocation, program expansion, or contraction. If the criteria for producing valid evidence and agency expectations are met, and the evaluation achieves its objectives, there should be a higher probability of influencing related policy and future funding.

## The Role of Program Evaluation or Evaluation Research in an Organization

The politics, mission, policies, and resources of a funding and/or implementing agency will play, in varying degrees, dominant roles in defining the following evaluation or research issues:

- The types of objectives to be evaluated for a specific population, problem, and practice setting;
- The evaluation design and type(s) of evaluation to be conducted;
- The selection of qualitative, process, impact, outcome, and cost baseline and follow measures;
- The types, amount, and periodicity of data collected; and
- The staff, resources, and time allocated to conduct the all types of evaluations.

Policymakers, managers, and evaluators need to agree in writing on these issues. Expected deliverables, timelines, and criteria of success need to be explicitly written in an evaluation plan.

The director or staff members may see program evaluation in different ways. Evaluation may be seen by many as a management tool to improve planning and resource allocation or to improve population health program policies and practices. Others may believe it is a way to gain insight into what happened and why. Almost all participants will view an evaluation as a method to ascertain a program's level of success or failure. The "worth" or "merit" and strengths and weaknesses of a program will be defined. Some individuals, however, may believe that an evaluation, especially a randomized clinical trial (RCT) or group randomized community trial (GRCT), is a waste of time and money: "They already know the program works." Regardless of the philosophical or political perspective, an evaluation team needs to meet scientific, evidence-based criteria. When it prepares and implements a program and its evaluation that meet these criteria, an evaluation team should meet the funding organization's purposes and expectations.

Agencies such as the NIH, CDC, NICE, WHO, AID (the Agency for International Development), or global health foundations typically fund an evaluation (in theory) to provide evidence about quality, feasibility, behavioral impact, and/or improved health. Unfortunately, a large proportion of funded national and international development programs that purport to be implemented to improve the health of target populations have serious methodological flaws. Although the opportunity usually exists to conduct cost and economic analyses of HP-DP programs as a routine component of almost all evaluations, methodologically sound cost-efficiency studies are also seldom conducted by domestic and international programs. It is important to realize that the interest in, expectations of, and funding from a unit of the federal government or an NGO will have a tidal quality. Enthusiasm and financial commitments for rigorous evaluations will ebb and flow and will be, at times, like the ocean, the weather, and politics—quiet or stormy, and unpredictable.

Evaluators must recognize the politics of decision-making and resource allocation, and have the technical and leadership skills (emotional intelligence) to negotiate realistic objectives, given the available funding, staffing, and time constraints. In practice, fiscal, philosophical, and political issues frequently play a dominant role (often greater than science issues) in policymaking and budgetary allocations to a program and its evaluation. Frequently, a local-, state-, or country-level HP-DP program is launched with much publicity, but there is limited evidence of efficacy to document behavioral impact, and to improve health status indicator rates.

Another common, serious mistake is to transplant an HP-DP program from one state to another state, or worse, to another country, without explicit plans and adequate resources to tailor and field test all methods and procedures of the new program to the new target population, program setting, staff capacity, and infrastructure. Funding agencies need to establish transparent, rigorous peer review policies and procedures to increase the probability that methodologically sound HP-DP programs and evaluations are planned and implemented. A commentary on politically driven domestic and international programs is presented in this chapter.

## Planning an Evaluation: Defining Realistic Objectives

Program and evaluation staff needs to determine, through a meta-evaluation (ME) and meta-analysis (MA), evaluability assessment, and consensus discussions, what an HP-DP program and its evaluation probably can and cannot achieve. Drafting objectives, discussing them, and agreeing on a small number of core objectives constitute the basic process that a team should implement in order to set realistic targets. A methodologically sound, detailed written evaluation plan is essential to assist the program and evaluator in defining and resetting objectives (if needed) during the implementation and evaluation of a project. Representatives of the scientific community, in or outside an organization, have a responsibility to inform decision-makers if a valid evaluation cannot and should not be performed for this "program" with its current methodological deficiencies, inadequate resources, and unrealistic task and timeline. *Saying "no," however, will always be a difficult task, because of politically driven leadership.* In general, agency leadership (and politicians) and program managers of state and national organization should define a smaller number of more realistic objectives and expectations of impact from HP-DP programs and policies.

Evaluation teams need to approach the drafting and revision of a plan with insight about how different program components and methods relate to one another conceptually and operationally. When compromises, adjustments, and changes are made, a team needs to know and define what impact these modifications will have on achieving objectives and evaluation validity. Evaluation and program staff need to recognize, given a science base, that there may not be a "perfect" HP-DP intervention, or definitive measurement methods to apply at this time to this population and this problem. The best and most complete evaluation insight will most likely be produced, however, when rigorous methods and designs are matched to the objectives, task timeline, and available funds.

When an evaluation plan is prepared, a "theoretical or logic model" will typically be selected to guide conceptual discussions. The Social Cognitive Theory (SCT) is a common framework used to plan HP-DP programs (Bandura, 1986). Whatever theory is selected, the "model" should describe how the program and "model" components are interrelated and tailored for each program. The PRECEDE-PROCEED model by Green and colleagues, presented in Chapter 2 (Planning an Evaluation), is an excellent example of how to systematically plan and evaluate an HP-DP program. Not all dimensions of a program and its evaluation, however, are clear during the planning and early implementation stages. Negotiation, compromise, and consensus development are typical activities in the development of a plan. Opportunities to examine and modify selected components of an HP-DP program may exist prior to or in the early stages of program implementation, but frequently will not exist once a program has started.

It is essential to ask the following question during planning-implementation analyses, and during preparation of an evaluation report: Does our evaluation plan meet external, global methodological standards and critical peer review? An evaluation team must also ask, Do we have adequate political-organizational support, budget, and resources, program staff, and sufficient time to deliver the program and conduct a valid evaluation?

A primary purpose of this book is to improve an evaluation team's ability to confidently participate in the preparation of a plan, realizing as fully as possible the alternatives and consequences of each change during planning and implementation.

An evaluation also needs to take a common-sense approach and to define reasonable expectations. Each individual program component cannot and, in most cases, may not need to be evaluated. *A randomized clinical trial (RCT) or group randomized community trial (GRCT) should not be automatically planned for an HP-DP program.* Trying to evaluate what cannot be evaluated with inadequate resources and time, or evaluating with a limited evidence base, or before the program has been tailored and pilot-tested for a population and a program infrastructure, are examples of common, serious planning deficiencies. Priorities must be set because resources are always finite. An evaluation team needs to focus energy and resources on achieving core objectives, and needs to allocate adequate resources to deliver the program. Even a complex evaluation, led by a well-trained group of experienced scientists, with adequate resources, staff, and time, will not always produce a definitive answer for specific program evaluation and evaluation research questions.

Multiple examples of successfully implemented RCTs and GRCTs are presented in Chapter 3 (Efficacy and Effectiveness Evaluation) of this volume. Although challenging, they present valid evidence that an HP-DP intervention can produce significant changes in a behavioral impact or health outcome rates. The serendipity of unanticipated, desirable or undesirable, consequences and impacts during program implementation and evaluation must also be acknowledged. *All evaluations experience implementation problems.* Assuming a sound evaluation plan, the best an evaluation may be able to do is to rule out a few plausible reasons for significant or non-significant changes and support one or two good, evidence-based explanations of why the program worked or did not work.

## Professional Competence in Program Evaluation

Evaluation has been identified for over 60 years as an integral component of public health, clinical care, school health, worksite, and community health programs by standard-setting organizations such as the WHO, the American Public Health Association (APHA), the European Union (EU), and the US Association of Schools of Public Health (ASPH). Academic programs and professional leaders in health education throughout the world have typically defined evaluation competency as an essential skill of MPH-MSPH-MS trained public health professionals. In 1988 the Institute of Medicine (IOM) created the Committee for the Study of the Future of Public Health. Representatives from the federal government, national health and medical professional organizations, public health agencies, and nonprofit public health groups defined three core functions of public health. Each, as noted in Table 1.1, has a global application and an application to program evaluation.

The IOM also noted that these three broad categories of functions require specific planning and evaluation competencies in 10 areas:

- Assessment and investigation of health risks, problems, and health and safety hazards in the nation, province or state, and community;
- Enforcement of laws and regulations to protect and promote health, prevent disease, and ensure and improve safety;
- Public education and empowerment of people about health risks and solutions;
- Mobilization of community partnerships to plan solutions to health problems;
- Development of health policies, programs, and plans to support individual and community health efforts;
- Linking people to public health and primary care programs and services;
- Assuring a competent public health and personal healthcare workforce;
- Evaluating the availability, accessibility, quality, cost, and effectiveness of personal, primary care, and population health programs in providing services; and

TABLE 1.1 Core Functions of Public (Population) Health

| CORE FUNCTION | DEFINITION |
| --- | --- |
| Assessment | Regularly and systematically collect, synthesize, analyze, and make available epidemiologic information on the community, including statistics on health status, health-related behavior risks, community health needs, and needed studies of health problems. |
| Policy Development | Develop comprehensive health policies based on epidemiological and behavioral assessments and the application of the current science, knowledge, and practice base. |
| Assurance | Assure that basic services are provided to achieve defined health objectives. |

- Conducting research and program evaluations to monitor progress and to provide new scientific evidence and solutions to population health problems.

Curricula in accredited MPH programs or schools of public health throughout the world should be providing graduate academic courses and mentored field experiences designed to develop competencies in all 10 areas, especially "program evaluation." *Currently, with the exception of many graduate programs in health education–health promotion, MPH programs in public health in the United States do not require a core course in "Evaluation of HP-DP Programs."*

## Credentialing and Professional Preparation for HP-DP Specialists

The master's degree (MPH-MSPH-MS) competencies and credentialing process for program planning and evaluation of HP-DP programs have existed in North America for over 40 years. The US Society for Public Health Education (SOPHE), established in 1951, is the standard-setting professional organization for undergraduate and graduate professional preparation in the field of health education and promotion. Since the 1970s, the US Coalition of Health Education Organizations, representing academic and practice leadership in the field of health education-promotion, has consistently called for improving academic training programs and increasing the planning and evaluation competencies of health education specialists. Information in Table 1.2 defines 10 "Areas of Responsibility" for certified health education specialists (CHES). Specialist staff with these skills, and experience are produced by an accredited graduate degree curriculum.

In 1978, a National Task Force on Professional Preparation was established, which led to the creation of a National Commission for Health Education Credentialing (NCHEC). The two current primary programs of the NCHEC to promote improved competency are (1) professional certification of health education specialists (CHES), and (2) promotion and application of "A Guide for the Development of Competency-Based Curricula for Health Educators" by BS and MPH, MS, and MSPH programs in the United States. The NCHEC has two publications describing these initiatives: *A Competency-Based Framework for Professional Development of Certified Health Education Specialists* (1996), and

TABLE 1.2 A Competency-Based Framework for Graduate-Level Health
Education Specialists

| | |
|---|---|
| Area of Responsibility I: | Assessing Individuals and Communities |
| Area of Responsibility II: | Planning Effective Programs |
| Area of Responsibility III: | Implementing Programs |
| Area of Responsibility IV: | Evaluating the Effectiveness of Programs |
| Area of Responsibility V: | Coordinating the Provision Services |
| Area of Responsibility VI: | Acting as a Resource Person |
| Area of Responsibility VII: | Communicating Health, Behavior, and Education Needs |
| Area of Responsibility VIII: | Applying Appropriate Research Principles and Methods |
| Area of Responsibility IX: | Administering Programs |
| Area of Responsibility X: | Advancing the Profession |

SOURCE: US National Commission for Health Education Credentialing, Inc., and SOPHE (1999).

*The Certified Health Education Specialist: A Self-Study Guide for Professional Competency* (1998). A CHES is expected to be able to perform multiple evaluation functions and to be skilled in specific technical areas (SOPHE, 1999).

In June, 2008 the Galway (Ireland) Consensus Conference on Credentialing in Health Promotion–Health Education was held to promote global exchange and understanding about core competencies, professional preparation, and accreditation. It was conceived as one of the first steps to promote the development of global standards of health promotion practice. Although invitations were extended to colleagues engaged in graduate professional preparation and senior governmental entities representing all WHO regions, most of the 35 attendees at the conference were primarily from Europe and North America. Multiple papers on credentialing were delivered to inform the participants on conference deliberations. A major conference outcome was the drafting and dissemination of an international consensus statement for review and comment.

Approximately 80 contributors had an opportunity to provide their perspectives and make philosophical and editorial comments. "Planning, Implementation, and Evaluation," including a need for more emphasis on the measurement of impact and outcomes, emerged as one of five salient themes in a content analysis of the conference draft recommendations. A special section of *Health Education and Behavior*, in June 2009, edited by J. Allegrante and M. Barry and a Guest Editorial Board, provided a comprehensive discussion of the proceedings of the conference. The dissemination and application of core competencies by the Galway Conference, especially in graduate programs, should promote global evaluation standards of practice.

# Systematic Reviews: Meta-Evaluation and Meta-Analysis

An evaluation team needs to review what is known about how to assess and to intervene to help change behaviors and environments of specific populations and identify implementation barriers. A team needs to have insight about successful and unsuccessful programs for specific health problems and practice settings. Although guidelines to conduct systematic reviews and ratings of evaluations have existed for decades, a large percentage of published HP-DP program "evaluations" do not meet standards of professional practice. A review of numerous reports about the reasons for intervention failure reveal that many HP-DP programs proposed and funded by various agencies (especially international aid agencies) had serious methodological deficiencies. They had limited and invalid evidence to support intervention delivery, effectiveness, or cost.

A written comprehensive, systematic review using standardized methodological criteria, a *meta-evaluation (ME)*, of the peer-reviewed literature (and other available valid reports), is one of the first products a team must produce to plan an HP-DP program and evaluation. In planning a program, an evaluation team needs to know what must be measured (the gold standard) and how to define what core data to collect. An ME includes evaluations that have applied experimental or quasi-experimental designs. An ME should inform a team about the range and multiple types of typical challenges, problems, and mistakes made by previous evaluations and evaluators during planning and implementation. An ME (systematic review) would include qualitative evaluations, providing discussions about a range of contextual issues that a meta-analysis typically excludes.

If a sufficient number of evaluations of high quality exist to confirm the validity of an HP-DP program for a specific problem and well-defined population, a *meta-analysis (MA)* would be performed. A meta-analysis applies a mathematical formula to aggregate data from independent RCTs to produce the most statistically robust, aggregated estimates of levels of impact-effect size. The challenge for all reviews of HP-DP program evaluations is that a meta-evaluation frequently provides only one or two examples of rigorous evaluations for the seemingly infinite number of health and safety problems, target populations at risk, cultures, and program practice settings. For example, how can we improve the mortality and morbidity rates of mothers and infants in Chicago, Illinois, or Jackson, Mississippi? How can we increase the management and control of high blood pressure, high cholesterol, diabetes, or asthma among black adults in community-based, primary care clinics in Birmingham, Alabama, Birmingham, England, or

Cape Town, South Africa? How can we reduce water-borne diseases in rural towns/villages in Xian Province, China, or the Yukon-Kuskokwim Delta Region, Alaska? A meta-evaluation is the most likely systematic review to be useful in answering these questions in planning a new or revising an existing HP-DP program.

*Meta-evaluation (ME) and meta-analysis (MA), however, are frequently used interchangeably. As the different definitions indicate, this is an incorrect use of two very distinct terms. A meta-evaluation describes the overall science-base of an HP-DP program. An ME answers the question, What were the many lessons learned about assessment and intervention methods attempted by programs that failed?* An ME applies a broader inclusionary and more practice-focused perspective in deriving insight and guidance, in addition to evidence, data, and insight from an RCT or GRCT evaluation.

The *Cochrane Collaborative Review* is a recognized scientific review process to evaluate the universe of an HP-DP program for specific health problems and populations. The *Campbell Collaborative Review* is a recognized scientific review process for educational and social and behavioral sciences literature. The methods and results from these two sources are complementary and should be primary sources of data and insight to an evaluation team. In addition to the Cochrane Reviews, evaluation teams should also use the Consolidated Standards Of Reporting Trials (CONSORT) Statement developed for RCTs, and the Transparent Reporting of Evaluations with Non-Randomized Designs (TREND) Statement and procedures to plan and report evaluation methods and results. These sources use standard methods with specific ME criteria in multiple categories to help synthesize and produce a report on the "state of the science-practice" about evaluated interventions.

The *International Initiative for Impact Evaluation* (3ieimpact.org) is another informative resource for evaluations in low-income countries. It has augmented and adapted the CONSORT review methodology for RCT "impact evaluations" of social, educational, and economic policy interventions. The 3ie checklist is called CONSORT Elaborations for Development Effectiveness (CEDE). These resources can be accessed to provide a broader perspective.

## Evaluation PHASES: Documenting the Validity of Results

A meta-evaluation (ME) and, if appropriate, a meta-analysis (MA), combined with current Practice Guidelines, define the quality, strengths, and weaknesses of the evidence base for HP-DP intervention ($Xn$) and observation-measurement ($On$) methods for a specific health problem and target population. As noted above in the definition of terms, a meta-evaluation is a systematic methodological review and rating of the internal and external validity of HP-DP program evaluations, using specific criteria in eight categories (listed above).

A meta-evaluation review and rating by two independent reviewers of each evaluation report for a specific problem typically ask a set of standardized questions within each category. This review tells the evaluation team how many evaluations were successfully (and unsuccessfully) implemented, with valid or invalid results. It provides data and should produce insight to make conclusions about the quality of HP-DP implementation methods and the internal-external validity of results for each and all evaluations.

*The internal validity and external validity of an HP-DP treatment are always slowly developing targets, varying by the stability or volatility of multiple interactive characteristics that may predict behavioral or environmental changes over time for a specific intervention, population, problem, practice setting, and system of services.* It is important to emphasize that validity is always population-problem-setting-place-time-period specific. An evaluation team needs to be cautious about the interpretation and generalization of results to its population and setting (external validity) from a meta-evaluation of an HP-DP intervention. While an ME and MA, in combination with the experienced judgment of an evaluation team, are the rational place to start, a common mistake in planning an evaluation is to over-generalize weak of bodies of evidence.

When this information is synthesized into a review by evaluation leadership and staff, depending on the number and quality of studies, a summary statement can be made about the state of the science and the practice of assessment and intervention procedures for a specific problem and population. If there are a sufficient number of rigorous evaluations, a meta-analysis should provide informative data and insight about the range of impacts of a program for a specific population and practice setting. The summary data and insights from an ME and MA define what can be called the "Evaluation PHASE for an HP-DP program." The Evaluation PHASE defines the internal and external validity and knowledge base and scientific horizon of an HP-DP program. This includes definitions of salient variables and rates for a specific problem, population, and program setting.

Table 1.3 identifies four Evaluation PHASES to categorize the science and practice bases for an HP-DP program for each health problem.

TABLE 1.3 Evaluation PHASES for HP-DP Programs: Defining the Science Base

| PHASE I EVALUATION | PHASE II EVALUATION | PHASE III EVALUATION | PHASE IV EVALUATION |
|---|---|---|---|
| Evaluation Research (Theory-Based > Feasibility) | | Program Evaluation (Practice-Based > Translation) | |
| Formative Evaluation | Efficacy Evaluation | Effectiveness Evaluation | Dissemination Evaluation |
| Short Term Impact | Mid-Term Impact | Long Term Impact: Behavior + Health | |
| Internal Validity | | Internal + External Validity | |
| Core Types: Meta + Process + Qualitative + Cost Evaluations and Analyses | | | |

As noted, *four evaluation methods, (1) meta-evaluation + meta-analysis, (2) process evaluation, (3) qualitative evaluation, and (4) cost and economic evaluations and analyses, should be planned and applied as CORE methods in all evaluations, regardless of the PHASE of maturity of an intervention.* When these CORE methods are not applied by an evaluation, a major opportunity is lost to gain empirical evidence and insight about one of more salient characteristics of a program and evaluation for a problem, group, and setting.

In introducing this "Evaluation Typology" that categorizes HP-DP Evaluation PHASES, two primary references provide helpful background discussions: the NIH-National Cancer Institute Model for Cancer Control, Greenwald and Cullen, *Journal of the National Cancer Institute* (*JNCI*, 1985), and the report by Flay, *Preventive Medicine* (1986). More current thoughtful commentaries about internal and external validity gaps in evaluation planning are presented by Green and Glasgow, ". . . : Issues in External Validity and Translational Methodology," *Evaluation and the Health Professions* (2006), and by Steckler and McLeroy, "The Importance of External Validity," *American Journal of Public Health* (2008). Although multiple federal agencies and professional organizations have stressed the need for greater emphasis on reducing the science to practice gap, the NIH is arguably the primary funder of large, peer-reviewed trials to address the issues raised here and in the literature.

The following is a description of the two Evaluation CATEGORIES: **Evaluation Research** and **Program Evaluation**, and four Evaluation PHASES: **Formative Evaluation, Efficacy Evaluation, Effectiveness Evaluation**, and **Dissemination Evaluation**. The epidemiological and statistical evidence, documenting the relationship between behavioral risk factors and population attributable risk/fraction (PAR) for a specific problem and population, is needed for all PHASES. A detailed epidemiological-statistical profile for multiple years should be prepared by all evaluations documenting current and past behavioral and health outcome rates and trends for a target group.

## PHASE 1 (Formative Evaluation) and PHASE 2 (Efficacy Evaluation): Evaluation Research

**PHASE 1 and 2 Evaluations** are theory-based, developmental studies to determine the feasibility-fidelity of delivery of major HP-DP program measurement and treatment procedures and to document estimates of behavioral impact or health outcomes for a specific problem-population-practice setting. These two types of evaluation can be grouped into a category called **Evaluation Research**. The scientific Aims of PHASE 1 and 2 Evaluations are designed to primarily document the internal validity of an HP-DP program and answer four questions:

- *Aim 1*: Can the new, untested HP-DP program be delivered by specially trained staff under optimal practice conditions to a representative sample of the target population? (*process evaluation*);
- *Aim 2*: Were the intervention and observational-assessment methods acceptable and used by the target group of providers and clients? (*qualitative evaluation*);
- *Aim 3*: What level of significant change in behavioral or health status indicator rates (effect size estimates) were documented? (*behavioral impact-outcome evaluation*); and
- *Aim 4*: What resources were expended and efficiencies were documented? (*cost-effectiveness/benefit economic evaluation*)?

These evaluations are the first set of rigorous studies designed to answer specific questions about the value-validity of a proposed theoretical model of behavior change, and the feasibility of new interventions to change behavior and improve population health in a specific practice setting.

In PHASE 1 Formative Evaluations and PHASE 2 Efficacy Evaluations, specialized intervention and assessment staff, trained-supervised by faculty/scientists at academic research centers, supervise the implementation of a plan, including intervention and observational-assessments procedures for the Experimental (E) Group and usual care, or Control (C), Group. As noted in the definitions, this evaluation category documents the initial feasibility of the delivery of a program. It produces, if successful implementation is documented, the early evidence about the level of impact and intervention costs for specialty staff for "ideal" practice conditions.

If several PHASE 1 Formative Evaluations, typically smaller scale studies, 2–4 sites and > 200–400 participants, have been successfully implemented and have produced valid evidence of significant changes attributable to an intervention, then PHASE 2 Efficacy Evaluations, with larger samples/sites, for example, 4–10 sites and > 500–1,000 participants, would be planned and conducted to replicate all major PHASE 1 methods with a comparable population. As each PHASE and type of evaluation are successfully implemented, there is an opportunity to add to an evidence base. Through the successful application of rigorous methods to produce evidence with high internal validity, the science base for specific HP-DP program interventions becomes more mature.

Unfortunately, meta-evaluations of the literature indicate that many PHASE 1 and 2 Evaluations did not conduct (or conducted inadequate) qualitative, process, and cost analyses. National HP-DP Program Guideline Report Committees that perform reviews and produce MEs for federal agencies frequently document incomplete portraits and invalid evidence bases for problems and specific populations. Many evaluations had not conducted one or more of the core types of evaluation. Cumulatively, this is how large gaps in evidence are created in all HP-DP areas.

## PHASE 3 and 4: Program Evaluation

**PHASE 3** Effectiveness Evaluations and **PHASE 4** Dissemination-Translational Evaluations can be grouped into an Evaluation Category called **Program Evaluation**. They should be designed to answer salient questions about the *internal validity* and *external validity* (the degree of generalizability of results to large target populations at risk). PHASE 3 and 4 Evaluations should not be conducted unless the evidence base of feasibility and efficacy from multiple PHASE 1 and 2 Evaluations is positive and, with few exceptions, consistent and valid. *Quality, process, efficacy, and cost should have been well documented by PHASE 1 and 2 Evaluations, before planning PHASE 3 and 4 Evaluations.* PHASE 3 and 4 Evaluations answer five questions:

1. Can the intervention/program be delivered with fidelity by regular staff at an adequate number of sites and clients representative of practice settings for a defined population?

2. Are the HP-DP intervention methods effective when delivered by the trained, regular staff to the target population under normal practice conditions?
3. Were the evaluation samples of sites/clients sufficiently large and representative to meet statistical power assumptions and to provide new, additional evidence to support the internal and external validity and generalizability of the methods and results to the target population at risk?
4. What was the cost, cost-effectiveness, and, if appropriate, cost-benefit associated with the existing and new HP-DP program?
5. Does the available science, program, and practice base confirm that the HP-DP program is sufficiently effective, efficient, and ready to be disseminated as a Practice Guideline and Population Health Policy for routine delivery by trained regular staff who provide routine services for defined populations in communities, cities, counties, states, or a country.

Two core questions in planning PHASE 3 and 4 Evaluations are the following: Has the efficacy—internal validity—of an intervention from PHASE 1 and 2 Evaluations been confirmed, and was this judgment based on a sufficiently large number of peer-reviewed studies among multiple samples of the target group? Transplanting an HP-DP intervention confirmed as efficacious from only one or two evaluations for a specific problem and population in one state to another state, or to another "comparable" high- or low-income country, without adequate time and resources to tailor and conduct rigorous Formative Evaluations, is a common problem noted in the evaluation literature.

PHASE 3 and 4 Program Evaluations should include large, representative samples of a defined population with specific health problems for which behavioral and population attributable risks (PAR) are well defined, for example, > 1,000–2,000/per study and > 500–1,000 experimental (E) participants and > 500–1,000 control (C) participants. They might typically involve 10+ to 40+ sites, for example, 5+ to 20+ experimental (E) sites and 5+ to 20+ control (C) sites. Defining the minimum number of units, sample size/unit, and representativeness of the population are critical analysis and methodological issues. The sample size and number of units for matching, random assignment, treatment, and analysis should be based on insight from a meta-evaluation (ME). The sample size and estimated effect sizes and the number of sites will always vary by the problem. Sample sizes should be based on the ME and preliminary evaluations at the evaluation study sites.

Inadequate sample size and poor statistical power are common, serious errors that compromise the validity of most HP-DP evaluations. Sample size estimation based on the validity of effect sizes of completed evaluations also have major implications for defining the number of sites, timeline, duration, and evaluation cost. Chapter 3 presents a description of the principles and methods to calculate the sample size requirements for an impact or outcome evaluation among individuals or groups of participants in an evaluation. Murray (1998) in "Group Randomized Designs and Analysis" presents a comprehensive discussion of the most salient issues that an evaluation must address when it plans to use the site as the unit of assessment, treatment, and analysis.

PHASE 3 and PHASE 4 studies, because they are Program Effectiveness Evaluations, should be designed to answer questions about the degree of both internal validity and external validity of results for an intervention for a population. A core objective of a PHASE 4 Program Dissemination Evaluation should be to confirm the degree of adoption of an HP-DP program by regular staff. They also are designed to confirm the behavioral impact or health outcome changes from routine delivery of evidence-based methods by regular trained staff "under normal conditions" for a defined system and population. PHASE 4 Evaluations typically assess the effect of a large, ongoing HP-DP program, for example, an injury reduction health communication campaign, a new health policy, a law for a city, county, province/state, or country, or the behavioral or health impact of "Best Practice Guidelines."

A randomized design should always be the first choice of all evaluation phases. However, if randomization is not possible, feasible, or appropriate, for example, organizational leadership decides to provide the evidenced-based HP-DP program to all eligible clients, or a new cigarette tax or speed limit change is made in a state, a time series design (TSD) may be a strong alternative evaluation design. Discussions and examples of the application of a TSD or a non-randomized comparison group design are presented in two case studies in Chapter 3.

## Internal Validity to External Validity: The Enduring Challenge

As noted in the definitions of evaluation terms and descriptions of Evaluation PHASES in Table 1.3, a primary but not exclusive objective of a PHASE 1 or 2 Efficacy Evaluation is to determine the internal validity of behavioral impact results for an HP-DP intervention(s). Having ruled out all salient threats to the internal validity of results, can you attribute statistically different changes to "X" for the defined population of clients who received "X" for a specific problem, at participating sites and locations, and during a specific time period? The objectives of PHASE 3 and 4 Effectiveness Evaluations is to determine the internal and external validity of behavioral impact or health outcome results for an HP-DP intervention(s). The challenges to PHASE 3 and 4 Evaluations is to produce evidence that has ruled out all salient threats to both internal validity (IV) and external validity (EV). PHASE 3 and 4 Evaluations, to produce valid, credible results, must be designed to be implemented under normal practice conditions by regular program providers to a large, representative sample of at-risk clients at an adequate sample of practice sites.

The primary challenge to documenting EV is the following: *Having ruled out threats to IV, can the evaluation results be generalized to a defined population with a specific problem and target group at specific service program delivery sites?* While there are multiple methodological issues to confirming the EV of the results of an evaluation of any HP-DP program, the first and most serious is the representativeness of an eligible sample of participants for a defined population at risk, for example, for a specific problem being served by a specific type of professional staff or urban versus rural public elementary schools. Beyond the salient issue of representativeness to be addressed (*who*) are critical issues such as the replicability and feasibility of routine delivery of the HP-DP program with fidelity: *what-where-how-when-how much* was delivered to *whom*? It should be obvious that there are no easy answers to planning and implementing an HP-DP evaluation that will produce results with both high internal validity and eternal validity. It is very rare that an evaluation will document both the internal validity and external validity of an HP-DP program.

Much has been written and said about the large "evidence to practice gap" and internal versus external validity challenges in the United States and globally for at least 50 years. Over the years, multiple discussions about this topic have been presented by Campbell and Stanley (1966) and Cook and Campbell (1979). As noted, Greenwald and Cullen (1985), Flay (1986), Green and colleagues (1977, 2004, 2006), and Steckler and McLeroy (2008) have identified the need to produce better practice-based evidence and to improve the external validity of HP-DP evaluations. In the last decade, NIH created its Clinical and Translational Science Award (CTSA) Program in 2006; the Agency for Healthcare Research and Quality (AHRQ), whose primary goal is research translation, implemented its

Translating Research Into Practice (TRIP) and produced multiple "Clinical Practice Guidelines Reports." All discussions emphasized the formidable challenges faced by an evaluation to assess the internal validity and external validity of its results. Expanded discussion of the issues related to external validity are presented in Chapter 3 (Efficacy and Effectiveness Evaluation) of this volume. Because of the design, scope, and duration of several evaluations in Chapter 3, the internal and external validity of evaluation results are examined.

## Practice-Based and Community-Based Participatory Research and Program Evaluation

The philosophy of practice-based and community-based participatory research (PBPR-CBPR) reflects a set of the core principles of health education–health promotion–disease management theory. The concepts of "participation," "community engagement," and "action research," are well-established ways to think about how to conceptualize the HP-DP program planning and evaluation process (Green, 1974). The complementarity of qualitative and quantitative principles and methods is also well established. For example, excellent discussions of multiple issues related to this topic can be found in a monograph edited by two acknowledged leaders in the field of program evaluation: Thomas Cook and Charles Reichardt (1979). *A major challenge to contemporary HP-DP program evaluation and research leadership will be to integrate PBPR-CBPR principles into a science and practice for planning and evaluation dialogue, that is, engaging participation by community members and practice-based professionals, building capacity, and sharing knowledge to produce a new evidence-base.*

Comprehensive discussions of CBPR are presented by Minkler and Wallerstein in *Community-Based Participatory Research for Health* (2003). Chapter 13, "Issues in Participatory Evaluation," by Springett presents a succinct reflection about the differences and complementarity of "Conventional Evaluation and Participatory Evaluation." Appendix C, by Green et al., presents "Guidelines for Participatory Research in Health Promotion." The NIH, in *Principles of Community Engagement* (2nd ed., 2011), discusses a range of salient content. This publication was a component of the NIH Clinical and Translational Science Award Consortium. Chapter 7 (Sofian, Chair, et al.), "Program Evaluation and Community Engagement," identifies five types of evaluation: formative, process, summative, outcome, and impact. The roles of scientists and community stakeholders are described, and assessment methods are presented.

Large bodies of insightful literature are available on PBPR and CBPR to use to plan HP-DP research and evaluation projects. A cautionary note, however, is needed about the CBPR philosophy and methods. An insightful report by Khodyakov, Stockdale Joens, et al., "Measuring Community Participation in Research," in *Health Education and Behavior* (2013), examines a variety issues related to the assumption of the impact of CBPR projects. They discuss the complexity and challenges of validly measuring "community participation," identify limitations of measurement strategies, and confirm the need for substantial, rigorous CBPR measurement research.

As noted in the introduction, more multilevel, complex interventions proposed by a trans-disciplinary team will be needed to increase the probability of successful process, impact, and outcome evaluations. In discussions about the philosophy of program evaluation, successful applications and evaluations of the Population Health Model will require stronger, direct linkages between public (population) health science, policy, and practice stakeholders. Selected partnerships with representatives of the clients, families, and communities served will enhance program success. Direct linkages with the local social and political infrastructure may also be an important ingredient for many (but not all) solutions to the complex problems. The judicious selection and rigorous application of methods of practice-based and community-based participatory research (PBPR-CBPR) by HP-DP programs and evaluations will be needed.

While CBPR represents an array of sound principles and methods useful to plan, implement, and evaluate an HP-DP program, the plan must have the opportunity to produce results with high measurement validity and potential internal and external validity for the problem-population-setting. Meta-analyses documenting the evidence base and the effectiveness of CBPR assessment and intervention methods are needed to guide future evaluation planning and collaboration. Excellent case study examples of evaluations using CBPR and PBPR are presented in Chapter 3. Each of these case studies and the methods and concepts reviewed in each chapter are designed to produce data, information, and *practice-based evidence*, which, if successfully implemented, should produce data and insight about *evidence-based practice*.

## Clinical Practice Guidelines for HP-DP and Management

The concepts of evidence-based medicine (EBM) and evidence-based practice (EBP) reflect a systematic review of the validity methods for patient-client assessment, diagnoses, and treatment. When a team conducts a meta-evaluation and meta-analysis to define a science base for an intervention, it should always review and reference Clinical Practice Treatment, or HP-DP Program Guidelines. The Cochrane Collaborative Review should also be a primary source to identify the "state of the science-practice" for the diagnosis, treatment, and management of all diseases and health and safety conditions. These reviews define the quality of the evidence base, or **Evaluation PHASE** of HP-DP program development and define its readiness to disseminate.

In the United States, Congress established the Agency for Health Care Policy and Research (AHCPR) in 1989, and its successor, the Agency for Healthcare Research and Quality (AHRQ) in 2000. AHRQ has two primary responsibilities: to review clinically relevant guidelines to assist physicians, educators, and healthcare practitioners in determining how diseases can be most effectively prevented, diagnosed, and managed clinically, and to establish standards of quality, performance measures, and medical review criteria. As mandated by the US Congress, each of the 27 US National Institutes of Health (NIH) also produce "State of the Science Reports" and "Treatment Guidelines" for specific diseases for which they are the lead agency. All national governments in high-income countries have a health agency or ministry with the same mission as AHRQ, for example, the National Institute of Health and Clinical Excellence (NICE) in the United Kingdom.

A large number of clinical practice guidelines and national and international consensus reports on specific diseases and/or conditions have been published and disseminated in the last two decades, for example for HIV/AIDS treatment; tuberculosis (TB) control; smoking cessation; oral rehydration; malaria control; and high blood pressure, asthma, cholesterol, and Type 1 and 2 diabetes control and management. These disease prevention and management guidelines define the process and outcomes of quality healthcare: all integral components of an HP-DP evaluation plan. Evaluators need to thoroughly review these sources and their methods to improve planning and evaluation practice for programs, professionals, patients, and families in healthcare settings. Reports from these national agencies provide guidance about the internal and external validity of treatments.

All evaluations will face challenges produced by the heterogeneity of clients and staff and programs for all health and safety problems. Evaluation specialists and teams need to be knowledgeable about the trends, politics, policies, and organization of disease prevention, diagnosis, treatment, and management programs in their local area, region, and country. Evaluation leadership and staff must also have up-to-date information about the infrastructure, capacity, and financing of health services, especially for all evaluation sites and area(s) for the HP-DP program.

## Evaluation PHASES: Translating HP-DP Science to Practice-Based Evidence

As noted, rigorous systematic reviews and MEs of the global peer-reviewed literature, and published clinical practice guidelines are needed to provide data and insight to help a program define the scientific or Evaluation PHASE of population assessment and intervention development. While experience and professional judgment are important predictors of successful planning, an evaluation plan needs to represent an accurate review of the evidence, as well as describe the Evaluation PHASE or *scientific horizon* for a problem. An ME review defines the minimum measurement and intervention methods for each evaluation.

An ME may also confirm that there is little (or no) valid evidence base supporting the efficacy or effectiveness of a specific type of HP-DP program for a population and problem. If there are successful evaluations, however, an ME and an MA may identify the most appropriate modifications of intervention and assessment methods for a comparable population at risk, in a different practice setting. With this insight, decisions can be made about what qualitative, process, impact, outcome, and cost evaluations should be planned and applied next. The systematic application of ME and MA principles and methods will present a current statement about the degree of internal validity (IV) and external validity (EV) of an HP-DP-Program. An enduring and complex challenge to an evaluation team is developing a plan to determine the level of EV.

A major global challenge in each decade is to concurrently and significantly expand the quality and quantity of PHASE 1 and 2 Evaluation Research (Formative and Efficacy Evaluations) and PHASE 3 and 4 Program Evaluation (Effectiveness and Dissemination Evaluations). We need to continue to produce a stronger science and evidence base for changing high risk behaviors of large populations at risk. Randomized clinical trials (RCT) need to be conducted to answer questions about interventions when individuals are the unit of intervention and analysis. This approach needs to be complemented by an increasingly larger number of evaluations of interventions for defined social and geographic units and groups: group randomized community trials (GRCT). We also need an increase in rigorous population-based research methods, including the use of time series designs-analyses and matched non-randomized comparison group designs. Well-planned and implemented **Comparative Effectiveness Evaluations** should produce knowledge about what HP-DP interventions work for target groups in families and communities, patients, children and adolescents in schools, clinics and primary care systems, and large, well-defined, high-risk populations.

It is also important to emphasize: the purpose of an evaluation, if sound methods are applied and successfully implemented, is to determine if a new HP-DP program or treatment methods $(X1 + X2 + X3)$ are better than an existing program $(X1)$. *A non-significant (NS) result is commonly referred to as a "failure." It is not deemed a failure if a program is successfully implemented, and the results have high validity.* While confirmation of a significant effect is preferred, if the evaluation involved a large, representative cohort of participants with a major condition and excellent measurement, an NS result provides important policy, program, and practice insight. It says that providing $X2 + X3$ treatment methods is not a good solution for *this* problem and *this* target group. Because $X2 + X3$ will be more complex to routinely provide, and will take more staff time and money, valid NS results, combined with an ME, should assist the HP-DP program leadership to make future program and policy decisions.

## Planning and Evaluation Domains and Stakeholders

Defining the evidence-base and PHASE of scientific development for an HP-DP program are essential planning activities. Planning an evaluation also requires an equal level of understanding of a broader set of science-policy-practice issues. An evaluation team needs to understand the contextual issues relevant to an evaluation for each local population and practice setting/sites. There are three salient planning and evaluation domains to consider in planning a program and its evaluation: **the Science Domain, the Policy Domain**, and **the Practice Domain.** Collaborators in each domain can be called stakeholders; they need to be partners during the planning process.

Individuals in each of these three domains, external and internal to a program, will view each aspect of a program and its evaluation from their perspective. They may or may not agree with the perspective of others within or between each stakeholder group. As part of an **Evaluability Assessment** (described in the next section), the perspective and issues of each domain of stakeholders need to be understood to plan a program and conduct its evaluation. Establishing a **Program Evaluation Policy and Management Committee** with stakeholder representation at the onset of planning will affirm and facilitate input from partners. Having direct, regular discussions with stakeholders, and conducting a review of the major issues to be addressed, an Evaluability Assessment is a standard procedure that an evaluation team needs to implement.

## Evaluability Assessment

Concurrent with the ME and MA, a series of consensus development activities, Evaluability Assessment Reviews, with participation of colleagues and representatives from each of the three major domains, needs to occur. An Evaluability Assessment review of a science and practice base refers to an examination of the quality of the evidence and knowledge produced from ME and MA reports for planning and evaluation. An Evaluability Assessment Report (EAP) should identify problems and recommend solutions to each. It may indicate that valid process-impact-outcome-cost evaluations may not be possible, given the time, resources, type of problems, and setting of an existing or new program. A draft EAP should be shared with managers and staff for review and discussion, especially focusing on feasibility and timelines.

An Evaluability Assessment identifies science, policy, and practice issues by gathering accurate information from domain representatives. Assessment of the enthusiasm, resources, and technical and operational capacity are critical for a realistic plan. These reviews should provide an accurate description of organizational, program, and staff readiness to provide a program at target sites, and to conduct an evaluation over a three- to five-year period. Examples of questions and issues are the following:

- What is the Evaluation PHASE and what is the level of clarity of the evidence base about interventions for our specific problem, our target population at risk, and our practice setting?

- What behavioral impact or health outcome levels (effect sizes) are realistic targets over what period of time for our target population and problem?
- What core indicators of progress are being measured now, what new indicators must be measured to document significant behavioral and health status changes, and what are the anticipated barriers to collecting "gold standard" measures/data at all program sites?
- What do the existing and new program components cost, and is there an opportunity or requirement for cost-effectiveness/cost-benefit evaluations? And how ready is a program and how capable and enthusiastic is its staff to implement the HP-DP program and an evaluation?

Failure to identify science, management, and practice concerns, providing inadequate staffing, training, and funding, and setting unrealistic time- and task lines are common flaws of plans. Setting unrealistic objectives and timelines with little or no relationship to the evidence base for a problem and population are typical characteristics of politically driven HP-DP programs. A plan with these deficiencies should raise questions about the competency of evaluation leadership.

The categories and rating scale for conducting an assessment are presented Table 1.4 in the Evaluability Assessment Form. A rating of ≥ 8 for each of the 10 categories, and an overall score of > 85 would typically confirm that a plan is strong in all categories. This form should be revised and adapted for use by an evaluation team for each program to review written plans and to interview key management and program staff and representatives of a target group. This review process will help a team identify issues to discuss and resolve, and methods to revise in a program and evaluation plan. The following sections present discussions about the types of issues that an Evaluability Assessment would examine for each domain and stakeholders group.

## Science Domain

The involvement of scientists, policymakers, managers, practitioners, and target audience representatives in a consensus development process at the onset of planning and during implementation is a fundamental strategy to contribute to problem definition, the creation of solutions, and selection of methods, designs, and procedures. The basic issues for a planning-evaluation team to discuss and resolve in an assessment of the Science Domain include

TABLE 1.4 Evaluability Assessment: Proposal Review-Rating Checklist*

| CATEGORY | RATING |
|---|---|
| 1. Meta-Evaluation/Analysis for problem/defined population | 0 1 2 3 4 5 6 7 8 9 10 |
| 2. Consultation: Staff/Local Officials/Agencies/Target Audience | 0 1 2 3 4 5 6 7 8 9 10 |
| 3. Needs Assessment Data and Pilot Study Analyses | 0 1 2 3 4 5 6 7 8 9 10 |
| 4. Realistic Staff Tasks and Timeline delineated/month/year | 0 1 2 3 4 5 6 7 8 9 10 |
| 5. Outreach Plan to recruit target audience by site/number | 0 1 2 3 4 5 6 7 8 9 10 |
| 6. Measurement-Assessment Instruments and Methods defined | 0 1 2 3 4 5 6 7 8 9 10 |
| 7. Plans to Pretest-Evaluate Intervention and Assessment Procedure | 0 1 2 3 4 5 6 7 8 9 10 |
| 8. Performance-Process Evaluation-Monitoring system described | 0 1 2 3 4 5 6 7 8 9 10 |
| 9. Impact-Outcome Evaluation Design-Methods described | 0 1 2 3 4 5 6 7 8 9 10 |
| 10. Adequate Annual Budget-Cost Analysis Methods described | 0 1 2 3 4 5 6 7 8 9 10 |

0 = Not Available . . . 10 = Excellent (> 8 each + > 85 Rating = Excellent Plan).
* Adapt to HP-DP program plans.

the following: Is there a strong or weak consensus about the "state of the population health science" for the target problem? Is the empirical evidence valid, reliable, representative, and conclusive about feasibility, efficacy, and cost of a program-intervention for a population, or is the evidence equivocal? Data-evidence-insight from MEs and MAs reviewed by representatives in this domain define what methods need to be applied to produce valid evidence, and what is the best rate of improvement that a specific intervention may be able to achieve for a problem and population.

## Policy Domain

An assessment and review of the Policy/Program Domain refer to an examination of the philosophical, political, financial, administrative, and organizational level of support for a program and its evaluation. Examples of questions to be discussed and answered in this review are the following: Why are the program and evaluation being conducted? Who supports (or does not support) the program and its evaluation? What is the strength and duration of institutional-philosophical-financial commitments of the sponsoring agency and management? Who is defining the objectives and type(s) of evaluation to be conducted or not to be conducted? Data-evidence-insight from representatives of this domain should define the policies/politics of an agency or organization that are related to the intervention and its evaluation: what a program says it wants to do, or should be doing, according to written organizational policies and procedures.

## Practice Domain

An assessment and review of the Practice Domain refer to an examination of the operational reality of an existing HP-DP program. Examples of questions to be discussed and resolved in this review are the following: What are the primary objectives and current structure, process, methods, and content of the current program? What are the characteristics of the "old," in contrast to a proposed "new," best practices program, for example, intervention and assessment time, intensity of contact, complexity, frequency, and cost? What resources are available each year for the program and staff training, pilot testing, and ongoing technical assistance? What are the competencies and attitudes of staff about the existing or new proposed program, the population, and its evaluation? Are program staff, target population, and community leaders included in planning the intervention and evaluation (participatory evaluation)? What do the staff and public think about the problem and the existing and proposed program-intervention? Data-evidence-insight from people from this domain will tell you what is happening at the local program delivery level: it says what the staff are really doing or not doing and what clients and the community really think about the HP-DP program.

## Science-Policy-Practice Partnerships: Domain Consilience

Stakeholders in each domain will have a major influence on what types of programs and evaluations will be planned. The importance of enduring, productive relationships between scientific-academic and non-academic scientists, managers, and colleagues/practitioners who provide insight and leadership is self-evident. Making progress in evaluating the impact of a national, state, or local program requires implementation of science-policy-practice partnerships. Each person (colleague or competitor) in each domain can inhibit or reach agreement about program and evaluation purposes. The evaluation planning and implementation process and the quality of an evaluation plan will be significantly enhanced if staff actively participates in planning and evaluation. Ideally, staff should view an evaluation as an opportunity for program improvement and professional growth.

An evaluation leader and team need to ask the following: How do we reduce the gaps and concerns within and between each domain? Evaluators-scientists, colleagues in practice, policymakers, managers, program staff, and clients need to recognize that the principal reasons for conducting a program and evaluation will differ from area to area, agency to agency, and program to program. Thus, it is essential to know the areas of agreement and differences in the perspectives of each group of stakeholders at the onset of planning. Solutions to the issues and differences within and between Science-Policy-Practice stakeholder(s) need to be identified as early as possible.

A contemporary evaluation philosophy, based on transparency, good communications, and partnerships, will bridge the science-management-practice gap. *The Science Domain, however, must be the foundational domain in an evaluation.* It defines what core HP-DP methods must be applied to produce valid (accurate), reliable (consistent), and representative (generalizability) results. The biggest challenge to HP-DP leadership (director or principal investigator) is to balance the natural, competing interests of people in each domain, achieving a "win-win" situation, without compromising (1) the validity of an evaluation, (2) the political support for the HP-DP program and evaluation, and (3) the successful delivery of the program by staff to a target population.

## Evaluation Progress Review: The 1960s and 1970s

Evaluation is an enduring, global concern of human services professionals. In the 1960s and 1970s, HP-DP program evaluation in the United States paralleled a societal interest in evaluation of medical care, education, and social services. In the 1960s, Rosenstock (1960), Hochbaum (1962, 1965), Campbell and Stanley (1963 and 1966), Suchman (1967), and Campbell (1969) stressed the need to improve the quality and quantity of evaluation research designs and methods. A typical concern expressed in the literature and conferences of this period were that evaluations *only* measured staff effort and resource expenditures: process evaluations. Significant changes reported to be attributable to a program, if documented, were often of questionable validity.

A large number of epidemiological studies during this period documented the role of behavioral and environmental risk factors associated with population incidence and prevalence rates. They confirmed attributable and relative risks for multiple diseases and behaviors. Several large-scale efficacy studies, representing first-generation evaluation models of clinic and community-based health promotion programs, were initiated in the 1970s: the North Karelia (Finland) Cardiovascular Risk Reduction Projects of 1972–1978 in Finland (Puska et al., 1979), and the Stanford

Heart Disease Prevention Study of 1973–1976 in California (Farquahar et al., 1977). Initial reports from each study documented the complexity of designing and implementing a health promotion program evaluation for total communities and large samples of high-risk subjects. The global evidence base confirming the efficacy of HP-DP interventions to change behavior and to reduce population health risks, however, was very limited in the 1960s and 1970s.

The problems of applying social and behavioral science theory and methods to evaluations of public health programs were extensively discussed in the literature. Rigorous evaluation designs and quantitative methods, cited in evaluation research methods texts (Campbell and Stanley, 1963; Campbell, 1969; Weiss, 1972 and 1973; Cook and Campbell, 1979; and Rossi et al., 1979) were rarely employed in HP-DP evaluations. Qualitative evaluation methods, from the foundation work of Glaser and Strauss (1967), Scriven (1972), and Patton (1980), received much attention. Glass published one of the first articles (1976) and book (1981) on meta-analysis.

Green and colleagues (1974, 1977), with the PRECEDE (*P*redisposing, *R*einforcing, and *E*nabling *C*onditions for *E*ducational *D*iagnosis and *E*valuation) Model, were the first group of academic professionals to define a coherent philosophy and a logic model, describing core global principles for health education program evaluation. In 1978, the WHO convened its member countries at the Alma-Ata (USSR) Conference. The "Health for All by 2000" declaration and supporting WHO documents established the need for all countries to establish an evidence base for defining national HP-DP objectives. Alma-Ata was the foundation initiative for the development by most of the developed WHO member states to begin in the 1980s to define the epidemiologic and behavioral evidence about problems and populations, and to develop national HP-DP objectives.

## Evaluation Progress Review: The 1980s and 1990s

The need to develop an HP-DP program knowledge base through the standardization of procedures, strengthening of designs, and replication of evaluation studies in diverse settings was a consistent theme in the 1980s. Salient follow-up contributions about how to systematically plan health education and health promotion programs were introduced by Green and Kreuter in "Health Promotion Planning: An Educational and Ecological Approach (1987). The "PROCEED" Model, published by Green and Kreuter in 1999, expanded the PRECEDE Model to include policy, systems, and environmental factors. Green and Lewis published "Evaluation and Measurement in Health Education" in 1986. Windsor, Baranowski, Clark, and Cutter (1984) published the first comprehensive text in North America, *Evaluation of Health Education and Health Promotion Programs*, for use by graduate professional preparation and training courses. A condensed version of the first edition of the 1984 book was translated into Chinese in 1990 and was disseminated to many other schools of public health throughout the country by the Shanghai Medical University-School of Public Health. A second edition of the Windsor et al. text was published in 1994.

Multiple federal agencies in the United States, especially the National Institutes of Health (NIH), and NGOs, such as the American Lung and Heart Associations, Cancer Society, and March of Dimes, funded prevention, behavioral, demonstration, and HP-DP research programs in the 1980s and 1990s. The National Heart, Lung, and Blood Institute (NHLBI), the National Cancer Institute (NCI), the National Institute for Drug Abuse (NIDA), the CDC, and the Robert Wood Johnson Foundation (RWJF) served as major sources of support for evaluation studies in multiple behavioral risk-factor areas in health promotion–disease prevention. A significant expansion of more rigorous evaluation literature began during this period.

During this period, second-generation reports became available from three NIH-funded evaluations of large-scale community health promotion programs designed to document the efficacy and impact of community health education–health promotion programs on cardiovascular disease (CVD) risk. The Minnesota Heart Health Project (MHHP; Blackburn and Leupker, 1980–1990) evaluated the reduction of cardiovascular disease using a comprehensive, community-wide risk factor reduction approach. The Pawtucket Heart Health Project (Carlton and Lassiter, 1980–1991) in Rhode Island used a variety of community-based interventions, including citizen participation at worksites, religious organizations, schools, grocery stores, and restaurants, in screening and planning. The Stanford Five City Projects (Farquahar and Fortman, 1978–1992) in California used mass media, broadcast and print interventions, and a variety of health education methods and materials and organizational development in their community-based programs to mobilize involvement to improve heart health. Each population-based program represented developmental models for community health planning and evaluation. Multiple project reports demonstrated the complexity of measuring and evaluating population behavior change and CVD risk reduction over 10–15 years. Stone et al. (1992) and Shea and Basch (1995) presented excellent discussions of the issues faced by community-based CVD evaluation studies.

During this period, the HIV/AIDS epidemic was recognized as a local and global public health problem. *Preventing AIDS: A Guide to Effective Education for the Prevention of HIV Infection* by Freudenberg (1989), one of the first reports about the state of the art and science of interventions and role of evaluation, noted, "Evaluation is the single most valuable way to learn what works and what does not work. It is the only way HIV/AIDS educators can develop a body of knowledge that can guide their practice." Two conclusions from the first decade of data-experience were made:

> No single intervention appeared to have maximal effectiveness, even within a single geographic area; and documentation of the effectiveness of interventions was compromised by plans that do not include rigorous process and impact evaluation methods.

Numerous current reviews of the literature confirm the enduring validity of these two conclusions about HIV/AIDS interventions, and for most chronic disease interventions. It is difficult to change the behavior of any population, and it is a complex process to evaluate the reasons for changes.

## Process Evaluation: Linking HP-DP Programs and Impact

All programs need to achieve a high level of process implementation, or delivery of program components with fidelity, to have an opportunity to produce salient changes among populations at risk. Excellent examples of the methods and utility of a process evaluation applied to programs of national scope were described by several researchers: Stone National Heart, Lung, and Blood Institute, 1994), "Process Evaluation in the Multi-Center Child and Adolescent Trial for Cardiovascular Disease (CATCH); Baranowski and Stables (National Cancer Institute, 5-a-Day, 2000), "Learning What Works and How: Process Evaluations of the 5-a-Day Projects"; and Windsor, Whiteside, Solomon, et al. (Robert Wood Johnson Foundation, Smoke Free Families-National Program Office, 2000), "A Process Evaluation Model for Patient Education Programs for Pregnant Smokers." In 1999, the CDC developed an Evaluation Framework. Steckler and Linnan (2003) completed one of the first books on the subject, *Process Evaluation for Public Health Interventions and Research*.

## Evaluation Progress Review: Objectives for the Nation and States

This section presents a synopsis of the US HP-DP Objectives for the Nation Reports: 1990 to 2010. These Reports are salient contributions to the evaluation progress review literature. The US Reports were developed in response to the 1978 Alma-Ata World Health Organization, "Health for All by the Year 2000" Declaration. The 1990, 2000, 2010–2020 HP-DP Reports (1) applied sound epidemiologic and statistical methods and expert assessments of historical trends in each area of high population risk for each objective over a 5- and 10-year period, (2) synthesized available HP-DP databases and intervention literature, and (3) used peer review methods to define the science base. Each decade Report (1990, 2000, 2010, 2020) and 1985, 1995, and 2005 HP-DP Mid-Course Progress Reviews are primary country- and state-(provincial) level references for planning program evaluations. The development of the Healthy People Objectives was one of the most important national (and state) level activities for HP-DP program evaluation in the United States.

Preparing an HP-DP Report is one of the first steps in systematically planning and evaluating programs for a country, state/province, or large metropolitan area. Next, the government decides what national or state/provincial agency will be responsible for preparing the Report and collecting valid and representative data to establish baselines and monitor progress every 3–5 and 10 years. At the same time, national governmental leadership decides which will be the coordinating federal agency, in partnership with other governmental entities and NGOs, to conduct Progress Reviews.

As part of its National Health Interview Survey (NHIS), the National Center for Health Statistics (NCHS) of the US CDC initiated in 1985 the first national HP-DP Study to collect data and monitor national progress. The Office of Disease Prevention and Health Promotion (ODP-HP) was established by the Congress in the DHHS Secretary's Office to coordinate national HP-DP Progress Reviews. Every two to three years and at the end of each decade, a lead federal agency, for example, the National Heart, Lung, and Blood Institute (NHLBI) of the NIH and its National High Blood Pressure and Cholesterol Control Programs, establishes and convenes its national advisory committee, in partnership with other federal and non-federal agencies and professional organizations. The HP-DP Committee conducts and presents a Progress Review Report to the DHHS Secretary, US Congress, and the public. The Progress Review identifies what specific health and behavioral objectives (1) have been met, (2) are moving forward, or (3) are moving backward. A draft Report is routinely made available for public and professional review, critique, and written comments, electronically or by mail. The following is a synopsis of the 1990, 2000, 2010, and 2020 Reports.

## Healthy Objectives for the Nation: 1990, 2000, 2010, 2020

In September, 1980, the Secretary of the DHHS prepared and published the first national Report: *Objectives for the Nation* (1980). It included baseline data and identified 227 objectives and 15 health priority areas in three program areas: (1) Health Promotion Services, (2) Preventive Health Services, and (3) Health Protection. The DHHS published a Mid-Course Review in 1985 to document the status of the 1990 objectives, and to make projections about their accomplishment by 1990: 108 (48%) objectives were likely to be met by 1990. It is worth noting that 227 objectives were specified; 58 (26%) were written without baseline data. Thus, the number of measurable objectives of the 227 was 169; the percent achieved was 108/169, or 64%. In the absence of data, professional judgment by a panel of experts and consensus to define objectives was used.

In September 1990, the DHHS presented *Healthy People 2000: National Health Promotion and Disease Prevention Objectives*, with 22 priority areas and 336 objectives. Priority areas were grouped into the three categories. A new category of importance to program evaluation was created in the 2000 Report: Priority Area 22: Surveillance and Data Systems. A Mid-Course Review was disseminated in 1996: 25% of the measurable objectives were met by 2000.

In January 2000 the DHHS released the *Healthy People 2010 Objectives*, with 28 program areas and 467 objectives, as the US contribution to the WHO "Health for All" strategy. Examples of different objectives are presented in Table 1.5. The *Healthy People 2010 Objectives* were distinguished from the *2000 Objectives* by stronger data systems. The experiences from 1980 to 2005 demonstrated that a systematic process and planning framework was essential to identify where data/information were missing and where improvements were or were not occurring. Approximately 20% of the measurable objectives were met over a two-year period.

### HP-DP 2020 Objectives for the Nation

The National Center for Health Statistics developed an interactive database that defines the wide range of objectives and contains a comprehensive discussion of the objectives by category and monitoring data for the 2020 Objectives.

TABLE 1.5 *Healthy People 2010*: Examples of Types of Objectives

| TYPE | OBJECTIVE |
|---|---|
| Health Status | To reduce the infant mortality rate to no more than 4.5 per 1,000 live births. |
| BASELINE: | 7.2 per 1,000 live births in 1998 |
| Risk Reduction | To increase use of occupant protection systems, such as safety belts and child restraints, to a subsequent 92% and 100% |
| BASELINE: | 69% of the total population used safety belts and 92% of motor vehicle occupants < 4 years used child restraints in 1998 |
| Service and Protection | To increase to 95% the proportion of adults who have had their blood pressure measured within < 2 years and can state whether HBP was normal or high |
| BASELINE: | 90% of people < 18 had their blood pressure measured within the < 2 years and were given the systolic + diastolic values in 1998 |

SOURCE: US Department of Health and Human Services, *Healthy People 2010.*

## A Global Health Progress Review: The Millennium Development Goals (2010)

In 2000, representatives of the International Community, led by the UN, defined targets to improve the development and economic conditions of low-income countries. Sub-Saharan Africa was a special target region. Substantial reductions in poverty, a primary determinant of health, were perceived to be the core mechanism to promote health and prevent disease among those in greatest need. Through significantly enhanced financial and capacity-building partnerships between high-, middle-, and low-income countries, commitments were made to improve economic growth.

In September 2000, leadership from 189 countries defined eight Millenium Development Goals (MDGs): (1) eradicate extreme poverty and hunger; (2) achieve universal primary education; (3) promote equality and empower women; (4) reduce child mortality; (5) improve maternal health; (6) combat HIV/AIDS, malaria, and other diseases; (7) ensure environmental sustainability; and (8) develop a global development partnership. A set of 18 targets and 48 progress indicators were used to monitor progress. Four new targets were added in 2007. The MDG Report 2014–2015 is available at mdgs.un.org. Excerpts and examples of progress from the most recent MDG Report are presented in Table 1.6.

### Millenium Development Goals Progress Review

The following is a Progress Review of the MDGs. Conducting valid assessments of progress in meeting the 22 targets and the validity of Aid

TABLE 1.6 Millenium Development Goals, 2015

Goal #1: The number of people in extreme poverty decreased from 47% (1990) to 22% (2010). The percentage of underweight children under 5 years old dropped from 25% (1990) to 16% (2010).

Goal #2: The number of primary school-age children out of school has dropped by 33 million, but 72 million were denied an education in 2007.

Goal #3: 95 girls were enrolled in primary school for every 100 boys vs. 91 girls in 1999. With only 53 of 171 countries reporting data, these parity rates are not valid. No progress was made.

Goal #4: The global mortality rate for < 5 was 51/1,000 in 2010 vs. 87 in 1990: a 41% reduction. Measles deaths dropped by 74% in this period and coverage increased from 73% > 83%.

Goal #5: Maternal deaths were 400/100,000 births in 1990 vs. 210/100,000 in 2010, a 47% decrease.

Goal #6: The estimated number of AIDS deaths < by 2 million (2007) and new infections < 16% (2001–2007). The % of the population with safe drinking water increased: 76% to 89% (1990–2010). The use of treated bed nets for children increased from 2% in 2000 to 20% in 2006.

Goal #7: Per capita $CO_2$ emissions increased 31% above 1990 levels. Ozone depleting substances among 195 participating countries achieved a 97% reduction. From 1990 to 2011, 1.9 billion people gained access to latrines, flush toilets, and other sanitation facilities.

Goal #8: Net disbursement of development assistance Increased from $114 billion in 2007 to $126 billion in 2012: highest recorded.

Effectiveness for specific countries and regions have been recognized as contentious issues by the global population health science community. While some progress has been made in many of the Goals for many people and for many countries, tens of millions of people and a large number of countries and regions, especially in Africa, have experienced little progress. If the data from these rates are valid, one interpretation is that some improvements have been and are being made in some Targets, and in all eight Goal areas. But there is considerable heterogeneity between and within regions in the magnitude, consistency, and type of impact. The lack of progress in most of the 18 target areas was consistently documented in Sub-Saharan Africa. Measurement issues, including no data and data of poor quality, continue to compromise MDG evaluation progress (and AID Effectiveness). As the MDG 2009 Report acknowledged, no simple answers exist for any of these problems.

While the debate about the need to expand or compress targets and indicators needs to continue, and data quality needs to improve, MDGs and Targets, like other global or national objectives, can be viewed as general guides to set global HP-DP program and policy goals. Until each country produces valid, reliable, and complete and current data, all reports about current and past status, trends, and especially progress need to be interpreted with considerable caution.

MDG progress, like beauty in art, will vary by viewer criteria, experience, and especially the political perspective and type of government in power. Unfortunately, corruption, theft, and poor management practices are well documented in the regions and countries of greatest need. A variety of characteristics of each individual country, such as the lack of integrity and commitment by national leadership, instability, and a lack of infrastructure, eliminate the opportunity for improved conditions. They predict a lack of improvements in the targets. The evaluation of MDG progress was significantly affected by the global economic recession of 2007–2009. The large, variable impact of the recession on individual countries and citizens needs to be recognized. If the per capita income is $30,000–40,000 versus $300–400, the dramatic differential impact is self-evident.

The solutions are a continuing commitment to work with the political, economic, and policy leadership to improve the capacity and infrastructure across national sectors in the health, education, and development sectors, especially for women and children. Part of the solution to the enduring issue of a lack of host country stewardship of the millions of dollars for HD-DP projects is to significantly increase the monitoring and oversight of development aid. A rational system of progress benchmarks and data for a timeline to document legitimate use of funds would reveal levels of success and failure. Some projects should be terminated and others substantially revised.

In 2015, the United Nations will develop a list of MDGs. While many MDGs have been met, and the UN and member nations are to be applauded for their support, it is clear that the UN and its leadership seem to have learned few lessons. Future projects must be far more focused: fewer achievable and cost-effective objectives are needed. In addition, almost all projects should be not be funded unless serious data quality and implementation (Process and Impact Evaluation) deficiencies are substantially reduced or eliminated. Much has been written and presented on the problems with the MDGs. An excellent review and discussion of the Millennium Development Goals is presented by J. Waage et al., *The Lancet* (September 13, 2010).

The following reports present two perspectives: one for a public audience and one for a professional audience. Both are critical. "Dead Aid: Why AID is not Working and How There is a Better Way for Africa" (Dambisa Moyo, 2009) provides an insightful explanation about reasons for decades of massive failure and a rational road map for potential progress. A recent book by the Copenhagen Consensus Center provides guidance about *How to Spend $75 Billion to Make the World a Better Place*. This report, based on a rigorous review of 40 proposals by a group of senior economists, identified several areas as excellent candidates to be the primary focus of the MDGs: (1) reduce malnutrition, (2) reduce malaria and TB, (3) increase pre-primary education, especially for girls, (4) increase universal access to sexual-reproductive health, and (5) expand free trade. These are the most likely candidates to produce optimal improvements to the health and lives of people, especially children and women. While it is reasonable to debate the areas, and adjust to regional needs, unless the science base is a stronger guide to UN decisions (rather than politics), in 2030 the failure of the UN to achieve optimal levels of impact is likely to be well documented again.

## The Health Promotion Movement and Evaluation

Since the Alma-Ata Conference, the WHO and a large number of member countries, as an extension of the "Health for All" Principle, have supported a variety of inter- and intra-country HP-DP initiatives over the last 30 years: Healthy Cities, Health-Promoting Schools, Health-Promoting Hospitals, and Healthy Workplaces. The Ottawa Charter for Health Promotion (WHO, 1986), the Adelaide Recommendations (WHO, 1988), The Sundsvall Statement on Supportive Environments (WHO, 1991), the Jakarta Declaration on Leading Health Promotion into the 21st Century (WHO, 1997), and the Mexico Charter in 2000 continued to promote expansion, at the national and global level, of a "Health Promotion Philosophy." A new Health Promotion Charter was adopted by the 700 international health participants and officials from 100 countries at the Sixth Global Conference on Health Promotion in Thailand (2005). The Bangkok Charter for Health Promotion highlighted the challenges facing global health, including the growing double burden of communicable and chronic diseases. The Charter called for a commitment to making health promotion a core responsibility for all governments, a key focus of communities and civil society, and a requirement for good corporate practice. The Charter calls on local, regional, and national governments to make investments in health as a priority and to provide sustainable financing for health promotion activities.

While there has been general agreement and support among a significant proportion of the domestic and global public health policy, science, and practice communities for a "Health Promotion Philosophy," the cumulative body of valid empirical evidence from behavioral impact evaluations and economic analyses of a "Health Promotion Program Model" is very limited. A criticism of the health promotion field has been the tendency of its proponents to focus on the advocacy of the philosophy and breadth/scope of activity, for example, 500 Healthy Schools, 200 Healthy hospitals, and 100 Healthy Cities, but to place insufficient emphasis and commitment of resources to conduct rigorous scientific evaluations of individual "Health Promotion Programs."

Unfortunately, when a program is based primarily on political advocacy and purports to be focused on sociopolitical determinants of health, is planned with little empirical evidence, and does not collect valid data to measure progress, it misses the opportunity to document health impact and health improvement. Evaluation results and evidence, for example, significant changes in behavior and health status, supporting the "Health Promotion Program Model," have typically documented no significant impact. Systematic reviews, using meta-evaluation criteria, typically confirm that very few Health Promotion Program evaluations had adequate internal or external validity. The advocacy approach has produced much skepticism among the population health science community. These issues are discussed in greater detail in the next section.

## The Science-Policy-Practice Gap in Health Promotion and Population Health Science

Twenty-first-century planning and evaluation of HP-DP programs requires a trans-disciplinary mixed model and team in order to have any real opportunity for success and impact. Although no one model can be expected to provide a universal answer to designing HP-DP interventions that will always work, the "Health Promotion Model" can be contrasted with the evidence supporting a "Population Health Science Model." Future evaluations need to blend the qualitatively oriented focus of the Health Promotion Model with the quantitatively and qualitatively focused methods of the PRECEDE-PROCEED Model developed and applied by Green and colleagues, and many others through the world. Their approach stresses a planned application of a logic model, use of mixed quantitative and qualitative methods, and engagement of science, practice, and consumer stakeholders, for example, PBPR, to plan and evaluate tailored interventions for specific problems, populations, and settings.

The application of well-established principles and methods of epidemiology, biostatistics, behavioral science, health education, and multiple related population health disciplines must be considered and applied by future HP-DP evaluations. Future evaluation planning needs to apply these disciplines, but also place a broader and equal emphasis on organizational change and the participation of target groups to gain their support for a program and its evaluation. The next generation of HP-DP evaluations needs to significantly reduce the existing science-policy-practice gap. Achieving this goal requires explicit and implicit commitments to significantly improve public policy decision making. "A Framework for Mandatory Impact Evaluation to Ensure Well Informed Public Policy Decisions," by Oxman, Bjorndal, Becerra-Posada, et al., in *Lancet* (January 2010) provides a cogent discussion on this topic. They define an approach, "A WHO Framework," that governments in all countries need to consider to make the best use of finite resources.

While our knowledge base about how to plan and evaluate is comprehensive, there continues to be a very large gap between the science bases of HP-DP planning and evaluation, and the routine application of these principles by evaluation teams and program leadership. Numerous evaluation reports from individual projects, meta-evaluations of specific bodies of evidence by Cochrane and Campbell Collaborations, and reports from national evaluation units consistently confirm the poor quality of many HP-DP program evaluations. A very large number and overwhelming proportion of published evaluations or disseminated project reports for low-income countries do not meet the most basic standards of evaluation practice. Many HP-DP program evaluations in high-income countries also failed to meet standards of evaluation practice.

The following are three commentaries on the large, existing HP-DP science-to-practice gap. One represents the low-income sector, and two represent the high-income sector. *When Will We Ever Learn: Improving Lives Through Impact Evaluation* by the Evaluation Gap Working Group in Washington, D.C. (Savedoff, Levine, and Birdsall, Center for Global Development-CGD, 2006) presents an excellent synthesis of the state of the science and practice of program evaluation. The Evaluation Gap Working Group, supported by the Gates and Hewlett Foundations, reviewed over a two-year period the methodological rigor of impact evaluations of social programs in developing countries supported by international aid through 2005. After a comprehensive review by over 100 senior policymakers, agency staff, and evaluation specialists, the Evaluation Working Group concluded that it was rare that a methodologically sound "Impact Evaluation" was conducted. When an evaluation was conducted, the quality of it was almost always poor. This report poignantly noted:

> Poor quality evaluations are misleading. No responsible MD would consider prescribing medications without properly evaluating their impact or potential side effects. Yet in social programs ... no such standard has been adopted. While it is widely recognized that withholding programs that are known to be beneficial would be unethical, the implicit corollary—that programs of unknown impact should not be widely replicated without proper evaluation—is frequently dismissed. (p. 3)

Roger Vaughen, associate editor, Statistics and Evaluation, *American Journal of Public Health*, in a special Issue of the journal in 2004, indicated that evaluation has many meanings, but whatever the definition, it is the business of public programs to find out what works. Consistent with the commentary and reports cited throughout this book, he noted:

> Evaluation is an essential part of public health: without evaluation's close ties to program implementation, we are left with the unsatisfactory circumstance of either wasting resources on ineffective programs or, perhaps worse, continuing public health practices that do more harm than good. The public health literature is replete with examples of well intentioned but unevaluated programs ... that were continued for decades, until rigorous and appropriate evaluations revealed that the results were not as intended." (p. 360)

The Health Committee, UK House of Commons, prepared a report entitled "Health Inequalities" (2009). It presented a synthesis of the evidence to the government, public, and scientific community about the impact of health policies and funded HP-DP programs since 2000. The UK Report dispelled the myth that poor evaluations are *only* conducted in low-income countries. The Report and testimony to the House of Commons by multiple senior UK academics at public sessions confirmed that very little progress had been made to determine which HP-DP programs were effective. There was strong, unanimous agreement by all contributors. Almost all evaluations had serious methodological problems, applied very poor designs, and/or failed to appreciate the complexity of evaluation. The Report, especially Chapter 3 ("Evaluation"), indicated:

> " ... despite a ten year push to tackle health inequalities and significant government effort and investment, we still have very little evidence about what

interventions actually work. This is in large part due to inadequate evaluation of the policies adopted to address the problem.... (p. 28)

In addition to the technical deficiencies, the report also discussed "[t]he ethical case for evaluation." It raised the same issue as the above Report from the Center for Global Development: addressing health inequalities with a poor evidence base. The UK report noted:

While lack of research is not a justification for inaction ... the Nuffield Council of Bioethics' recent report on public health interventions puts forward a strong ethical case for the obligation to research interventions. Introducing unevaluated interventions into communities to risks, in much the same way as participating in trials of new drugs or surgical procedures are to exposed to risk ... the intervention may have unintended consequences. ... (p. 34)

These three discussions have explicit, current implications for many health promotion program advocates, especially the zealots and politicians in many countries who frequently lobby for initiatives and substantial resources with limited evidence of efficacy. They loudly assert that rigorous evaluation methods and randomized clinical trials (RCT) are unnecessary, and that evaluations are not a good use of resources. While an evaluation of HP-DP programs is complex and an RCT should not be automatically conducted for all programs, future evaluations and evaluators who do not apply well-established evaluation methods, especially in many countries of greatest need, need to address the ethical implications and gross inefficiencies of their activity.

The Evaluation Working Group Report (2006), the House of Commons Health Inequalities Report (2009), and many other commentaries and Reports cited throughout this text represent important reference guides to academic programs, evaluation teams, and organizational leadership. These sources provide an enduring insight and comprehensive discussion about the array of conceptual and methodological issues that future evaluations and evaluators must consider. The global literature clearly tells us in 2015 how to conduct rigorous qualitative, process, impact, outcome, and cost evaluations of population health programs. We know how to plan and evaluate, how to potentially improve population health, and how to improve the science, policy, and practice base for major chronic and infectious diseases in any country or region.

Accordingly, both the leadership in government and NGOs, especially units in international development agencies that fund programs and so-called Offices of Evaluation that have the responsibility of evaluating these initiatives, must decide to accept the responsibility for failing to plan and conduct valid assessments of program impact. In the last decade alone, hundreds of agencies have spent and wasted billions of dollars on hundreds of programs that failed to be implemented and evaluated. All too frequently, little or no data were collected on salient process, cost, impact, or outcome rates, or vast amounts of data were collected, only to be ignored.

## An HP-DP Evaluation Paradigm Shift

It is not naiveté, but wisdom from 50 years of literature reviews and the breadth and depth of training, experience, and performance of the authors of the first to fifth editions of this book that define clear solutions to the multiple problems noted. Without an explicit political and policy paradigm shift, without clear guidelines that demand rigorous, ethical impact/outcome evaluations that focus on internal and external validity, most future HP-DP initiatives, especially global AID, will again waste billions of dollars of resources. The opportunity to help those who will almost always need the most help will be lost. Governmental agencies and NGOs in both high- and low-income countries need to stop funding methodologically deficient HP-DP programs that have little or no evidence to support their replication, fidelity of delivery, or effectiveness. Methodologically weak evaluations will not produce valid results, and cannot benefit participants. The leadership and professional staff of funding agencies must recognize that methodologically weak evaluation plans do not meet ethical standards for human participation. As the Nuffield Council on Bioethics (UK, House of Commons, 2009) noted: "It is unethical to propose, fund and conduct an HP-DP Program evaluation that cannot yield internally valid results."

One of the first steps to reduce these enduring problems is to establish and routinely implement a transparent peer review process that consistently applies global standards of science and ethics. Using existing program proposal review procedures applied by the NIH or UK NICE, and Cochrane Review criteria, will significantly address the issue. Peer review groups also have the explicit responsibility to decide on the acceptability or non-acceptability of evaluation plans. Institutional Review Boards (IRB) need to be established and must accept the responsibility to approve only new HP-DP proposals that demonstrate explicit protection of human subjects.

Improvements in the technical quality of HP-DP program and evaluation proposals and peer review and IRB policies and procedures, although rational strategies, are, however, only the beginning of the process of addressing the myriad of serious problems cited. A stronger professional and societal commitment is needed to improve this situation. Political and professional leaders in national organizations whose mission is to serve the public, the scientific community, and especially public representatives, need to speak out. They need to demand that salient scientific and ethical issues be resolved well before funding decisions are made about all new programs.

## Program Evaluation Leadership: Future Challenges

A comprehensive array of conceptual and methodological guidance about all aspects of program evaluation for almost any problem and population are readily available in the published literature. Rossi and Freeman published their seventh edition of *Evaluation: A Systematic Approach* (2004). Patton has provided cogent discussions of *Qualitative Research and Evaluation Methods* (2000). Methods to systematically plan health education and promotion programs are thoroughly described by Green and Kreuter in *Health Promotion Planning: An Educational and Ecological Approach* (2005; the "PROCEED" Model). Prior editions of this book were published in 1984, 1994, 2004, and 2010. *Evaluation of Health Promotion-Health Education-Disease Prevention Programs* was published in Chinese in 1990 and Korean in 2005. The fifth edition of this book represents input from a large number of senior public health faculty from the first. second, third, and fourth editions. Although sharing considerable content of the earlier editions, this edition reflects a comprehensive vision of program evaluation standards for professional practice, regardless of where they are applied.

Multiple rigorous evaluations were conducted in the 1990s and throughout the world in the first and second decades of the twenty-first century. The global scientific literature provides explicit guidance about how to define evaluation targets for any problem or population. This collective experience, insight, and wisdom provide a complete range of complementary discussions about the technical complexity and political and programmatic issues related to evaluation. An abundance of references exists for the advanced, master's, and doctoral trained evaluators and population health program planners and directors. Comprehensive descriptions of theoretical and methodological issues and practical problems to plan and conduct evaluations are readily available. Although all evaluations will be complex, regardless of the PHASE, how to evaluate HP-DP program feasibility, effectiveness, and costs for all major health problems and risk factor has been well defined.

Throughout the world, especially at the federal level in high-income countries, the perceived need for more "comparative effectiveness research" and "health impact evaluation" has been voiced by political leadership and discussed in a large number of professional documents. It is important to emphasize that neither of these concepts is new to the program evaluation community. However, given the continued emphasis on the concept of evidence-based programs, it would seem more likely that the political, scientific, and health professional leadership of governmental and non-governmental agencies will demand that future HP-DP programs set more realistic objectives, plan more feasible programs, and apply more rigorous methods. Political leaders, however, need to stop making absurd demands or promises for immediate results from public health/healthcare policies and related HP-DP programs. Political and professional leaders need to start responding to the loud voices that demand resources and action without evidence by demanding (as loudly) sufficient resources and planned, rigorous, evidence-based solutions.

Future HP-DP program evaluations need to embrace this philosophy. Assuming sufficient resources and time, they should be expected to apply more rigorous scientific methods to document improvements in program quality and to have an impact on behavioral and health status indicators. Particularly in periods of competing, finite, and/or diminishing budgetary resources, program leadership should be held more accountable for conducting rigorous impact evaluations of the initiatives they direct. If a domestic or international aid organization is truly committed to program quality and social equity, it will not compromise its standards of practice.

The maturation of the HP-DP science base is complex, challenging, and continuous. The measurement and intervention science base, however, will only improve from well-designed evaluation studies. Each sound PHASE 1 to PHASE 4 Evaluation has the opportunity to contribute to the global HP-DP and population health science, practice, and policy base. Proposed and funded projects need to be grounded, however, in evaluation methods and to meet global methodological standards to produce valid and representative qualitative and quantitative results. Proposals to conduct each type of evaluation should be rigorously and independently reviewed by a peer review group of scientists and an independent IRB to protect the rights of participants.

All HP-DP program evaluations provide numerous opportunities to bridge the typical gap between science- or academically based and practice-based professionals. Program evaluation should be perceived as a fertile opportunity for collaboration among scientists, managers, practitioners, and the people they serve, regardless of problem and setting. An evaluation should also serve not only as an opportunity to test new interventions and disseminate evidence-based innovations, but also as an important channel for the improvement of professional practice. The development, implementation, and adaptation of a complex evaluation plan to unanticipated situations, although at times stressful, are creative exercises for members of an evaluation team. Staff mentored on projects where "best practices" and "trans-disciplinary" philosophies are not only preached, but applied, will have their professional growth significantly enhanced.

Academic programs that prepare HP-DP specialists have a responsibility to translate and apply "global" principles and methods of measurement and intervention science in their teaching, research, and individual practices. While there are enduring methodological and resource issues that each evaluation must address, too many contemporary evaluations reflect very poor practice. *The multitude of poor examples in published, supposedly peer-reviewed journals, inform the public, the HP-DP profession, and especially graduate students about how not to plan and conduct an evaluation.* For new, higher quality programs to become an integrated part of the public health, healthcare, worksite, or community-social system, stronger graduate level training leadership, increased standards of professional preparation, and improved methodological sophistication are essential. These activities are essential to expand our knowledge, science, and practice base.

There is no mystery today about how an excellent evaluation should be planned and conducted. A gradual, incremental increase in the routine application of more rigorous standards and methods, and the production of stronger empirical evidence documenting feasibility and impact, should increase the probability of improvement in health indicators and rates for the high-risk populations in greatest need. These improvements should (but may not) increase the probability of resource allocation to HP-DP initiatives and improve a program or an agency's ability to affect health-related policies. Population health science and practice professionals who develop the technical and leadership skills to collaborate with agency policy and community stakeholders and citizens they serve are more likely to achieve greater professional success. They are more likely to play a more significant role in achieving their local, state, and/or country "Health Promotion–Disease Prevention and Management Objectives." Most important, the health of individuals, families, and communities will significantly improve.

# 2 | Planning an Evaluation

PRECEDE and PROCEED work in tandem, providing a continuous
series of steps or phases in planning, implementation, and
evaluation.

—*Larry Green*

N THIS CHAPTER, WE DESCRIBE methods to develop the HP-DP program
to be evaluated. As noted in Chapter 1, almost all individuals who will
use this book will have taken several three-credit courses. Discussions
about the application of HP-DP planning and evaluation methods assume
graduate-level knowledge and skill in the application of principles and
methods from biostatistics, epidemiology, health education–health promotion, and social-behavioral science. In almost all organizations, a graduate trained member of the staff will prepare an HP-DP program plan and
direct its implementation, and evaluation. A plan should be a detailed road
map: a blueprint that defines program structure, process, content, methods,
materials, and staffing. It should describe how its objectives, intervention
components, and each type of evaluation are logically connected. A sound
plan reflects "best practices": a synthesis and application of the state of the
science and practice for a problem, population, and practice setting. A plan
should provide specific guidelines for staff implementation and should
enable program description and future replication. It should also reflect a
consensus among staff about what should be done by whom, how, when,
and where.

HP-DP program and evaluation staff needs to determine, through a
meta-evaluation (ME) and meta-analysis (MA), evaluability assessments,
and consensus discussions, what an HP-DP program should be able to

achieve and what it probably cannot achieve for a specific problem and target population. Drafting objectives, discussing them, and agreeing on a small number of core objectives form the basic process that a team should implement to set realistic evaluation targets. Evaluation should be perceived by all contributors as an integrated component of planning.

Initially, we discuss in this chapter important basic concepts for program developers: the organizational context for planning, planning network, and specific procedures to develop the evaluation plan. Besides ensuring that a program is well grounded, good planning also helps to synthesize data and information, and to mobilize people and resources critical to program success. A detailed, methodologically rigorous evaluation plan is also essential to assist the program and the evaluator in resetting objectives (if needed) during the implementation and evaluation phases of a project. A detailed program and evaluation plan and justified budget are always necessary to obtain internal or external funds.

## The Organizational Context for HP-DP Programs

When evaluations of interventions are planned, scientists and program staff try to define the causes and solutions of a problem for a specific group of people. As part of the process, scientific leadership selects a theoretical model, and creates an intervention based on hypothesized relationships of concepts in the model. An evaluation plan is prepared to determine the efficacy of a theory-based, tailored/targeted intervention in modifying the salient concepts of the theory and changing the behavior of a target group. Successfully planning and evaluating a theory-based program will always be challenging.

While a fundamental standard of practice is that a program should be based on valid principles and theories, testing the validity of a theoretical model necessitates the acceptance and adjustment to the day-to-day operational realities of an HP-DP program. In practice, program management, operational, and evaluation staff need to try to come as close as they can to theoretical conditions in order to enable positive changes to occur. For example, existing theory suggests that developing peer support groups, with the same members meeting over time, may enable chronically ill people to acquire the social support, confidence, and motivation to manage their illness better. But, given patient work schedules, available meeting places and time, patient costs, a limited budget, or other factors, it may not be feasible to fully apply these principles. Program staff will need to continually try to bring about needed changes in organizations and communities to enhance conditions for behavior change among a target group.

Evaluation research, or PHASE 1 Formative Evaluations and Phase 2 Efficacy Evaluations, should be Theory-Based Evaluations (TBE). Each is designed to manipulate the social and physical environment to test hypotheses about causes and solutions. Program evaluations, or PHASE 3 Effectiveness Evaluations and PHASE 4 Dissemination-Translational Evaluations, contribute to the HP-DP knowledge base by assessing and describing the application of tested methods in similar settings and situations for large, well-defined populations at risk. Ultimately, valid program evaluations conducted as part of an ongoing program may contribute to the basis on which a theory becomes accepted as generally valid. The enduring challenge for the HP-DP field is to develop programs and to conduct evaluations to bridge the theory-practice-policy gap.

## Philosophy of the Organization

HP-DP specialists are employed by health, education, and social services agencies and organizations to plan, manage, and evaluate programs. Although this book has broad utility for a wide range of professionals, it is primarily written for graduate-level trained health education–health promotion professionals. Working with an organization means that staff must represent in programming not only its view, objectives, and philosophy, but also those of the parent organization or agency. At times there is conflict between what an individual believes is sound practice or well-grounded philosophy and the policies of the organization. Program staff and evaluators must recognize the politics of decision-making and resource allocation, and must have the technical and leadership skills to negotiate realistic objectives, given the available funding, staffing, and time constraints.

Unfortunately, local and state-level HP-DP programs are often launched by an agency with much publicity, but limited evidence of efficacy. As noted in Chapter 1, a newly developed or existing program may lack sound scientific methods. In general, agency leadership and managers (especially politicians and organization leadership) should define a smaller number of objectives and more realistic expectations of program impact or outcome.

## Program Justification

There are multiple reasons that an HP-DP program exists or is being proposed. Organizational or program leadership may see the need to design or significantly redesign a program, for example: "We really need to improve our hypertension control program for the elderly in our community health centers. We need to improve the quality and cost effectiveness of services." Or, according to organizational community partners or its advisory board, HP-DP program staff may be asked to design a program that agency clients need: "Given the data on the low percent of elderly with their hypertension control (40%) in our county-wide program, the board of directors feels we need to expand our existing program. We need to significantly increase high blood pressure control rates. Please draft a plan and budget to present at our monthly meeting." Or, HP-DP staff may be asked by an agency director or the HP-DP program manager to design a program on the basis of what its clients want: "What kind of health education program do our elderly clients need and want? Prepare a draft plan to find what they think, and prepare a budget and timeline for discussion at our next meeting."

## Mission and Goals of the Organization

A new program or its revision is likely to be organized in one of two ways: as part of ongoing activities providing related programs and health-related services directly to clients, or as a project by groups that provide no direct medical or nursing service. For example, a hypertension education and management initiative may be part of the senior citizen program of a local community health center. Clinical service providers may be available to assess and treat program participants with hypertension. Similarly, the program may be part of the services of a general medical clinic in the community that has a large elderly population and where physicians, dentists, physician assistants, nurse practitioners, or pharmacists routinely see clients with high blood pressure. The HP-DP program is often part of or is developed as an integrated component of ongoing health or social services of an organization with a wider set of health and human services activities.

On the other hand, a hypertension program might be developed as an activity of all senior citizen centers in a county where the aim is to assist elderly clients with many concerns, including health. In this case, participants might be referred elsewhere, if they need medical or nursing services. Similarly, a community education program may be developed by a private voluntary agency, say Citizens for a Better Community, and directed to all the elderly in an area. Such a program might recruit staff, if they are needed, or refer people to available services when necessary. The important aspect to note about these latter two examples is that the HP-DP program is part of a community-wide effort, and is not directly part of medical/nursing services.

Both the goals of health promotion and health education and the goals of evaluations are greatly influenced by the orientation of the sponsoring organization. The type and level of emphasis on evaluations conducted by an organization will depend on how it defines it mission. Organizations give priority to programs that further their primary goals. Healthcare organizations tend to be oriented primarily toward communities or individuals and toward disease treatment, management, or prevention. If an organization serves individuals, it will tend to focus on what people can do to improve their health. Such an organization (e.g., a hospital) might develop patient education to assist diabetic patients to manage their condition, assessing their signs, administering appropriate medications, and adjusting their caloric intake. The focus may be primarily on the individual and an individual solution to the health problem or condition.

For the program planner and evaluator, a basic principle is to fully appreciate the organizational mission before starting or revising a program. What are the organizational goals and mission related to the problem in question? As you consider your program in light of the organization that sponsors it, you may ask a question frequently posed: Is the objective of intervention always behavior change? An HP-DP program almost always tries to stimulate organizational and community changes to enable people to acquire the resources and services necessary for healthful living. This is particularly apparent when a program has a community-action orientation, but it is also the case when the program is oriented toward individual change.

All programs operate on the assumption that people will be different as a result of their participation. This assumption is easy to understand when a program focuses on individuals and disease management. Reducing falls among an elderly woman, for example, should enable her to increase her flexibility and walk 30 minutes each day. It is more difficult to see behavior change as the goal if the program focuses on communities and prevention. Assume, for the sake of discussion, that a program wants to help people improve inadequate public safety in a community. A goal may be to organize groups to demand service from the city housing authority, bring suit against recalcitrant landlords, or improve community policing to decrease vandalism.

## The Health Promotion Planning Network

Regardless of the type of sponsoring organization, planning and evaluation should never be a unilateral activity. A guiding principle of program development is that to be effective, development should always be planned with the participation of major interest groups. The design, implementation, and evaluation of a program should always involve a network of people (stake-holders): representatives of the target group, program planner/evaluators, others in your organization, and representatives of outside organizations who provide needed services and resources. If a program fails to account for the clients' perspective, it cannot possibly appeal to potentially change their motives or enable them to see the relevance of the behavior change to their situation.

Without the participation of potential participants, a program may be planned that misses the vital ingredient to enable participants to behave in a new way or to change environmental conditions that inhibit healthful behavior. Without the views of those who provide needed related services, it will also be difficult to mobilize the resources and cooperation to carry out a comprehensive program. Program planning needs agreements with all major stakeholders. Volumes of papers and books describe sound meth-ods of "Community-Based Participatory Planning and Evaluation" that should be routinely applied in planning and evaluating HP-DP programs. Discussions and case studies in Chapter 4 (Measurement and Analysis in Evaluation) of this volume provide additional insight about the utility of participatory methods.

## PRECEDE/PROCEED Planning Model

Although a variety of frameworks exist to plan and evaluate HP-DP pro-grams, the most widely recognized and successful is the PRECEDE/ PROCEED Model developed by Green, Kreuter, and colleagues. PRECEDE/PROCEED is a comprehensive model used in virtually all settings, for example, community, school, medical/clinic and worksites. The Model is data driven, recognizing that defining the causes of health problems and behaviors requires the application of quantitative and quali-tative methods. Primary causes of target behavior must be systematically assessed to identify and tailor specific intervention components. Principles and methods of epidemiology, biostatistics, and anthropology-ethnography are blended to describe a target population.

Green, Kreuter, Deeds, and Partridge (1980) presented the PRECEDE/ PROCEED planning and evaluation framework in the 1970s as PRECEDE. As noted in Chapter 1, PRECEDE is an acronym for *P*redisposing, *R*einforcing, and *E*nabling *C*onstructs in *E*ducational *D*iagnosis and *E*valuation. It was developed to enable health education practitioners to design interventions using a planning process based upon a thorough assessment of each component's antecedents or underlying causes. In the late 1980s, the PROCEED part of the framework was added, in recognition of the need for health promotion interventions that go beyond traditional approaches in changing unhealthy behaviors. PROCEED stands for *P*olicy, *R*egulatory and *O*rganizational *C*onstructs in *E*ducational and *E*nvironmental *D*evelopment. PRECEDE and PROCEED work in tandem by allowing the planner to implement a continuous series of steps to plan, implement, and evaluate programs. In PRECEDE, planners identify priorities that form the basis of quantifiable objectives: they become goals in the implementation of the project in PROCEED.

Green and Kreuter updated PRECEDE/PROCEED in 2005. As noted in Figure 2.1, its application now involves an eight-step process. This framework utilizes guidelines for prioritizing objectives so the resources needed to develop an intervention can be identified and used. For example, a naïve program planner may think: all we need to do to change health behavior is to inform the public about the consequences of a health threat, develop a readable booklet on the topic, and disseminate program materials. Twenty-first-century planning needs to avoid such archaic and simplistic solutions. A meta-evaluation, quantitative and qualitative population and staff assessments, and a consensus development process and prioritization are essential to plan and implement all phases of the PRECEDE/PROCEED Model.

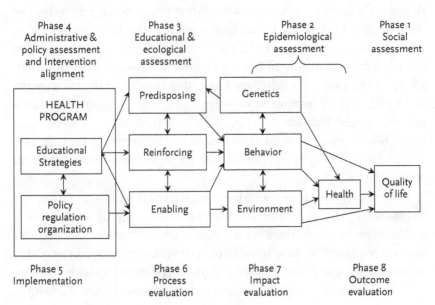

FIGURE 2.1 PRECEDE/PROCEED Model.

The application of PRECEDE/PROCEED in all Phases is based on the principle of participation and consensus. This principle assumes that success in achieving behavior change in any population is enhanced when individuals in the target population have the opportunity to actively assist in the prioritization of problems and in developing and implementing the solutions. The idea of participation is rooted in the community organization and empowerment philosophy. In the application of each Phase of the Model, planners must take considerable effort to include the target population in all aspects of program planning, implementation, and evaluation.

PROCEED highlights the importance that the social environment plays in health and health behavior. While a significant proportion of health is attributable to individual behavior, planners also need to consider the role that the social environment plays in contributing to healthy and unhealthy behaviors. Although many individual behaviors lead to serious health consequences, many behaviors are influenced by strong factors in the physical and social environment. The acknowledgment of the impact that the environment plays in behavior is a central component of the ecological approach to health promotion. A brief description of the application of the PRECEDE/PROCEED Model is described below.

## Phase 1: Social Assessment

A planner's first task is to assess the target population's perceptions of their quality of life. There are many reasons to understand why the social assessment is important. Green and Kreuter (2005) indicate that perceived health and quality of life are reciprocal concepts. They acknowledge that the notion of health is not an end in itself, but rather is a means to an end. It is an instrument of value that allows individuals to reach personal goals. Individuals value their health because of what good health brings. Planners need to understand target group concerns related to a quality of life to enable them to design programs relevant to a target population.

When a programs is developed to meet the needs of a target group, this increases the chances that the group will embrace the program and that it will be more effective. There are multiple ways for planners to collect different types of social data. In addition to typical demographics available for most target groups and areas, there are several useful social assessment methods: discussion groups; Nominal Group Process, Delphi Technique; focus groups; and surveys.

## Discussion Groups

A discussion group should discover how social problems are perceived, or which problem is most important to a group. A mixture of representatives of the target groups should participate. Group members are volunteers who agree to discuss the issues they find most pressing or that concern them most. Participants might be people who hold positions with community groups or other organizations, or they may simply be interested individuals who experience the problems and are likely to know the viewpoint of their peers. A discussion group has the advantage of allowing people to discuss and even vote on a problem of immediate interest.

When conducting group discussions, it is important make clear what actions your sponsoring organization is prepared to take in light of the perceptions and concerns of the group. If your organization can provide little or no assistance for the problems directly uncovered by discussion, sometimes you can help group members locate appropriate assistance. Indeed, the whole domain of community organization and action within the field of health education is based on this role on function. By examining available data, community representatives explore how the particular problem occurs in their area and then select one aspect of the problem to address.

## Nominal Group Process and Delphi Technique

In situations where varying points of view must be reconciled, staff frequently use the Nominal Group Process, Delphi Technique (Delbecq 1974), or a similar approach. The Nominal Group Process is an interactive method for determining needs by having opinions listed without critique from the group and then rated by secret ballot. Some meetings are convened by HP-DP staff to discuss specific priorities of individuals or community groups. In such a meeting, group members, facilitated by a trained member of a staff, determine which problem or aspects of the problem are most important. These techniques enable group members to select problems and to reach consensus on aspects of problems without letting individuals' views dominate. The secret ballot minimizes the influence of interpersonal dynamics on the ratings themselves.

The Delphi Technique (Delbecq, 1974) is a method of sampling opinions of a small group of individuals, usually experts, community leaders, or key informants. This method uses a succession of mailed questionnaires with the request for the individual to rank a series of issues. The results are mailed to the individuals to refine the initial list of issues and priorities.

A disadvantage of discussions by volunteers is that you never know whose views the group represents. Some representatives of organizations may have clear-cut constituencies. Statements by them may accurately present the case for their constituencies—but not always. Similarly, concerns expressed by unaffiliated individuals may be uniquely felt. The views of one suburban mother of young children do not necessarily reflect those of similar women. It is difficult to know how far to generalize the opinions and experiences of volunteers. If a disparity eventually emerges between the views of representatives and a target population, fundamental problems may affect a program. Nonetheless, discussion groups can generally shed light on problems, and can provide rich insights about dimensions of the problems.

### Focus Groups

A focus group is a discussion among people similar to the target population you wish to reach about specific aspects of a problem or program. The term is borrowed from marketing, where consumer groups are convened and paid to tell manufacturers or advertisers the characteristics of products they prefer or elements of advertisements that capture their attention. The use of the focus group technique is a standard HP-DP program planning method. The primary difference between a focus group and a discussion group is the specificity of issues or questions concerning the program planners. The intention is to discover useful information about issues of most concern to the group. No consensus is required. As in discussion groups, focus group members may not represent the opinion of all members of a community.

### Surveys

The purpose of a survey, whether a mailed questionnaire, telephone questionnaire, or a face-to-face interview, is to elicit specific information from a particular group of people. Almost all surveys have a specific set of questions with a fixed response structure: yes or no, or strongly agree to strongly disagree. Like information collected from discussion and focus groups, survey data are used to delineate the problem and describe the population. If the survey sample is large and representative of the target group of an HP-DP program, the answers and data may also be used as baseline data for measuring change.

In conducting a survey, HP-DP staff will define the target population, if it is accessible, and select a random sample of target participants at each eligible site. Sampling is the process of making observations that will serve as the basis for general conclusions about a specific problem and population at risk. Sampling is used to overcome the problem of lack of representativeness associated with discussion and focus group methods. By selecting people at random (e.g., women who come to clinics) or using systematic procedures (e.g., every fifth woman who visits the clinic for a four-week period), if the response rate is > 80% at each observation, the data are likely to be representative of typical clinic users.

The sample of women's views is likely to be similar to women not surveyed, whereas volunteers might be different in some respect from a larger target population. Sampling and techniques for conducting different types of surveys are described in Chapters 4 (Measurement and Analysis in Evaluation). Following data collection, planning staff analyze the data and use the findings to determine the strength of the association between the psycho-social characteristics identified in the assessment and community health problems. These data and insight should be useful to develop and tailor HP-DP interventions to a target population and communities.

## Phase 2: Epidemiologic Assessment (Health-Genetics-Behavioral-Environmental)

*Health assessments* identify the incidence, prevalence, and trends, preferably over at least a three- to fiveyear period, of the primary health problems or conditions in the target population's community. At this stage of PRECEDE/PROCEED application, one of two approaches is utilized: reductionist or expansionist. In using a reductionist approach, planners use data on the most important quality of life concerns found in the social assessment. They identify the contributing health problems that appear to be causally linked with these social concerns. In the expansionist approach, the planner begins the initial planning with an important health problem and then attempts to link it with quality of life concerns among members of the target population.

Individuals planning HP-DP interventions and evaluations will typically utilize the expansionist approach far more often than they will the reductionist approach. This is because funding opportunities are more often associated with health problems or health-risk behaviors in various populations of interest. When beginning with the expansionist approach, answers to at least four questions should be sought by health education and health promotion specialists: What is the problem? Who has the problem? Do they see the problem as a priority? Do they believe that they play a significant role in the reduction of the problem?

In conducting an epidemiologic assessment, you should consider conducting secondary data analyses with existing data, for example, vital statistics from the state and local data sets, results of local, state, national health surveys, and medical and administrative records. Data from these sources will provide you with information on morbidity and mortality in the target population. Analyses of these data will show which subgroups are most affected and who is at greatest risk. Data will usually be organized into the following categories: gender, age group, educational status, income levels, family structure, occupation, and geographic location. Each level of data should be analyzed by sub-group to determine its contribution to the health problem. You must be aware that although information from the national and state surveys provide information on a larger perspective, original data must be collected in samples of the local groups to ensure that the information obtained from the larger data banks are applicable for your setting.

## Writing Health Objectives

Once the factors of the major health problems have been defined in terms of risk levels, staff should be ready to develop objectives. This step is essential and one of the first to the program planning, implementation, and evaluation process. Objectives should be written with specificity and should answer five questions:

1. Who is the target population of the HP-DP program?
2. Where is the target population and program located?
3. What are the primary potential benefits, behavioral impact, and health status outcomes to the target population?
4. How much benefit in behavioral impact or health outcome rates is achievable?
5. When should the benefit be achieved?

The information collected and analyzed in the health assessment needs to be valid and reliable data in order to write measurable objectives for the program. Although these decisions will be guided by the needs of the target population, the program goals will be a statement of the program's ultimate benefit in changing health. For example, a health-related objective for a highway safety program could be to reduce alcohol-related driving morbidity and mortality. The program objective in this instance would be to answer the question, "What health improvements would be achieved in whom, by how much, and by when?" This might be answered in the objective that follows: "Alcohol-related traffic injuries and/or deaths will be reduced by 20% among drivers ≤ 18 years of age in County X between 2010 and 2015."

Measurable program objectives are essential to evaluate the program's success and to guide appropriate allocations of resources to achieve the objectives. HP-DP plans and evaluations should utilize national and regional public health consensus documents to guide setting reasonable targets for change. For example, the US Public Health Service document *Healthy People 2020*, which identifies national health promotion–disease prevention objectives for the nation, is a good reference to begin this process. State-level companion documents of *Healthy People 2020* are examples of other excellent references for establishing measurable objectives. The most important source, however, to establish realistic objectives is a meta-evaluation. It should inform the evaluation team about what level of impact or outcome has been produced over what period of time by completed evaluations with high internal validity.

### Genetics, Behavioral, and Environmental Assessments

The purpose of this step of PRECEDE/PROCEED is to identify genetic, behavioral, and environmental risk factors strongly associated with the health problems identified in the social and health assessments. The relative risks and attributable risks for the target population and accurate estimates of the percent of a health problem associated (caused) with each major behavioral or environmental risk factor must be established.

Genetics is a new construct in Phase 2 of PRECEDE/PROCEED. Molecular epidemiology has advanced the state of the science in the field of genetics and has discovered a number of genes associated with numerous health risk factors and various illnesses. Genes and their influence on health and disease involve complex interactions of genes and behavior, genes and environment, and genes with other genes. In many instances, these genetic associations are not well understood. At this point, a number of genes have been discovered that have been shown to be associated with increased risk for lung cancer, breast and cervical cancer, sickle cell anemia, cystic fibrosis, Tay Sachs disease, and obesity, to name a few. Currently, the science is not sufficiently developed for use in HP-DP program development. However, as science continues to unravel the genome, these complex associations will become better understood. Their utility in planning health interventions for target populations will be clarified.

Behavioral factors are the lifestyle of the target population that contributes to the incidence, prevalence, and the severity of the health problems. Environmental factors are external to the individual: some may be beyond personal control. However, in many instances, factors in the social environment may need alteration by policies, laws, and regulations to support behavior change in the neighborhood or community's social or physical environment associated with a health outcome.

This Phase should answer the question, What are the main causes of the health problem for our target population? Planners need to consider an inventory of salient behaviors that contribute to the social and health problems identified in Phase 1 and 2. Behavioral and non-behavioral causes should be defined in the assessments. Documentation of the primary behavioral causes of disease and death are usually available. There are also many non-behavioral causes of problems. Although many non-behavioral causes are not changeable, they should, nevertheless, be considered in planning. Once an inventory of influential behavior factors has been developed, your next task is to rate each in terms of its importance to the social concerns/health problems.

Two considerations are important in this evaluation. The importance of the behavior is evident when data show that (1) it occurs frequently, and (2) it is clearly associated with the health problem. The next step is to rate the changeability of behaviors. Even if a behavior is strongly associated with a health problem, it may not be appropriate to target unless you can reasonably expect it to change through an intervention. Green and Kreuter (2005) identify several rules of thumb to assess changeability. A behavior is considered changeable if the behavior (1) is still in its developmental stage, (2) has only recently been established, (3) is not deeply rooted in culture and lifestyle, and (4) has been found to change in previous intervention attempts. Selection of which behaviors to target in an intervention is based on importance and changeability.

The quadrant shown in Table 2.1 provides a useful method to consider which individual behaviors should be targeted in the intervention. Intervention targets should be chosen by combining importance and changeability ratings. Identify only those behaviors that are important, that contribute significantly to a health problem, and that are considered highly changeable.

## Writing Behavioral Objectives

The final task is to write measurable objectives for each of the major behaviors that the HP-DP program will be designed to change. To estimate levels of behavior change for writing objectives, data and insight from a

TABLE 2.1 Dimensions of Importance and Changeability

|  | MORE IMPORTANT | LESS IMPORTANT |
|---|---|---|
| MORE CHANGEABLE | High Priority (Quadrant 1) | Low Priority Except for Political Purposes (Quadrant 3) |
| LESS CHANGEABLE | Priority for Innovations Assessment Critical (Quardant 2) | No Program (Quadrant 4) |

systematic review of the literature and a meta-evaluation will define the levels of possible behavioral impact observed in evaluations in comparable settings. As described in writing health objectives in the Epidemiologic Assessment, write objectives using the following criteria: Who in the target population is expected to change? What behavior in the target population is expected to change? How much of the behavior is expected to change? When is the behavior impact rate expected to change?

### Environmental Assessment

Like a behavioral assessment, an *environmental assessment* requires an evaluation of several criteria. The first step is to identify which social or environmental factors causing health problems are changeable. When the behavioral assessment was conducted, behavioral factors were identified. By separating the non-behavioral factors, you identify organizational, economic, and environmental factors that impact health and/or quality of life. The second step is to rate these factors by their relative importance. This involves analyzing each on the basis of the strength of the association of the factors' impact on health and quality of life and the incidence, prevalence, and number in your population that are affected by the factor.

The third step requires rating the environmental factors in terms of changeability. This differs from the task completed in Step 1. Whereas you eliminated non-behavioral factors that are not environmental factors, in this step you delete from your list other environmental factors that would be least likely to change through policy, regulation, or organizational change. This task will be easier if only the factors that emerged in Step 2 are considered.

The fourth step is to choose the environmental factors that will become targets for change. Apply the quadrant that was utilized in the behavioral assessment to prioritize behaviors to complete your evaluation of environmental factors. Factors that are rated more important and more changeable should become the priorities for environmental change (see Table 2.1).

After the environmental factors that need to be changed have been determined, the last task is to write environmental objectives. The criteria for writing health and behavioral objectives are slightly altered. In most instances, you will not use the "who" in writing these objectives. These objectives address the following: What environmental factor will change? By how much should the factor change? When—timeline of the project—should the change occur? For example, an HP-DP program may intend to reduce environmental tobacco smoke (ETS) exposure of bartenders in restaurants by reducing the number of restaurants that allow smoking in their establishment as a part of a city-wide or county-wide comprehensive tobacco control project: The proportion of restaurants that allow indoor smoking will be reduced by 50% of the baseline rate within three years of the initiation of the project.

Another ETS effort may seek to reduce childhood exposure to ETS in city-wide and county-wide homes. A possible environmental objective could be the following: The proportion of homes with children < 5 years of age in County A that will not allow smoking inside the residence will be increased from 60% to 80% by 2015. A case study in Chapter 3 presents an example of the effectiveness of a city-wide ban on ETS in restaurants on January 1, 2007, by the Washington, D.C., City Council.

## Systematic Reviews and Rating of the Validity of the Evaluation Literature

How much behavioral impact can an HP-DP program produce? The answer is critical and can be answered by a meta-evaluation and a meta-analysis. One of the first steps that all evaluators should take in the development of an intervention and evaluation plan is a thorough review of the literature. This review will help to estimate effect size and sample size for different types of interventions. In reviewing the literature, there are two methods to use: meta-evaluation (ME) and meta-analysis (MA). ME and MA are methods that the contemporary evaluator must understand and must be able to apply. The distinction between the two methods rests primarily with the degree to which the literature base has sufficient maturity. In the early stages of literature, documentation of the efficacy of an intervention is usually limited. Often, only a few published evaluation studies exist to provide insight about the estimated impact of intervention methods or programs for a defined population and a risk factor. In this case, only an ME is performed.

## Meta-Evaluation

Meta-Evaluation (ME) is a systematic methodological review and rating of the internal and external validity of completed HP-DP program evaluations using specific criteria in eight categories. It applies standard rating criteria to estimate the internal validity of the impact of HP-DP programs: (1) program evaluation design; (2) measurement validity, reliability, and completeness; (3) sample size, effect size, and statistical power; (4) sample eligibility and representativeness; (5) definition, tailoring, and replicability of intervention and measurement procedures; (6) performance measurement and process evaluation; (7) behavioral impact and health outcome rates; and (8) cost effectiveness–cost benefit analyses.

Windsor, Boyd, and Orleans (1998) presented a detailed example of the application of ME methods. Only studies with a quasi-experimental or experimental design and a biochemical verification of self-reports of smoking status were included. The following minimal standards were recommended for future evaluations of health education methods for pregnant smokers:

- Only use an experimental design with an inception cohort of >80% of smoking patients at all prenatal care sites;
- Confirm the representatives of study participants at all sites;
- Estimate sample size and documented effect size needs based on power = 0.80, including at least 100 subjects in each E and C group;
- Provide complete baseline demographic, behavioral, and clinical assessments with standardized definitions using minimal exclusionary criteria;
- Use self-reports based on patient knowledge of the test combined with independent biochemical tests, saliva or urinary cotinine (COT) or carbon monoxide (CO) measures, using specific cutoffs at baseline, end-of- pregnancy, and at the first postpartum visit;
- Document a 90% or more follow-up rate for all patients for each observation;
- Provide a complete cessation intervention description to enable replication and documentation of pilot testing of procedures and training to staff to deliver the intervention; and
- Conduct a process evaluation to document intervention exposure and costs, including exposure by type, frequency, and duration for each program procedure.

It is essential to systematically apply well-established meta-evaluation standards to determine the extent to which the HP-DP literature provides insight about the intervention science and practice base. Windsor (2010) provides additional examples of a meta-evaluation and meta-analysis in this area of health education–health promotion in primary care.

### Meta-Analysis

Meta-analysis (MA) is a statistical analysis of the results of completed empirical research. The objective of the MA is to provide accurate and impartial quantitative description from completed experimental studies of the impact of an intervention for samples of populations for a specific risk factor and setting. MA differs from ME in that it presumes publication of a large number of completed experimental evaluation studies with sufficient rigor to define the evidence-science base for a specific HP-DP program.

The first step is to comprehensively review the literature to identify published studies through a meta-evaluation. At this stage, a serious bias may occur if an incomplete review of the literature is performed. An explicit set of ME rules should be established to exclude studies with serious methodological flaws; for example, (1) review only experimental studies with an E & C group, (2) use only studies that have sample sizes in both the E & C groups with baseline and follow-up data in excess of 100 subjects in each group, and (3) use only studies that provide confirmed evidence of measurement validity and reliability of the impact or outcome rate used to document change. In addition, the intervention for a specific population at risk and the effect size (ES) need to be specified, and replicable for each evaluation study. ES, as previously noted, refers to the difference in impact rate between the E and C groups.

The MA aggregates prior studies into a quantitative estimate of the impact of an intervention. It is a weighted average of the individual results, providing more weight for larger studies and less weight for smaller studies. The methodology for combining findings from studies is not new, and the techniques are straightforward. The primary difficulty of the MA is, typically, the selection of the studies to be used. Information from one study is rarely a replicate of another: populations, research procedures, and settings differ. The use of published literature can also lead to biased results: most journals choose not to publish negative/statistically non-significant results. Thus, an MA based on published literature alone may produce biased results.

Performing an MA is an essential step for all evaluations. Researchers and evaluators fail to adequately use available information, thus continuing the proverbs "history repeats itself" and "reinventing the wheel."

Even though an MA is a sophisticated analytic process, much can be learned with this method. Snyder and Hamilton (2002) provide an excellent discussion of the application of the MA methods to studies to estimate the effect of media campaigns on behavior change. Among a review of 48 studies, the average short-term campaign effect size (ES) of behavior change was 0.09. In persuasive campaigns that did not use a legal enforcement message, the average campaign behavioral effect size was 0.05. For campaigns with an enforcement message, the average campaign effect size was 0.17. This review provides a detailed discussion of the study selection criteria, sampling methods, measures, message content, campaign reach, control group trends, campaign length, outcomes, and ES.

Some MA techniques combine the results of studies based on whether they were successful: statistically significant. The implicit assumption when performing this type of summarization is that lack of significance is equal to a zero effect; this may not be valid. In addition, just counting statistical significance can also cause problems. Fleiss and Gross (1991) provide four primary uses of properly performed MAs: (1) to increase statistical power for important endpoints and subgroups; (2) to resolve controversy when studies disagree; (3) to improve effect size estimates; and (4) to answer new questions not posed by individual studies.

These rules cover several situations. A situation for the use of rule 1 might be to estimate whether the intervention was effective among women in a worksite smoking-cessation study. In a single study, there may be insufficient numbers of women to demonstrate a statistically significant result, but pooling results by performing the MA for several studies may provide an answer or conflicting results. Performing an MA may enable the answer to be more clearly seen. Rule 3 is used in planning an evaluation. Basing sample size decisions and estimated impacts on a single study, however, is risky. Even though an effect may be valid, there is a chance that the observed outcome was an overestimate or underestimate, because of the differences in population: the published study versus your study. The MA may help you to provide a better estimate. Mullen et al. (1997 and 2001) present additional discussions and examples of MA. Methods to calculate individual or group, sample size, are presented in Chapter 3.

In some situations, the use of available data related to a new question may bring some insight into previously unspecified questions. For example, suppose you are interested in the potential for smoking cessation to increase infant birth weight. From studies of smoking cessation among pregnant women where birth weight or percentage of low birth weight is reported and where smoking status is recorded, estimating the impact of tobacco use and non-use from recorded data might be possible. If this information were available from a variety of sources, the MA of this information might be used to infer potential health benefit for future studies.

Planning staff must have a clear idea of the potential impact of an intervention to establish realistic objectives. This is accomplished in two ways: (1) perform an ME and/or MA to define the maturity of the literature, and (2) conduct a formative evaluation that represents an application of the best intervention and evaluation methods synthesized from the ME and program experience by staff. The application of these two procedures, ME and MA, and a Formative Evaluation will provide the best evidence to initiate a program evaluation.

## Phase 3: Educational and Ecologic Assessment

At this point, HP-DP staff should be knowledgeable about the social, health, and behavioral and environmental problems that affect the target population. This Phase determines the major causes of the behaviors and environmental conditions identified in the Behavioral and Environmental Assessment. The products of the assessment will become areas for planning an HP-DP program. Green and Kreuter (2005) identified three factors that influence behavior:

1. Predisposing factors, which are strongly associated with a target behavior;
2. Enabling factors, which are strongly associated with the target behavior to allow for individual and group motivation to be realized; and
3. Reinforcing factors, which are strongly associated with a target behavior and that provide the reward for the target behavior to be repeated.

Predisposing, reinforcing, and enabling factors, individually and collectively, predict, in varying degrees, rates of behavior of a target behavior of a population. Application of the PRECEDE/PROCEED Model is based on the premise that the causes of health-related behavior are multifactorial. Therefore, planning and evaluation of changes in rates of behavior(s) need to consider the influence that each causal factor plays in increasing or decreasing the likelihood of a personal action and its potential for an effect on the other factors.

**Predisposing factors** are primarily psycho-social in nature. They include cognitive and affective aspects such as knowledge, literacy, personal feelings, beliefs, values, personality, and levels of self-confidence or self-efficacy. There are a host of other factors that could predispose behavior, for example, socioeconomic status, age, gender, and ethnicity. These other factors, because they are unchangeable, are not the focus of interventions (e.g., age, gender, ethnicity). All of the demographic factors, however, should be considered in planning an intervention and evaluation.

Predisposing factors commonly addressed by interventions include knowledge, health beliefs, values, attitudes, self-efficacy, behavioral intentions, and existing skills. Some or all of these factors may be relevant to the target population. On the other hand, some may play a more important role in influencing behavior than the others. A careful review of the influences of each of the factors is essential in helping you understand what to target in your intervention.

**Enabling factors** facilitate the action of an individual or organization. They include the availability, accessibility and affordability of health-related services and community resources. They may include living conditions that act to prohibit action and skills that are needed to enact a behavior. Enabling factors are frequently the focus of community organization, organizational development, and training components of a new HP-DP program. They include the identification of new resources and skills necessary to perform a desirable behavior and organizational actions needed to modify the community environment. Resources include the organization and accessibility of the health facilities, personnel, schools, outreach centers/clinics, or any similar resource. Personal health skills may be taught and may be used to enable specific health actions of a target population. Skills in influencing the community, such as those necessary to promote social action and organizational change, influence the physical and healthcare environment.

**Reinforcing factors** are either positive or negative feedback that individuals receive from others after taking specific action. This feedback typically influences whether a positive or negative behavior will be repeated or extinguished. Reinforcement may come from a wide variety of individual and combination of sources: a person's children, family members, social group, peers, coworkers, an employee's environment and supervisors, and healthcare and social services providers. The physical consequences of behavior need to be acknowledged as reinforcing factors. This may be the relief that asthmatics feel from the correct use of medication, or the positive feelings from physical conditioning and from participation in an exercise program.

There are three criteria to help select which predisposing, enabling, and reinforcing factors should be targeted for modification by an intervention:

- Identifying and sorting of factors into three categories;
- Setting priorities among categories; and
- Establishing priorities within categories.

The first task is to identify and sort the factors into three categories. This listing should be as comprehensive as possible. The data in this list may be obtained through either informal or formal methods. Informal methods may begin with planners using their knowledge, experience, and insight about why a category of behaviors exist. For example, you may suspect that knowledge, health beliefs, and lack of confidence are important predisposing factors related to the target behavior. Such estimates are most often confirmed through interaction with members of the target population. Additional insight may be obtained from use of focus groups, interviews, discussion groups, and questionnaires.

These same methods should be used to gather data from those who are involved in the delivery of intervention components and delivering services in organizations collaborating with the planning group. Based on these informal data, you may want to conduct a more formal assessment. Standard measures of many constructs are available in the literature to adapt for this purpose, including measures of beliefs, self-efficacy, attitudes, behavioral intentions, and social support. Results from a formal survey may be used to confirm findings from the informal approaches.

The second step is to set priorities among the categories. Even if you have a complete inventory of behaviors to target, you cannot analyze and prioritize them at the same time. You must determine sequencing of factors in your intervention. For example, consider a health promotion program that seeks to reduce prostate cancer among inner-city African American men. Consideration should be given to identifying priorities among the three factors for each step of development and sequence. Enabling factors to provide a prostate screening service must be in place before you can begin an educational campaign to address predisposing factors related to the use of the service. Once the enabling and predisposing factors are in place, attention can then be directed to reinforcing factors. The situation demands the following order of development: enabling, predisposing, and reinforcing factors.

The last is step is to establish priorities in the categories. In this step, planners will again use criteria on importance and changeability (see Table 2.1). As in the environmental and behavioral assessment, selection for targeting the three factors is based an emphasis on highly important and highly changeable variables. When evaluating importance, consideration should be to give the three criteria: prevalence, immediacy, and necessity. Prevalence refers to how widespread the factor is, while immediacy refers to the urgency of the factor. Necessity, on the other hand, gives consideration to factors that are low in prevalence, yet necessary for change.

When assessing changeability, you need to know how much change to expect. A systematic review of the literature may provide HP-DP staff with considerable or limited insight. Application of the meta evaluation and meta analysis methods described in this chapter should be applied to the literature that you identify. The product of this review should enable program staff to estimate the level of change in each of the prioritized factors.

### Writing Educational Objectives

At this stage, objectives can be drafted for each target predisposing, enabling, and reinforcing factor of an intervention. Objectives should be drafted, discussed, and finalized, using the four criteria used in writing behavioral and health objectives: *who/where, what, how much,* and *when.*

## Phase 4: Administrative, Policy Assessment, and Intervention Alignment

In Phase 5, the intervention strategies and final plans for implementation are defined. The primary purpose of this step is to identify the policies, resources, and circumstances in an organization or program that inhibit or facilitate implementation of measurement and intervention methods. At this Phase, the intervention strategies are described based on the previous steps in the PRECEDE/PROCEED Model assessment. HP-DP staff needs to assess the availability of necessary time, staff, and resources. Barriers to implementation, such as lack of staff or space, should be identified and resolved. In addition, any organizational policies or regulations that could affect implementation should be considered and addressed. An Administrative and Policy Assessment is specific to the context of the program and its sponsoring organization and thus requires political astuteness and experience as much as knowledge and credentials.

## Developing Interventions

Successful HP-DP programs are based on an understanding of why people behave relative to their health, and what causes or enables them to change or not. Program leadership should be familiar with the prevailing theories of behavior change so they can select the theoretical principles most relevant to the people, problem, practice setting, and program objectives. The available theories considered in light of the data from the educational and ecologic assessment, the behaviors selected as important and changeable, and the characteristics of the target group will dictate intervention methods most likely to be effective in the program being developed. Two levels of concern are important when designing an intervention: the content of the materials, and the processes by which people learn to behave differently.

When evaluating programs, evaluation researchers think that it is "cleaner" to assess different interventions separately (Green 1991). Discern whether rehearsal of skills is a more effective intervention than problem-solving groups or individual counseling. In the daily practice of health education, this separation of approaches makes sense only if previous studies and experience say it is the most effective way to proceed. Answering the effectiveness question is currently an important area for evaluation research. Theoretically, combined approaches should be better. In designing learning events, however, the behavior to be learned dictates the approach and determines the resources and materials needed to support the approach.

HP-DP materials and methods, for example, DVDs, audiotapes, power-point slide presentations, self-help guides, computer-generated tailored communications, and interactive voice response systems may be used as typical components of an intervention. Learning is a process supported by materials. Materials can provide information, stimulate discussion, and reinforce the information provided in a learning session. Selection of the methods and materials occurs after a decision has been made about the educational and behavioral objectives.

For each intervention contact, you must determine how members of a target population will demonstrate that they learned the behavior. Sometimes this is simple. For example, nutrition program participants might simply complete a checklist of low-fat foods at the end of a session on menu selection. For each learning event for which there is a specific objective, however, you need to determine whether the objective has been achieved. Monitoring provides important benchmarks of mastery for both the client and program personnel (Bandura, 1986).

The type, duration, and frequency of delivery of program intervention and assessment procedures are important issues for program developers: acceptability, appropriateness, and cost need to be considered. Current data suggest that programs of more than one session that are not overly long may yield the greatest degree of change. Highly focused, standardized, 10- to 15-minute counseling sessions and the provision of self-help materials can also be very effective for specific behaviors (Windsor et al., 1985, 1993, 2000). Unless specific data are available from evaluation research to suggest a particular time frame for the type of HP-DP program being planned, the determination of its structure and content should be based on the following criteria:

- What is best for the participants in their view?
- What have previous studies and similar programs shown to be effective?
- What is manageable, given the context in which the program must operate?
- What in your previous experience has been effective?
- How much content must be covered?

The location and availability of an HP-DP program is an important consideration. If the intervention site is not the place that the target group uses (i.e., school, home, and work), then you must consider a practical question: How often and how far can people be expected to travel to/from a site? If the program is part of other health services, then the location and frequency of sessions may be tailored to coincide with a routine pattern of contact.

The number of participants to include in a program is based on three criteria: the number matched to the intervention approaches selected, the number of populations to be reached, and practicalities of cost and manageability. Assume that you have decided on group discussion as a format for the worksite program on diet and exercise. From the review of literature, you know that 6–8 members in a group are optimum to ensure full participation in discussion. However, there are almost 500 men to be reached. Therefore, you may decide to hold information sessions for medium or large groups (20–25) with numerous visual aids, self-tests, and a lecturer. These may alternate with in-person discussion and support groups of small numbers (5–20) of men. In this way you hope both to reach a big audience with information and to meet the necessary conditions of the more intensive approaches within a reasonable cost.

If you have involved members of the program network in the planning process, the resources and support needed to start the program must be evident and available. If, early on, the employee health service has agreed to give medical checkups to employees enrolling in the weight-loss program, now is the time to work out the details of referral, record keeping, and so on. If you have developed a program alone, without external input, expect problems in trying to secure assistance.

This is when you determine administrative and logistical details, from recruiting participants to program evaluation. What departments, people, and resources are needed and available? Which people must give their approval before the program begins? Which facilities are needed for learning events? Are all parties needed to implement the program committed. Where necessary, is participation in writing? Have all organizational and legal constraints been considered?

Consider, again, the asthma education example. Assume that you have decided to evaluate reduced school absences as a related outcome of better management. Will the local school let you use its records? Will parents sign releases? Assume that you have decided to invite tenant organizers to the clinic to talk with parents about improvements in housing. Will the organizers need passes to visit the clinic? Must these visits be noted as referrals in clinic records? Each step of the program you have designed must be reviewed while you ask, have we accounted for the administrative, legal, and logistical aspects of this element?

At this juncture, you must also determine what kind of staff training is necessary to implement the program. Each member of a staff who will have an influence on the participants needs an orientation. Many may need special training to implement routine assessment and intervention procedures of the HP-DP program. Those who will facilitate discussion groups will need to be trained. Each program and group of participants is different. Program staff must be prepared to work with the particular group of people in the specific context.

The design of personnel training, like the intervention program, operates on two levels: those who must be briefed and oriented regarding the content or health condition, and those who must be trained in the learning process. Physicians, who play a role as counselors in an asthma education program, may be very well versed in clinical aspects of asthma but may need training in counseling techniques. HP-DP specialists may be highly skilled in facilitating discussion groups, but may need a background in the clinical dimensions of asthma. Do not to assume that healthcare personnel possess the requisite information and skills to counsel patients. In most situations, personnel have uneven levels of skills and knowledge. Orientation and training should fill this deficit. If different groups of personnel will undertake different tasks, train them separately.

It is almost always necessary to bring all program personnel together for combined sessions or orientation. If tasks cut across types of personnel, for example, physicians, nurses, schoolteachers, and health education specialists, who provide the same basic treatment methods when counseling, it is reasonable to train them together. The extent of training is determined by the tasks performed, the information to be provided, and the existing skill level of the personnel.

### Developing a Budget and Administrative Plan

When a program is developed, specific costs and administrative needs occur simply because the program is new. Costs of planning and development of methods, materials, and assessment tools are usually, in large part, one-time expenses. The configuration of personnel needed to carry out initial planning and development may be different from the pattern needed when the program becomes institutionalized or is part of an organization's routine.

The elaborateness of an HP-DP program is likely to be proportionate to the resources made available. Failure to allocate sufficient money is a major reason for the limited success of some health education programs. A budget should provide justification for each person and major tasks to be implemented during program development and delivery. The budget justification should convince the sponsoring organization or funder that fiscal allocations are warranted and the program will be affordable over time.

It is important to carefully think through what staff is needed to develop the program and to carry it out initially. Job descriptions need to be written and staff costs estimated. The following kinds of personnel may be needed: a program director to assume overall responsibility, coordinators to manage logistics, consultants in particular areas (content specialists, methods specialists, etc.), staff to deliver the program, and secretarial-clerical staff.

Many of these people may be available in the organization or as part of a planning network. Individuals from other organizations may participate. Their services may be paid or may be in kind contributions in a budget. To determine personnel cost, the simplest method is to estimate the number of hours per week, month, or year a person will need (percentage of effort) to

TABLE 2.2 Budget for Program Development and Implementation: Year 1 (2003)

| PERSONNEL | HOURS/WEEK | PERCENT OF EFFORT | SALARY/ ANNUM | FRINGE BENEFITS[a] | TOTAL | AMOUNT |
|---|---|---|---|---|---|---|
| Program director | | | | | | |
| Susan Greenbaum | 40 | 100 | $120,000 | $24,000 | $144,000 | —— |
| Program coordinator/educator | | | | | | |
| (To be named) | 40 | 100 | $75,000 | $15,000 | $90,000 | —— |
| Program evaluator | | | | | | |
| James Sinclair | 8 | 20 | $90,000 | $3,600 | $21,600 | —— |
| Secretary | | | | | | |
| Robert Murphy | 40 | 100 | $45,000 | $9,000 | $54,000 | —— |
| Consultants | | | | | | |
| | | | | | | Contributed by Heart Association |
| Carlos Velez (educational materials) | 2 | 5 | —— | —— | —— | —— |

|  |  | Contributed by university |
|---|---|---|
| Rachel Polanowski (data analysis) | 2 | 5 |
| Total personnel costs |  | $309,600 |
| Costs other than personal services |  | $2,500 |
| Books, materials, and acquisition of background data |  | $5,000 |
| Printing of questionnaires and evaluation materials |  | $4,500 |
|  |  | $321,600 |
| Indirect:[b]  [Total direct costs (x .30)] |  | $96,480 |
| Total year 1 request |  | $418,080 |
| Total year 2 request (.04) |  | $434,803 |
| Total year 3 request (.04) |  | $452,195 |

[a] Computed as 20% of salary.
[b] Computed as 30% of total direct cost.

devote to program activities and to calculate the amount that person will be paid per week, month, or year.

A budget must show the direct cost of personnel, the money they will receive to spend, and also the cost of fringe benefits provided by the sponsoring organization. All organizations have established rates for these costs. There are also other unseen costs in a program. What is the cost of housing the program? What about services provided by other divisions or departments of the organization, such as the financial office and the personnel office, to support program personnel? The indirect cost of these services will be calculated, based on an established rate. Some staff will also have several program responsibilities.

The cost of expenses other than personnel services will be need to defined. Some will be ongoing expenses, but others will be required only during program development. Expenses likely to be incurred initially include space, if program housing is not available; equipment (personal computers, desks, and so on); supplies (paper, pencils, and other office needs); telephone, facsimile, and electronic mail services; postage; photocopying; acquisition of studies, articles, and books (i.e., secondary data); printing costs for primary data (collection and evaluation materials); printing costs for educational materials; computer costs for data analysis; travel costs to and from program sites; and training costs.

Once you have determined who and what are needed to carry out the program, the budget can be developed. Table 2.2 illustrates how you might show program costs for the first development year and the following two years. Table 2.2 shows that the formula the sponsoring organization uses to calculate fringe benefits is 20% of a person's salary. In this example, indirect costs are determined to be 30% of total direct costs. Outside contributions are included in the budget, with an indication that no funds are requested from the department for the services listed. Showing contributed time in the budget more accurately reflects the percentage of effort to be expended. The bottom of the budget notes that requests will be made in years 2 and 3. The budget rationale explains that, after the first year, the program director will spend 100% of his or her time administering program activities. This is likely to be considered a reasonable ongoing expense. The rationale also states: the program will be expanded in the next two years to four sites, with no addition of staff. Each year the budget has been increased by 4% to cover increases in salaries and material costs.

*Personnel Services*

**Program director**: Susan Greenbaum will devote 100% time during year 1 of program development. She will assume overall responsibility for the program, maintain links with all cooperation agencies, and oversee day-to-day program activities. The yearly department budget provides for the cost of the program director. In years 2 and 3, it is estimated that Greenbaum will spend approximately 10% time supervising ongoing program implementation.

**Program coordinator-educator**: A person will be hired at 100% time to coordinate all day-to-day aspects of program development and to carry out the actual teaching in the program. The cost of the coordinator-educator is requested at 100% for all years of the program. After the first year of program development and evaluation, the program coordinator-educator will devote 100% time to the ongoing program and to its expansion to four sites by year 3 of program implementation.

**Program evaluator**: James Sinclair will spend 10% time in all years of the program and will coordinate all evaluation tasks.

**Secretary**: Robert Murphy will spend 100% time handling correspondence and record-keeping tasks. The department budget provides for the cost of this position.

**Consultants**: Each program co-sponsor, the local AHA and the local university, will contribute the equivalent of 5% consultation time by Carlos Velez and Rachel Polanowski for development of educational materials and for analysis of initial survey data, respectively. In years 2 and 3, consultation will be provided regarding program expansion and evaluation.

*Other Program Costs*

**Books, materials, and background data**: Although many resources are available in our own resource center and the library of the nearby university, we will need to acquire special materials from outside sources. These materials will need to be updated yearly, such as printing of questionnaires and evaluation materials. Most of the materials that will be needed for the program are available from existing sources, such as the AHA and other cooperating agencies. However, some costs will be incurred in the printing of specialized questionnaires to be used for needs assessment and for evaluation; these costs are likely to be incurred yearly.

To calculate costs for years 2 and 3, the year 1 budget has been increased each year by 4% to cover inflation and salary increases. Once you have developed the budget and budget rationale, you need to outline the time frame for carrying out major tasks. Note that representatives of organizations and groups from the planning network will meet regularly over the first year of development. The program will also be monitored continuously during the first three months of operation and will only be expanded to the second site after evaluation and revision. With a program description, including the evaluation plan, an outline of personnel and their responsibilities, a time frame, a budget, and a budget rationale, you are ready to seek funding, or, if money is in hand, to implement the work plan. In addition, on completion of the evaluation, you should be able to conduct cost analyses (see Chapter 6) of your program

## Phase 5: Implementation

In Phase 5 the HP-DP program is implemented according to the plans specified in the Administrative and Policy Assessment (Phase 4).

## Phases 6–8: Evaluation

The final steps in the application of the PRECEDE/PROCEED Model are to a conduct a process evaluation (Phase 6), impact evaluation (Phase 7), and outcome evaluation (Phase 8). Process evaluation determines the extent to which the intervention was delivered as planned. Impact evaluation determines whether changes occurred in the predisposing, reinforcing, and enabling factors. In addition, impact evaluation assesses whether changes in took place in the targeted behaviors and in the environment. The outcome evaluation determines whether the program had an effect on health status and quality of life. In each of the Phases an evaluation uses the objectives written in the planning process (Phases 2–3) to serve as standards for comparison of observed results and to make a decision about whether the project succeeded. For a complete discussion of the methods to conduct a process evaluation, impact evaluation, and outcome evaluation see Chapters 5 and 6, respectively.

## Case Study: *Clear Horizons*—A Community-Based Quit Smoking Program for Midlife and Older Smokers

This case study describes the methods used by program planners/researchers at the Fox Chase Cancer Center in Philadelphia, Pennsylvania, to apply the PRECEDE/PROCEED Model to plan, implement, and evaluate a smoking cessation program for midlife and older smokers (Rimer, Orleans, Fleisher, et al., 1994). When the project began, there was new epidemiologic evidence showing that smokers of all ages benefited from quitting. However, there were no programs or smoking cessation materials specifically designed for older smokers. This was due to a common misconception among lay and professional groups that it was "too late" for older smokers. *The objective of the project Clear Horizons was to develop a program to dispel misconceptions about whether it is beneficial to quit smoking in the later years and to address the "unique" barriers and facilitators to cessation in this vulnerable, underserved population.*

## Epidemiologic Assessment

The project planners applied the expansionist approach of PRECEDE/PROCEED in developing *Clear Horizons*. The first step was a literature search to gather epidemiological data to document the health consequences of smoking for older people and the benefits when older smokers quit. About 94% of smoking-related deaths occur after the age of 50 years, making smoking a problem that affects older people. At that time, smoking was a risk factor in 7 of the top 14 causes of death for those aged 65 years and older (Special Committee on Aging, 1986).

Twice as many older smokers and 1.5 times as many older female smokers died from stroke than older nonsmokers of both genders. In addition, spouses of older smokers are more likely to have lung cancer, emphysema, and other lung conditions. Smoking also complicates many illnesses and conditions common among older people, including heart disease, high blood pressure, circulatory and vascular conditions, duodenal ulcers, osteoporosis, periodontal disease, age-related macular degeneration, cataracts, lens opacities, and diabetes (Boyd & Orleans, 1999). In addition, smoking interacts with and restricts the effectiveness of many medications that are used to treat many of these conditions (Moore, 1986). For example, an older diabetic who smokes typically needs twice the insulin as an older diabetic nonsmoker.

The literature review also documented that quitting, even in the later years, is beneficial. In 1990 the Surgeon General's Report (DHHS, 1990) reviewed the existing medical and epidemiologic data and concluded, "it is never too late to stop." This document provided evidence that smoking cessation leads to significant health benefits, regardless of how long a person has smoked. Although the improvement in health that results from quitting smoking is well documented, many older smokers were unaware of the benefits. Stopping smoking can reduce or prevent the likelihood of such diseases as heart disease, cancer, and respiratory disease. The literature also showed that quitting can also stabilize chronic obstructive pulmonary disease (COPD). A review of large clinical trials concluded that cessation, even during one's sixties, increased both longevity and independent functioning.

While smoking leads to physical damage, the body responds immediately to cessation. Within one month of cessation, the body begins to repair itself. Data from the Coronary Artery Surgery Study demonstrated that subjects who quit smoking at age 55 years or older immediately began to reduce their chances of a heart attack. In comparison with nonsmokers, smokers had a 70% higher risk of death. Other findings revealed that survival benefits were more pronounced in moderately ill patients.

## Social Assessment

Given the unequivocal epidemiologic evidence that documented the health consequences of smoking and the considerable health benefits that result from quitting, program planners began to gather literature to connect the health data with issues of quality life to complete the social assessment. The literature revealed that an overlooked benefit of quitting smoking is the improvement in the quality of life that takes place when older smokers quit. Fries, Green, and Levine (1989) advocated that the most important outcome from smoking cessation may not be a longer life span but a longer *active* life span. This result would become most apparent in the delay or compression of chronic diseases and illnesses to later years of life. Another important outcome of smoking cessation is that quitters are more likely to remain living independently for a longer period of time. Planners confirmed these findings and their importance in the lives of older smokers through numerous focus groups completed with the target population.

## Behavioral Assessment

When the project began, over 13 million Americans over age 50 smoked. Approximately 32% of men aged 50–74 were smokers: 27% of the women in the same age range smoked. This group of smokers had for the most part smoked for many decades, some for more than 50 years. Most smoked heavily and were highly addicted to nicotine. Many began smoking when it was considered a glamorous part of the American social culture—long before its health consequences were well known.

## Environmental Assessment

An evaluation of the environment revealed two significant issues. First, there was a lack of targeted smoking cessation programs and related materials for midlife and older smokers. Second, there was a lack of no-smoking policies in community dwellings for older citizens. The lack of available targeted cessation materials, combined with the absence of no-smoking policies, contributed to the continuation of the smoking behavior among older citizens.

## Educational Assessment

Focus groups with 61 older smokers with a diverse socio-demographic composition recruited from communities and worksites in the Philadelphia, Pennsylvania, area specifically included questions on predisposing, reinforcing, and enabling factors. The participants were equally divided by gender and between midlife (50–64 years of age) and older (65 years and older) adults. Only 22% had a high school education and one-fourth were minorities, predominately African American.

A facilitator's guide was written, to ensure consistency among the groups, with targeted questions designed to test older participants' positions on these variables and how they affected their smoking behavior. Topics included positive and negative aspects of smoking, attitudes toward quitting, personal experiences with quitting, and reactions to specific smoking cessation programs and methods. Also, focus group participants responded to a structured questionnaire prior to group discussions. The survey form included items on smoking behavior, motivation to quit, sources of health information, program preferences, and socio-demographics. This tool produced key background information on participants. It served as a pretest for a large mailed survey among older smokers identified by the American Association of Retired Persons.

## Predisposing Factor

Several factors were considered important in the development of the health education program for midlife and older smokers. The following predisposing factors were suggested by the focus groups: a lack of perceived susceptibility to smoking-related illnesses, lack of belief in the benefits of quitting, low self-efficacy, and tobacco addiction.

Data from a target population acknowledged and confirmed a lack of belief in the benefits of quitting. Over one-half (51%) did not believe the health consequences of smoking. In fact, 52% reported that they believed smoking did not pose as much of a health threat as being 20 pounds overweight. Almost one-half (47%) reported that they were skeptical about the benefits of cessation. Also, 59% indicated a lack of confidence in their ability to quit smoking. Almost all said that they were highly addicted to cigarettes. Members of the target population informed the project planners in focus groups that they wanted methods they could use on their own.

## Reinforcing Factors

An essential dimension assessed by the project planners was reinforcing factors. A number of reinforcing factors were addressed, including social support, cessation messages from physicians, and improved sense of well-being from reduction of smoking-related symptoms by quitters. Data revealed that 62% reported that significant support systems from family and friends existed to support smoking cessation efforts by the target group. Focus group information also confirmed that 64% of midlife and older smokers had never been advised by their physician to quit smoking. However, 58% of older smokers did say that a physician's advice to quit would be a compelling reason to attempt cessation.

## Enabling Factors

Several major factors were apparent in the assessment of enabling factors. The most important of these was that there was no smoking cessation program designed specifically for midlife and older smokers. Another important factor was data that revealed most (77%) of the target population lacked sufficient smoking cessation skills. Most (82%) indicated that they were interested in self-help smoking cessation approaches, specifically methods that were tailored to the specific needs of an older population.

Only 7% reported that they would be interested in a group smoking cessation program. Reasons for not using a group program included lack of transportation, lack of privacy, too structured, and the burden of record-keeping. Also, the majority of the participants reported that they rarely listened to audiotapes (68%) or used a videotape player (67%). However, the majority reported that they "sometimes" or "often" read the newspaper (87%) or magazines (75%). These data provided additional support for developing a tailored, self-help publication as a viable health communication medium with this population. Regulations were designed to advocate the adoption of smoking cessation as an issue by regional and national organizations for midlife and older smokers. Another closely related component was the identification of older smokers as a high-risk group by national policy and governmental agencies.

## Administrative and Policy Analysis

Program planner's utilized information obtained from focus groups and the national survey of older smokers on predisposing, reinforcing and enabling factors to create a new smoking cessation program for midlife and older smokers (). This program included a new self-help guide and telephone-based counseling to support smoking cessation efforts.

## Health Education Methods

Program planners decided to develop *Clear Horizons* to fill the void of cessation programs for mid-life and older smokers. The new guide filled the older population's preference for a program they could use on their own. *Clear Horizons* was a four-color, 48-page guide targeted to the smoking habits, quitting concerns, and lifestyle of older smokers (Orleans, Rimer, Fleisher, et al., 1989). A magazine-style format, similar to the AARP publication *Modern Maturity*, was adopted to provide additional appeal. The guide's content blended entertainment and information, used large, clear type, and was written at an eighth-grade reading level. Multiracial smokers in their fifties through seventies were depicted in photographs to provide information and inspiration.

The content was based on the data retrieved from focus groups and survey participants. Information in the guide highlighted the specific health harms of smoking for older adults and the health benefits of quitting. The guide also described how smoking interacts with many common medications to restrict their efficacy. Prochaska's and DiClemente's Transtheoretical Model (1983) was used to present relevant self-change methods that are appropriate for smokers in various stages of quitting. Tips on the use of pharmaceutical adjuncts (e.g., nicotine gum) were also featured.

A final important step in the development of the *Clear Horizons* guide was a pretest with potential users in the target population. In-depth interviews were conducted with 29 smokers who were at least 50 years old.

These smokers were recruited from Philadelphia, Pennsylvania, area community groups and organizations. Interviews assessed smokers' perceptions of the guide's appeal, acceptability and relevance of its content, including cover art, realistic nature of the characters depicted in the photo-vignettes, information that was new, and overall usefulness of *Clear Horizons*. Eighty-six percent of the interviewees overwhelmingly endorsed the guide and confirmed its format, style, and size of print as appropriate for midlife and older smokers. Three-fourths of those interviewed agreed that the guide was written for persons like themselves and that the size of the print was appropriate for older readers.

Telephone calls were added to the program because of their influence in facilitating behavior change in other smoking cessation projects. Telephone counseling consisted of two 10–15 minute calls spaced 4–6 weeks and 16–30 weeks after the smoker received the guide. Call content was based on the social learning theory of Bandura (1982) and the theory of short-term counseling developed by Janis (1983). Calls were designed to bolster motivation and confidence and to promote adherence to the quitting strategies in the guide by (1) providing positive non-judgmental feedback and reinforcement geared to stage of change; (2) addressing the individual's unique quitting motives and barriers; and (3) following the individual's preferences regarding methods and commitment to a personalized quitting plan using the strategies of *Clear Horizons*.

Each call was tailored to the needs of the older smoker. Counselors assisted participants to identify their strong quitting motives and to overcome unique quitting barriers. Counselors also boosted self-efficacy and provided timely reinforcement and social support. These calls combined tailoring and support elements and served as cues to action. The counselor mediated the guide by encouraging the smoker to try the recommended strategies and providing personalized advice.

## Implementation

*Clear Horizons* was a PHASE II Evaluation Research project, and was implemented as a randomized community trial. Smokers aged 50–74 were recruited from across the United States through an advertisement placed in *Modern Maturity* magazine. Interested seniors were directed to return a postage paid postcard with their name, address, and telephone number. There were 1,867 respondents, who were mailed a brief recruitment survey that contained questions about smoking history, barriers to quitting, and demographics.

All respondents were randomly assigned to one of three groups: (1) a control (C) group who received the NCI *Clearing the Air* (USDHHS, 1991) a 24-page non-tailored cessation guide, (2) an experimental group who only received the *Clear Horizons* guide, or (3) an experimental group who received a *Clear Horizons* guide plus two telephone counseling calls at 4–8 weeks and 16–20 weeks, after the mailing of the guide. Group 3 was also offered the *Clear Horizons Quitline*, a helpline for further quitting assistance if smokers needed more help.

## Evaluation Methods

Process, impact, and outcome evaluation methods were applied in the *Clear Horizons* project. Baseline smoking and socio-demographic characteristics of the population are shown in Table 2.3 and Table 2.4. No statistically significant between group differences were documented by Rimer, Orleans, Fleisher, et al. (1994).

## Process Evaluation

At the three-month follow-up telephone interviews, the three groups were asked to rate the quality, satisfaction, and their use of their respective guides (see Table 2.5). Respondents provided ratings to the guides on several dimensions, including whether the information contained was new; whether the guide depicted people like the ones they knew; whether the content in the guide was useful; whether the guide was written for someone like them; and whether was the guide easy to use.

TABLE 2.3 Smoking-Related Baseline Characteristics of Program Participants

|  | CONTROL (N = 537) | CLEAR HORIZONS (N = 511) | CLEAR HORIZONS (N = 505) |
|---|---|---|---|
| Mean number of CPD | 26 | 27 | 27 |
| Heavy smoker | 51% | 54% | 55% |
| Smoke < 30 min of arising | 90% | 91% | 90% |
| MD Advised quitting < Year | 65% | 64% | 67% |
| Tried quit-smoking clinic | 39% | 39% | 36% |
| Tried Nicorette | 44% | 44% | 41% |

Chi-square or Krustal-Wallis test. All variables not significant. P > 0.05.

TABLE 2.4 Baseline Characteristics of *Clear Horizons* Participants

| | CONTROL (N = 537) | CLEAR HORIZONS: GUIDE ONLY (N = 511) | CLEAR HORIZONS: GUIDE + CALLS (N = 505) |
|---|---|---|---|
| Mean age: years | 62 | 61 | 61 |
| Education: H.S. graduate | 33% | 34% | 36% |
| > H.S. graduate | 59% | 62% | 54% |
| Female | 62% | 63% | 64% |
| White | 98% | 96% | 96% |
| Marital status: married | 55% | 56% | 57% |
| Employed: No | 62% | 59% | 57% |
| Region: Northeast | 32% | 31% | 31% |
| Midwest | 23% | 23% | 23% |
| South | 26% | 28% | 30% |
| West | 19% | 18% | 15% |

Overall, the groups who used *Clear Horizons* rated the guide higher than the group who used *Clearing the Air* on four of the five dimensions. The only variable that did not favor *Clear Horizons* was "depicting people like ones they knew." There were significant differences on the other four ratings. Compared with control subjects, higher proportions of subjects in both the tailored guide groups rated their guide highly (quite/completely).

As noted in Table 2.5, there was a significant difference in the distribution of guide rating scale scores; higher proportions of controls had low or medium guide rating scores, while higher proportions of tailored guide alone and tailored guide and calls subjects had high scores ($P < 0.001$). For example, 28% of the C group gave their guide a high overall score compared with 36% of the tailored guide alone subjects (#2), and 41% of the tailored guide and calls subjects (#3). Study groups also differed significantly in the amount of the guide they read ($P < 0.001$). The amount read may reflect the intensity of treatment. The control group had the highest proportion of subjects who read none of their guide (14%) compared with 12% of the tailored guide alone group and 5% of the tailored guide and calls group. The tailored guide alone group had the highest percent who read some of the guide. The tailored guide plus calls group had the highest percent who read the entire guide.

There was also a significant difference among the study groups in whether a subject read the guide ($P < 0.001$). Compared with the control subjects, larger proportions of subjects in both tailored guide groups re-read *Clear Horizons*. Whether a subject re-read the guide was significantly associated

TABLE 2.5 Participant Ratings by Group

| RATING CATEGORY | CONTROL (%) | CLEAR HORIZONS GUIDE (%) | CLEAR HORIZONS GUIDE + CALLS (%) | |
|---|---|---|---|---|
| Ideas are new | | | | 0.001 |
| Not at all/A little | 46 | 36 | 30 | |
| Somewhat | 29 | 29 | 33 | |
| Quite a bit/Completely | 26 | 35 | 37 | |
| People you know | | | | 0.861 |
| Not at all/A little | 14 | 14 | 16 | |
| Somewhat | 26 | 23 | 24 | |
| Quite a bit/Completely | 61 | 62 | 60 | |
| Helpful | | | | 0.001 |
| Not at all/A little | 11 | 7 | 4 | |
| Somewhat | 22 | 16 | 14 | |
| Quite a bit/Completely | 67 | 77 | 82 | |
| Written for you | | | | 0.005 |
| Not at all/A little | 8 | 8 | 7 | |
| Somewhat | 23 | 18 | 14 | |
| Quite a bit/Completely | 69 | 74 | 80 | |
| Easy use use to Use | | | | 0.001 |
| Somewhat | 19 | 12 | 9 | |
| Quite a bit/Completely | 74 | 81 | 86 | |

with the guide ratings scale (P < 0.001). A higher proportion who re-read their guides rated them highly. A process evaluation of telephone counseling received by those in the group using *Clear Horizons* and follow-up phone calls also revealed high ratings (not shown). About three-fourths of those who were interviewed about the calls rated them helpful (70%), that the counselor understood how they felt (77%), and that the counselor was encouraging (88%). To explore the characteristics of subjects responding favorably to the calls, a summary call rating scale form consisting of the four items was calculated. The Cronbach alpha = 0.73 indicated that the measurement scale was good.

Significantly more subjects under age 65 years rated the counselor calls highly (41%) compared with those over age 65 (P < 0.05). Subjects who rated the calls highly had significantly higher scores on the variable "how much do you want to quit" (P < 0.05) and a composite "how much will quitting help your health" and "how much will continuing to smoke hurt your health" (P < 0.01). In sum, the process evaluation showed high levels of program delivery and high program acceptance of the tailored intervention materials.

## Impact Evaluation

The impact of the intervention on smoking cessation was assessed at 3 months and 12 months post-baseline. As noted in Table 2.6, quit rates at the 3-month follow-up were significantly higher for the *Clear Horizons* plus telephone counseling group (13%) than for either groups receiving *Clear Horizons* alone (9%) or *Clearing the Air* (7%). By the 12-month follow-up, however, the quit rate of the group receiving *Clear Horizons* guide alone (21%) had edged ahead of the rate of those who had received *Clear Horizons* plus telephone counseling (19%), and was significantly higher than the quit rate of the participants receiving the non-targeted *Clearing the Air* guide (14%). These findings indicated that a targeted self-help guide alone may benefit older smokers more than generic quitting guides.

The cessation rates in this community trial increased over time. This is not unusual in self-help smoking cessation programs and is, in fact, one of the highly attractive features of self-help quitting. A possible reason for this increase in cessation over time is that those who do not succeed with their initial quit attempt often put aside their self-help materials and then use them again in another quit attempt. Research in quitting success confirms that the more times those who fail try to quit, the more likely it is they will eventually succeed. *Note:* A second randomized controlled trial evaluated the *Clear Horizons* guide in conjunction with the tailored physician interventions with older smokers in primary care practices in Pennsylvania and New Jersey. Statistically significant outcomes were observed for the *Clear Horizons* group. (See Morgan, Noll, Orleans, et al., "Reaching mid-life and older smokers: Tailored intervention for routine medical care," *Preventive Medicine* [1996] for a discussion of the methods and results of the project.)

TABLE 2.6 Quit Rates by Group

| | CONTROL | CLEAR HORIZONS GUIDE ONLY | CLEAR HORIZONS GUIDE + CALL | P-VALUE: CHI SQUARE |
|---|---|---|---|---|
| 3-Month Quit Rate | 7% | 9% | 13% | NS |
| 12-Month Quit Rate | 14% | 21% | 19% | < 0.05 |

## Outcome Evaluation

In this phase of the PRECEDE/PROCEED assessment of changes in health status, indicators and quality of life are evaluated. It was not possible to measure improvements in morbidity and mortality from smoking-related diseases due to cessation in the older age group because of time limitations and budget constraints. However, the latest medical evidence on the health benefits from cessation among older age groups suggested that the benefits from quitting may be greater for older quitters than younger age groups (Boyd and Orleans, 2002).

## Lessons Learned

The PRECEDE/PROCEED model was effective in planning the design and evaluation of *Clear Horizons*, a self-help smoking cessation guide for midlife and older smokers. This project, however, has some limitations that warrant discussion. The project was limited by its choice of a marketing strategy to recruit older smokers for evaluating the new intervention. The placement of a recruiting advertisement in *Modern Maturity*, a magazine published by the AARP, did not result in a large number of older minority smokers, including older African American smokers. Those who did respond to the advertisement were well educated. In fact, more than 50% completed high school. In retrospect, perhaps other methods of recruitment should have been employed to ensure that older minority smokers and older smokers with less education were recruited. It is possible that *Clear Horizons* may not have been appropriate for those with lower literacy levels.

The goal of the process evaluation was to determine older smokers' reactions to various aspects of the *Clear Horizons* guide. It was not possible to relate the quit rates to a single aspect of the ratings. The ratings of the guide showed that midlife and older smokers responded more favorably to a tailored educational smoking cessation guide than to the more general guide. That is, users rated *Clear Horizons* more highly and were significantly more likely to have quit smoking at 12 months but not at 3 months. From an intervention perspective, tailored guides, or any tailored health education materials, may encourage more behavior change because they facilitate more use and exposure. In this project, this advantage may have been to increase repeated use and reference over time. Repeated use of the methods and materials most likely affected the increase in quit rates at 12 months follow-up.

# 3 | Efficacy and Effectiveness Evaluation

Success depends on knowing what work.

—*Bill Gates, co-chair, Bill & Melinda Gates Foundation*

## Introduction

Although a program evaluation will always have multiple objectives, its *primary objectives* should be to determine the level of fidelity of delivery of HP-DP program intervention and measurement methods by staff and acceptability by clients, and its efficacy or effectiveness in producing significant changes in salient impact rates. A *co-primary objective* should be to produce data and insight of sufficient quality to inform decision-making about the HP-DP program and related health policies. Unfortunately, most evaluations do not achieve these objectives.

Poor process, impact, outcome, and cost-economic evaluations are often conducted because of insufficient time and resources, and/or, unfortunately, poor technical expertise and lack of staff experience. Many invalid HP-DP evaluations occur because they are politically driven. They do not reflect the selection and implementation of sound methods. Before the allocation of significant resources to a new or ongoing program is made, a rigorous evaluation plan, adequate budget, and realistic timeline are essential in order to have any opportunity to produce valid results.

As discussed in Chapter 1, a meta-evaluation (ME) should be conducted as one of the first planning steps to determine the measurement and intervention evidence base for a target problem and population. An ME, a systematic review using standard criteria, defines the **Evaluation PHASE** for each HP-DP program and defines the feasibility of different types of evaluation for a specific health problem, population, and practice setting. A written program plan and budget with a description of the type, frequency, and intensity of intervention methods, and replicable definitions of measurement and data-collection procedures, based on a current ME, must be drafted and circulated for internal review and discussion. An **Evaluability Assessment**, defining the barriers to a rigorous evaluation and thoughtful internal staff review, needs to be completed to determine the level of readiness of a program and staff to conduct the program and its evaluation.

Formative Evaluations and pilot tests to identify barriers and solutions to program needs and to improve routine program implementation are standard, essential components of an evaluation plan. The experiences of the author over a 40-year period and MEs of HP-DP programs confirm that many components of an adequate evaluation plan are often missing, incomplete, or methodologically flawed. Evaluation consultants are often asked to evaluate programs for which multiple technical components are lacking, and/or are asked to evaluate a program that has existed for several years, and is nearing the completion of a implementation-funding cycle.

## Categories of Evaluation Designs

When preparing an evaluation plan, especially selecting an evaluation design, multiple methodological and practical issues, as discussed in Chapter 1 and 2, must be addressed. It is essential to identify and to attempt to control for numerous, possible sources of large biases that always attenuate, or compromise, the interpretation of results. *A thorough appreciation of evaluation design principles is needed to answer two questions about the validity of results: (1)Was a change in an impact or outcome rate statistically significant? and (2) Can the observed change be attributed to the HP-DP program, or were some or all results attributable to other plausible explanations?*

An evaluation design identifies over what period of time, for whom, when, and what intervention and measurement procedures were (or should be) applied during implementation. If well planned and successfully implemented, an experimental design should produce the most valid data and insight to support defensible conclusions about effects. A sound design should also enable a program to estimate, with some degree of confidence, what levels of change might have occurred, if participants were not exposed to a new HP-DP program. As noted in Table 3.1, there are three categories of design: *pre-experimental, quasi-experimental*, and *experimental*.

TABLE 3.1 Categories of Evaluation Designs

| DESIGN | DESCRIPTION |
|---|---|
| Pre-Experimental | Includes one group of participants with baseline and follow-up observations. It may assert variable control over the major biases to the validity of results. Used to establish the level of success and base rate of impact of an existing HP-DP program. |
| Quasi-Experimental | Includes an experimental E group and a comparison (C) group created by methods other than random assignment. It includes baseline observations of both groups prior to and after the application of intervention procedures. It may yield interpretable and supportive evidence of impact, asserting varying degrees of control over several biases, but usually not all biases to the validity of results. |
| Experimental | Includes random assignment to an experimental E and control C group. Observations of both groups, prior to and after application of the intervention procedures, are performed. If successfully implemented, it should yield the most interpretable-defensible evidence of impact. It should assert the highest degree of control over major biases that compromise the validity of results. |

## Evaluation Design Notation

Learning basic evaluation design notation (as shown in Table 3.2), like learning evaluation terms, is necessary for efficient and consistent communication. A small, common set of letters, designating different design elements, are used in diagrams and discussions in other sections of this chapter.

## Factors Affecting the Internal and External Validity of Results

A Meta-Evaluation defines the developmental PHASE of an HP-DP program for a specific problem and population. The internal validity of a program is defined by multiple, methodologically sound **PHASE 1** and **2 Evaluations**. If **PHASE 3 and 4 Evaluation** results from a large number of studies with high internal validity are consistent and positive, the **"external validity"** of an HP-DP intervention may be supported in varying degrees. Multiple, rigorous impact and outcome evaluations are needed, however, to produce a professional consensus **(Best Practice Guidelines)** about internal validity, especially the external validity of all HP-DP programs.

TABLE 3.2 Evaluation Design Notation

| NOTATION | DEFINITION |
| --- | --- |
| R | Random assignment of a participant, unit, or site to an evaluation group |
| E | Experimental—intervention or treatment—group. E1, E2, E3... ; indicates planned exposure of the group to different intervention and assessment Procedures (P) |
| C | Control (equivalent) group established only by random assignment; indicates no exposure to an intervention or exposure to standard intervention and assessment Procedures |
| (C) | Comparison group established by any method other than randomization |
| X | Intervention procedures applied to an E group. X1, X2, X3 ... ; indicates an intervention consisting of multiple, different Procedures |
| N | Number of participants in the E, C, or (C) group |
| O | Observation or measurement to collect data: tests, interviews, ratings, or record reviews O1, O2, O3... ; indicates multiple measurements at different times |
| T | Time when an observation, assignment to a group, or application of intervention procedures has occurred: T1, T2, T3... ; indicates specific times for Procedures |

People, staff, places, and program characteristics will always vary in small or large ways. An HP-DP program and its evaluation plan should be tailored to the unique structural and process characteristics and to personnel and participants in a specific setting (contextual factors). While the technical methods of an evaluation of a high blood pressure control program being planned to document effectiveness in Washington, D.C., or Sidney, Australia, should be comparable, each individual program needs to be concerned much more about how to optimize program acceptability to staff and clients, and effectiveness where the program and its evaluation are being conducted. Implementation success should be enhanced and the probability of positive change increased by adapting program procedures to the population and practice setting for which it is being delivered.

*Although in principle, an evaluation should be primarily concerned with internal and external validity, almost all evaluations will be concerned with producing results with high internal validity.* This enables a program to make optimal use of resources, time, and staff to increase the opportunity to produce desired changes at this time, for this population and practice setting. External validity, generalizability to a defined population, is almost always beyond the resources of an evaluation. Measles vaccination will, with rare exceptions, be effective for all children in any country and have high internal and external validity. Multiple, complex factors, however, need to be considered before an HP-DP program can say it has external validity. The issue is population heterogeneity, as well as variations in capacity, staffing, and resources where a program is delivered.

## A Contemporary Synthesis of Biases to Internal Validity

The evaluation literature in education, health education–health promotion, and the social and behavioral sciences for over 50 years has traditionally identified eight common threats (biases) to internal validity of an observed result based on Campbell and Stanley (1966). Each threat in Table 3.3 may confound or bias the interpretation of HP-DP program "efficacy" or "effectiveness" by independently or collectively producing all or part of observed changes in impact or outcome rates.

Contemporary evaluation methods and 30 years of HP-DP evaluation studies and research of high quality have produced a synthesis of the eight threats to validity from Campbell and Stanley (1963). Contemporary

TABLE 3.3 Threats to Internal Validity

| THREATS | DEFINITION |
| --- | --- |
| #1 History | Bias from significant, unplanned national, local, or internal organizational events or exposures occurring during the evaluation that may produce behavior change |
| #2 Maturation | Bias from biological, social, behavioral, or administrative changes occurring among participants or staff during the study period, e.g., growing older, staff becoming more/less skilled, or more effective-efficient in program delivery |
| #3 Testing | Bias from taking a test, being interviewed, or being observed |
| #4 Instruments | Bias from changes in the characteristics of instruments, observation methods data-collection processes, affecting the reliability + validity of instruments |
| #5 Statistical Regression | Bias from selection of an E, C, or (C) group on the basis of a high or low level of characteristic yielding changes in future measurements |
| #6 Selection | The identification of a C or (C) group not equivalent to the E group because of demographic, psychosocial, or behavioral characteristics |
| #7 Attrition | Bias introduced in impact data by non-random loss (> 10%) in the E, C, (C) group |
| #8 Interactive Effects | Any combination of the seven threats to validity |

TABLE 3.4 Primary Categories of Bias to Internal Validity of Results

| BIAS | DIMENSIONS | ISSUES |
| --- | --- | --- |
| Measurement (M) | Validity (V) | Quality + Completeness: Methods and Types of |
| | Reliability (R) | Data at O1 + O2 + On . . . for a Theoretical or Planning Model |
| Selection (S) | Participation Rate (P) Attrition Rate (A) | Representativeness: Eligibility (%/+) of the sample of the target population at risk at O1 + O2 + On . . . |
| History (H) | External Events (He) Internal Events (Hi) Intervention (Hx) | Exposures: Type- Intensity-Duration-Frequency of to a planned and unplanned HP-DP program events and salient external events during the evaluation |

evalution as noted in Table 3.4, the eight sources of bias to the internal validity of results were condensed by Windsor, Clark, Boyd, and Goodman in 1994 (2nd ed.) and 2004 (3rd ed.) into the three primary bias categories: **Measurement**, **Selection**, and **History (M-S-H)**. The literature confirms that these categories are the most frequent, serious sources of biases that compromise results. An evaluation team needs to know how best to control for each, and to select a design to apply to enable it to rule out plausible, alternative explanations of impact or outcome.

## Measurement Bias

As discussed in Chapter 4, the first and most salient category of bias to attribution of a significant change in an impact or outcome rate from an HP-DP intervention is **measurement**. This bias category combines threats #3 (Testing) and #4 (Instrumentation) of Campbell and Stanley. It has two primary sources of potential error and bias in an impact or outcome rate: poor validity (V) and poor reliability (R) of measurement. Elimination of these biases should always occur before an evaluator can accurately assess if, and how much, change has occurred in an impact rate.

A meta-evaluation (ME) of pertinent literature defines primary behavioral impact or health outcome rates and dependent variable(s). It identifies "gold standard" methods and describes how to validly and reliably measure each. In addition, an ME defines the most salient independent demographic variables, and/or psycho-social constructs that predict impact or outcome rates for a target population. An ME provides the evaluation with valid data and insight to define what types of bias may have been introduced by measurement error, and participants lost to follow-up rates. Appropriate psychometric analyses are essential to establish the validity of measures and data. Detailed discussions are presented in Chapter 4 (Measurement and Analysis in Evaluation) of this volume.

At the onset of planning, the objective of an evaluation should be to select the optimal set of data and focus on implementing methods, pilot-testing all observation-measurement methods to reduce error at O1 and O2, and achieve > 90% participant/data follow-up rates. *Validity, reliability completeness, and staff/participant burden, rather than the amount of data, should guide the final decisions about "core" evaluation data.* A basic concern is the extent to which an evaluation used replicable and standardized measurement methods. Were "gold standard" methods selected from a meta-evaluation of the measurement science for a specific problem or condition? Were "gold standard" measurement methods applied for salient predictor-process-impact variables?

An evaluation needs to present empirical evidence confirming the quality, accuracy, and stability of impact data, collected prior to, at the onset, and during an evaluation. *It is important to stress: a design "controls" for measurement bias only if the error is small and comparable for all evaluation groups. Random assignment of participants/data with poor measurement validity equally distributes large sources of bias; randomization does not control for large errors.*

## Selection Bias

The second category of bias to attribution of an HP-DP program effect is **selection**. This bias category combines threats #5 (Regression), #6 (Selection), and #7 (Attrition) of Campbell and Stanley. Participant inclusion and exclusion criteria will affect how representative an evaluation sample is of the population, before an evaluation begins. Eligibility criteria should be well justified, and should not exclude a significant proportion, for example, > 10%, of a target population, at the onset of the evaluation. The combination of demographic, psycho-social, and current behavioral data for E and C group participants enables an evaluation to establish equivalence at a baseline (O1) and the end-point assessment period (O2). This category has two primary sources of bias: low participation rate of eligible E and C group subjects at O1, for example, > 10% with different baseline characteristics, and a high attrition rate (lost to follow-up/LTF) of E or C group participants at O2, for example, > 10% with different baseline characteristics. An evaluation plan needs to describe the eligibility criteria for the target population (denominator) and present data documenting the total characteristics and number of eligible participants who participate (numerator) and refusals at each evaluation sites.

*Important questions not answered by many evaluation reports include the following:* What percent of eligible subjects participated and refused at each site throughout each year of the evaluation? Who, after initially agreeing to participate, decided, actively or passively, to withdraw, or drop out? Who among participants eligible for a follow-up were lost to follow-up (LTF)? Randomization, which may include stratification and matching prior to assignment, is the primary method to control for a large number of independent characteristics, **selection biases**, of a study sample that predicts the probability of a change in a dependent impact or outcome rate. The criteria and methods to address these issues are defined in Cochrane Review and ME procedures. *It is also important to emphasize: if a large percent of eligible participants do not agree to participate and a large percent are LTF, randomization does not control for these significant biases at O1 and O2.*

Unless there is a justifiable rationale, for example, E, C, or (C) group participants have moved to another non-study location, subjects randomized should typically be used to compute an attrition and impact rate: **"Intent to Treat Policy."** An evaluation needs to compare the baseline characteristics of participants who agree, and those eligible but who refuse to participate at baseline or who withdraw later during the evaluation. Each baseline participation and follow-up attrition rate defines how small or large a selection bias was in an evaluation. Because participation requires voluntary informed consent, enrolling > 90% of eligible participants, and following up on > 90% would be considered excellent participation and attrition follow-up rates for almost all HP-DP evaluations. Participation rates and/or attrition rates, however, lower than each of these two "Program Performance or Practice Standards > 90%" will reduce and may compromise the validity of results. *The core question to be answered by all evaluations is the following: To what extent can the results of our evaluation be applied to the target population at risk in this HP-DP practice setting?*

The ability to generalize evaluation results to a large, defined population at risk will be severely limited or impossible, if all selection biases are not addressed, especially during planning, pilot testing of methods, and implementation of the evaluation. It is essential to conduct a formative evaluation, pilot testing all measurement and intervention procedures by all staff at all sites, to enhance routine implementation. These methods should significantly reduce participant refusals at the onset and reduce E, C, or (C) group participant attrition rates during an evaluation.

## Historical Bias

The third category of bias to attribution of impact is **history**. This category combines the validity threats #1 (History) and #2 (Maturation) of Campbell and Stanley. It has three primary sources of bias. First, what transient or enduring external historical events (He) may be a plausible, independent cause(s) of observed significant changes? A powerful, nationwide "H" event that had a substantial external impact on the life of Americans and all evaluation studies in progress was the September 11, 2001, attacks. A more typical historical event for a state, county, or city that may have a transient effect on a program evaluation, for example, cancer screening rates, would be that the governor develops breast cancer, or a mayor develops prostate cancer during the evaluation.

Second, what internal historical programmatic events ($H_i$) may have occurred during the evaluation, for example, changes in policy, organizational or program structure, and loss of staffing, and/or resources? Third, what specific intervention Procedures (X1 + X2 + Xn) were delivered or not delivered to what percentage of eligible E group participants? The issue here is the extent to which exposure or non-exposure to specific intervention (Xn) procedures, intensity, duration, and frequency, was documented by a process evaluation. What was the degree of stability, consistency, and replicability of delivery of intervention procedures by staff (**Program Fidelity**)?

The economic recession > 2008 would be a salient example of an $H_i$ that affected programs.

## Evaluation Designs and Bias

While there are many types of evaluation designs, a very small number can be applied to assert sufficient control for the salient biases to the validity of results. Four design options are presented in Table 3.5, with information about the seven potential independent sources of bias to internal validity, and an eighth source (□), the interactive effects of biases 1 to 7. *Note: No notation is placed in Table 3.5 to signify that each design and bias needs to be examined by each evaluation.* Each bias may be an alternative, plausible explanation for an observed effect, instead of the HP-DP program. Even when a randomized design (#4) is used, evaluation results may be equivocal or compromised, unless plausible alternative explanations of change are ruled out.

An experimental design (#4) should be the first choice to rule out threats to validity and to produce a high degree of certainty about effectiveness,

TABLE 3.5  Biases to Internal Validity of Selected Designs

|  | (M) | | (S) | | (H) | | | ALL BIASES |
| --- | --- | --- | --- | --- | --- | --- | --- | --- |
|  | MEASUREMENT | | SELECTION | | HISTORY | | | |
|  | (1) | (2) | (3) | (4) | (5) | (6) | (7) | (8) |
| EVALUATION DESIGNS | V | R | P | A | HE | HI | XN | M + S + H |
| #1. One Group Pre-Post Test: E O X . . . O | | | | | | | | |
| #2. Non-Randomized Comparison (C) Group: E O X . . . O O (C) O O O O | | | | | | | | |
| #3. Time Series: (C) O O O   O E X . . . O . . . O X O X O X O | | | | | | | | |
| #4. Randomized Pre + Post Test + Control Group: R E O X . . . O O R C O O O | | | | | | | | |

V = Validity, R = Reliability, P = Participation Rate, A = Attrition Rate, O = Observation, Sum of M + S + H. . . He = External Events . . . Hi = Internal Program Events . . . X. . . = Interventions.

and cost-effectiveness or cost-benefit of an intervention. More complex multi-factorial designs involving three or four evaluation groups can be conducted to answer multiple questions about independent (X1) and interactive effects (X1 + X2 + X3) of HP-DP intervention procedures. Factorial designs would typically be applied in a PHASE 1 or 2 study, which would have adequate scientific expertise, resources, staff, and sufficient time to meet multiple/complex implementation, training and analytical demands. A group randomized clinical trial (GRCT) design, a multi-site study involving matching and randomization of schools-clinics-worksites-villages-communities-counties, may also be selected.

Examples of group randomized, non-randomized, and time-series evaluation designs are presented in this chapter. Planning and conducting a GRCT, however, presents an additional array of complex implementation, analytical, and fiscal issues. A comprehensive discussion of GRCT and analyses is presented by Murray (1998). A systematic review of 34 randomized cluster designs by Eldridge et al., *Lancet* (2008) confirmed that approximately 50% of the evaluations that applied a GRCT design had serious methodological problems. Many GRCTs also failed to report data/information especially about the feasibility and delivery of the HP-DP intervention.

The characteristics of a program, or practice delivery setting, and/or the target group may make it difficult to conduct an evaluation of high methodological quality. Nevertheless, an evaluation team should always start with the most rigorous design possible. Then, if necessary, modify the design or adjust to an unanticipated situation. If an evaluation plan starts by adjusting the rigor of its methods, an opportunity is usually lost to examine the program or program elements before all design possibilities have been explored. Unfortunately, because of a lack of training, experience, and especially political expediency/pressure, program and evaluation leadership frequently select a methodologically weaker evaluation design to asses impact.

Although compromise on the use of an experimental design when planning an evaluation should rarely occur, an RCT may not be feasible for some programs and settings. The evaluation literature confirms that a quasi-experimental design, a matched **historical non-randomized comparison (C) group design** may be applied in selected situations to assess impact. The (C) group design, however, will require applications of specific evaluation and analytical methods. Because of the inherent issues in interpreting results from a quasi-experimental design, when either is applied, implementation problems will compromise the internal and external validity of the evaluation. In some evaluations, a time series design (TSD) may be the most appropriate choice.

## Threats to the External Validity of Results

A meta-evaluation involving a comprehensive, systematic review and rating of peer-reviewed, published evaluations by an independent panel of experts and meta-analysis (if appropriate) are the primary methods used to define external validity. The NIH, AHRQ, and Cochrane Review use this methodology to evaluate and make judgments about the evidence base and internal and external validity of an HP-DP treatment program. As discussed in Chapter 1, external validity is defined as the degree to which a meta-evaluation has documented the level of confidence to which a statistically significant change in a behavioral impact or health status outcome rate from **PHASE 3** and **4 Evaluations** can be attributable to an HP-DP treatment and can be generalized to a large, defined population with a specific problem. The ME may provide documentation that the HP-DP program is more or less effective for specific populations or practice settings, for example, adults versus adolescents, or clinic-based versus home-based programs.

The multiple challenges and complexity to produce evidence from one or two well-designed evaluations generalizable to a health problem and large, well-defined population in the United States—for example, fall injuries to children under < 6, high blood pressure control among senior (> 65) citizens, or pregnant smokers supported by Medicaid—are self-evident. While rare exceptions exist, the external validity of the results from HP-DP evaluations for almost all problems and populations are based on valid, cumulative evidence from a large number of successfully implemented evaluations in multiple locations and in a variety of systems of care within the same country and language.

In addition to the threats (biases) to internal validity described in this chapter, four categories of threats to the external validity-generalizability of evaluation results are commonly identified: (1) selection-treatment interaction bias, (2) treatment-reaction bias, (3) multiple treatment bias, and (4) measurement reaction bias. The primary issue to resolve for **Bias Category #1** (selection-treatment interaction bias) is the extent to which the participants of completed evaluations were representative of the population to whom the results are being generalized. Examples of critical questions to be answered include the following: What were the eligibility criteria? What were the characteristics of participants who agreed or refused to participate, who continued in the evaluation, who dropped out, and/or who were lost to follow-up? Was the HP-DP treatment only effective for participants with a specific set of characteristics, for example, male versus female, low versus middle income, or middle aged versus senior citizen?

The dimensions of Bias #1 that need primary attention are the very large contextual-environmental variations in the demographic characteristics of participants and HP-DP program staff. Very large differences in the infrastructure, budgeting, training, and resource levels of clinic or practice settings within and between HP-DP programs and public health–primary care systems always exist. If consistent, positive results are produced, presentations of data about *where* (multiple geographic locations), *when* (time period-durability), and *how many* HP-DP evaluations were successfully conducted strengthen judgments about the degree of external validity.

Bias Category #1 is likely to be the most salient, complex threat to validity among the four bias categories. Confirmation that stratification, matching, and randomization of a large representative number of sites or participants at HP-DP program sites was successful may address the first level of generalization. Confirmation that the representative sample of evaluation sites and population at risk who agreed to participate and who completed planned follow-up assessments procedures from both the E and C groups may address the second level of generalization. If summarized ME and MA results are judged to be representative, this should mean that there is a high likelihood that the program can be delivered with fidelity across states and programs by regular staff during regular delivery of program services.

**Bias Categories #2, #3**, and **#4** are concerned about the extent to which measurement and treatment procedures of the HP-DP program were sufficiently unique to independently produce part or all of an observed significant treatment effect. Planning a **PHASE 4 Dissemination Evaluation** whose treatment and measurement methods have demonstrated feasibility and transferability from **PHASE 1, 2,** and **3 Evaluations** for the target population, problem, and practice setting will diminish, if not eliminate, possible threats from **Bias #2, #3,** and **#4.** Case studies 2, 4, and 7 in this chapter were evaluations designed to produce results with both internal and external validity.

## Evaluation Design Summary

An evaluation design describes how an HP-DP program has planned to minimize or eliminate major, systematic (non-random) biases for pre-existing characteristics of participants. An experimental design, if successfully implemented, typically asserts control over biases in three major categories, Measurement Bias, Selection Bias, and Historical Bias, by equally distributing error among the E and C groups of participants. Randomization of participants at each evaluation-program site, or stratification and matching of sites, equally distributes by chance (if successful), all measured and unmeasured participant characteristics. This process should establish at least two equivalent groups at baseline: a C group to typically receive a "basic" HP-DP intervention (X1) and an E group to typically receive a "basic + best practice" HP-DP intervention (X1 + X2 + X3).

*It is important to stress: a randomized design does not always "control" for the multiple dimensions of the three bias categories. E versus C group equivalence at baseline and at follow-up should not be assumed: it must be empirically confirmed.* Although rare, if the E and C groups significantly differ on a baseline viable(s), this difference will usually be due to random error, not systematic error. Analytical methods, for example, Analysis of Covariance, may be applied to the impact data to adjust for baseline differences. During the planning and formative evaluation phases, an evaluation team needs to train staff, prepare an implementation plan, and conduct pilot tests to identify and to address each source of bias. The methodological and implementation issues in selecting a design, shown in Table 3.5, are described in the following sections and case studies.

## Design #1: One Group Pre-test and Post-test

As a pre-experimental design, Design #1 is the most basic method for program assessment. *It should be not used to assess program behavioral impact or health outcome over any extended period of time,* for example, > *12 months.* In this design, baseline measurements are made (O1), an intervention (X1) is provided, and follow-up observations-measurements (O2) are performed. Attributing an observed significant change that occurred between O1 and O2 to the intervention (X) requires an evaluation to systematically explain how it controlled for Measurement, Selection, and Historical biases. For example, did other historical events, unplanned exposures, or unexpected activities of program participants between O1 and O2 partially or fully explain an observed significant change? The longer the period of time between O1 and O2, the more probable it is that an internal or external historical (H) event, unplanned exposures, or program changes may have influenced participant behavior and affected program results. Measurement or selection biases may also explain any observed changes between O1 and O2.

Design #1 can be very useful, however, in conducting an immediate/ short-term assessment of an existing HP-DP program. A program may decide to assess the immediate impact (1–6 months) of an intervention for a specific problem (elderly falls) or a specific condition (high blood pressure control). The interval between O1 and O2 must be short, and the evaluation planned and successfully implemented so that selection and historical biases are implausible explanations of a significant impact. If the baseline and follow-up measurements are valid and complete and occur prior to and soon after the intervention, for example, a few weeks/months before and after, historical bias may not be a plausible threat to impact results.

A process evaluation is essential to confirm successful implementation of intervention and assessment procedures.

Maximum control over measurement quality and data-collection processes must be asserted to control for this bias, regardless of the size or evaluation purpose. Confirmation of data validity and sample representativeness are essential in Design #1, and all designs. If measurement validity is confirmed and the time period is short, the first threat to internal validity for Design #1 will be *selection bias*. Did the program document high (100%) O1 and O2 assessment rates (> 90%) for evaluation clients? What is the extent to which evaluation participants are comparable or different from other users at HP-DP program sites? The following is an example of the use of Design #1.

### Design #1 Example

The director of a Medicaid-supported prenatal care program in Kansas City, Kansas, and her six clinic managers decide to document the prevalence of patient smoking status on entry and during care. They also want to determine the behavioral impact of existing patient counseling methods (X. . . ) of regular nursing and social worker staff. The director asks for a formative assessment report in six months, three months before the next fiscal year.

Because of resource and time constraints, the six clinic sites are matched into three dyads by patient entry-level demographic variables and monthly new patient census. Three clinics are randomly selected from the three dyads, and consecutive patients at each clinic who smoked are enrolled in the formative assessment study. During a one-month period at the three clinics, 100 of 115 pregnant smokers (87% participation rate), 30–40 patients per site who received normal prenatal care and counseling, completed a brief baseline assessment Form. Their current smoking status was documented on the Patient Assessment Form (O1). Because patients do not accurately report smoking status, an expired carbon monoxide (CO) test value was collected for each patient by regular staff as part of normal program procedures. These data informed patients and staff about prevalence rates and patient levels of tobacco exposure at the first prenatal care visit.

All 100 patients received the existing counseling program (X1): a 5–7-minute, one-to-one RN counseling session plus a brochure on risks. The MD of each patient also routinely provided very brief advice at each patient visit. At their third or fourth clinic visit, the same assessments procedures were performed (O2). A self-report of smoking status and CO test of 92 of the 100 patients were again recorded by the nursing staff as part of a routine follow-up (O2). A patient had to say she had quit and had a CO value of < 6 PPM (parts per million) to be counted as a quitter at O2. The cohort of smokers can be called a standard program E group or a comparison (C) group.

In this example, the following impact data might be documented among the 92 patients at O2: (1) a significant increase in perceived maternal-infant health belief risk score (tobacco use) from 70% to 95%, and (2) the number of self-reported quitters of the 92 O2 follow-ups with a CO confirmed quit was five. This level of impact, a 5.0% quit rate (5/100, not 5/92: Intent to Treat policy), would need to be examined for each primary bias to internal validity. Measurement of smoking status was very good (self-reports + CO test), and the time period between O1 and O2 was short. The sample of three clinics was randomly selected from the six matched dyads, 87% of eligible patients were enrolled, and 92% were followed up as part of normal care.

One important methodological question is this: How representative of the typical patient population at the six sites were the 90 patients at the three study sites? This can be confirmed by monthly clinic census reports at each site. Although it needs to be documented, the study cohort in this example is probably comparable to patients at the three clinics *not* selected, because of matching and random selection, and short time period. A participation rate of 87% and an attrition rate of only 8% at the clinics also provided very good support for a small selection bias. The short time period would indicate it was unlikely that patient exposure to other internal or external historical events/biases produced a 5.0% quit rate. *The most plausible explanation of the 5% quit rate would be that it was attributable to the counseling received from the patient's nurse and brief advice from other professional staff at the first, second, and third clinic visits.* If successfully implemented, an internal validity score (1 = very low to 10 = superior) for this study would be an 8.0 (very good). This study provides good data and insight for future planning. **Case study 2** in this chapter applied Design #1.

## Formative Assessment Evaluation

A study using Design #1 can be called a "Formative Evaluation." If Design #1 is used to determine the current level of program impact, it needs a short implementation period, an excellent level of implementation, valid measurement, complete baseline (100%), and an excellent level of follow-up data (> 90%) to be able to attribute observed results to an existing HP-DP program.

After a meta-evaluation of the evaluation literature is completed, this assessment should be one of the first planned evaluation activities for all HP-DP programs to document the normal, behavioral impact of an existing program. It provides immediate empirical data and insight about the level of success of the existing program, and implementation barriers for a practice setting.

This rigorous "Pilot Study" also provides an HP-DP program and agency with a defensible estimate of the typical impact of an existing intervention for a target population, using regular staff of an existing primary care program. Valid documentation of the normal behavioral impact rate of an HP-DP program is essential to estimate the sample size for the E and C group (discussed later in this chapter) in a future two-group evaluation proposal. A Formative Evaluation should also provide planning and site staff experience about how to plan and conduct an evaluation.

## Design #2: Non-Randomized Comparison (C) Group

Following completion of the Design #1 evaluation (or prior to planning), program leadership may ask the coordinator of Health Promotion and Education Programs (MPH-CHES) for their agency to present a 20-minute meta-evaluation report at the next monthly staff meeting. This person may be asked describe "best practice (BP)" client assessment and intervention methods for pregnant smokers. Design #2 might be considered by leadership, if they decide, after reading the meta-evaluation, that the 5% cessation rate is significantly lower than a rate from BP methods.

If program leadership decides to introduce a new "best practice" program to significantly increase the cessation rate, data and methods from the Design #1 Formative Evaluation can be used to plan Design #2. The agency can compare the existing program (X1), now referred to as the (C) group, versus a new, proposed program, X1 + X2 + X3 + X4, for an E group of patients. The original sample of 100 pregnant smokers used in Design #1 can be called either a **Standard Treatment group** or a **Historical Comparison (C) group**. The bracketed comparison (C) group notation confirms the creation of the group by a method other than randomization. The group that receives the new best practice intervention would be called an experimental (E) group.

## Design #2 Example

Assume that the MCH leadership team decided to introduce new, more efficacious, best practices counseling procedures (X1 + X2 + X3 + X4). Although a randomized study (Design #4) to compare X1 versus X1 + X2 + X3 +X 4 is a stronger option, they may have decided for practical reasons to systematically apply Design #1, and then apply Design #2. If well planned and successfully implemented, the addition of a second group (non-randomized) *may* improve a program's ability to rule out alternative explanations of behavioral impact.

As noted in Design #2, the same baseline (O1) and follow-up assessment methods (O2) must be applied to both the E and (C) groups of participants at all sites, or at an equal number of sites representative of all program sites. Each planned observation of patients must use the same standardized measures of high quality. Biases may also be partially dealt with by ensuring that neither the (C) nor the E group from the program sites is selected because of an extreme trait.

After staff has completed the Design #1 evaluation of the impact of X1, regular staff would then be trained to deliver the new counseling program procedures, X1 + X2 +X3 + X4, to all E group patients. In this way, regular staff behavior in the clinics would not be influenced by the counseling training program during implementation of Design #1. In this example, the two observation and intervention methods are performed by the same prenatal care staff at the same clinics to comparable cohorts of pregnant smokers, but at different times in a 9–12-month period.

Assume, for purposes of discussion, the application of the same measurement methods, very comparable baseline participation, and follow-up attrition rates in the application of Design #1 and #2. Assume a self-reported + CO confirmed quit rate of 14% (14/100) among the E group for Design #2 is compared to the old (X1) program (C) group impact rate of 5.0% for Design #1. A Chi Square test ($X2 = 6.82$) comparing the two quit rates indicates a statistically significant difference > 0.01 level. This provides encouraging results. The primary question to be answered by Design #2 is, therefore, Was the new E group intervention (X1 + X2 + X3 + X4) more effective than the (X1) intervention delivered to Comparison (C) group by the same nurses at the same sites, or are there other plausible explanations for the significant E versus C group quit rate difference?

If Design #2 is successfully implemented, the evaluation team will need to systematically rule out the three main categories of bias. The extent to which this design controls for selection biases is a primary issue: How comparable were the baseline characteristics of each cohort: Design #2 E group of 100 patients versus Design #1 (C) group of 100 patients? If the evaluation was conducted at only three of six clinics, how comparable were the patients at the evaluation clinics to patients in non-participating clinics? The internal validity of these results can then be described. The internal validity score of the Design #2 evaluation example would probably be 8.0 (very good).

Case study 3 in this chapter, *Maternal and Child Health Journal* (2013) is good example of a Design #2 application. *In addition to this example, a useful class exercise would be to have a group of three or four students review and rate a quasi-experimental evaluation not presented in this chapter*: "Evaluation of a Community-Based Intervention to Promote Rear Seating for Children," by Greenberg-Seth et al., *American Journal of Public Health* (2004), 1009–1013.

## Design #3: Time Series

Time series designs (TSD) and time series analysis (TSA) have been infrequently applied and generally under-utilized as a design to evaluate the "effectiveness" of HP-DP programs (Windsor et al., 2004). Biglan, et al. (2000) noted: "Greater use of interrupted times-series experiments is advocated for community intervention research." Time series designs enable the production of knowledge about the effects of state- and country-wide intervention health policies in circumstances in which a randomized trial is too expensive or simply impractical. Design #3 requires the availability and accessibility of an existing valid and complete data and information system for the target area, population, and problem. These data are essential to accurately describe past, current, and future incidence rates of a specific risk factor(s) or event(s) and impact rates for multiple years, for example, DUI rates, or motorcycle injury rates.

A **PHASE 4 Dissemination-Effectiveness Evaluation** is the most likely type of evaluation to use a TSD to assess the impact of a new state-wide or system-wide public health program. This design is especially appropriate for evaluating the effects of a new health policy, tax, law, or the system-wide dissemination and adoption by an agency and staff of a new "HP-DP Best Practice" intervention to be delivered to all eligible clients. Design #3 can be considered if a program can:

- Establish that a routinely reported data monitoring system exists for the HP-DP impact rate, is accessible, and is current;
- Establish the validity, reliability, completeness, and stability of impact measurement and rates;
- Establish the periodicity-pattern of the impact or outcome rate being examined for a large well-defined problem, system of care or services, population at risk, and a specific geographic area;
- Document at multiple monthly, quarterly, or annual data points at least two to three years before, and two to three years after the HP-DP intervention was introduced; and
- Introduce the HP-DP system-wide intervention at a specific time and, if well justified, to withdraw the intervention abruptly at a specific time period in the future.

The application of a time series design (TSD) requires that an adequate number of valid observations, data, and rates are available, preferably over a three- to five-year period before and after implementation of the HP-DP policy program, to document behavioral or health outcome rate trends. The observation points should occur at equal intervals—monthly, quarterly, semi-annually, or annually—and cover a sufficient time period to confirm pre-intervention and post-intervention variations for an impact rate. Observations and analyses of a behavior change trend over time, however, even with fewer data points (e.g., two to four baseline and two to four follow-up assessments covering a two-year period), may represent a significant improvement over Design #1.

*Although most discussions of this method refer to a TSD as a "quasi-experimental design," it is arguable that in some cases it should be referred to as an "experimental design."* An evaluation that applies a TSD, if successfully implemented, can produce results with high internal and external validity. Case study 4 in this chapter is an excellent example of the application of a TSD and analysis in the evaluation of the impact on surface miner injury rates of a national health and safety training policy and program. It had high internal and external validity for the US population of 110,000 miners and 10,000 mines. There are multiple examples in the literature.

If applying a TSD, a program needs to examine the extent to which the evaluation design can control for measurement, selection, and history biases. Because of the long duration of an evaluation, although selection and measurement are very important biases when a TSD is applied, historical biases are a central concern. People, places, environments, and conditions change over a 3–10 year period. The plausibility of the impact of factors such as weather, seasonality, major local or national historical events, and changes in health policies, taxes, or procedures must be examined. Because the principal issue in applying a TSD is to document the significance of a trend in an observed rate, the HP-DP treatment needs to be powerful enough to produce and sustain significant positive shifts in an impact rate beyond normal variations. The threat of external and internal historical events increases significantly with the duration of the evaluation.

An excellent example of the application of a time series design was published by the US National Bureau of Economic Research (2011) by Chen, Jin, Kumar, and Shi in "The Promise of Beijing: Evaluating the Impact of the 2008 Olympic Games on Air Quality." They used local Air Pollution Index (API) data and Aerosol Optimal Depth (AOD) particulate data from NASA satellites from 2000 to 2009. The researchers confirmed, from thousands of observations in multiple cities, that the air quality (API Index) improved from 109 in 2000–2001 to 77 during the Olympic Games in 2008. It reverted to 83 one month after the games and to 96 within 12 months in 2009. The program to improve air quality in Beijing was one of the largest natural experiments in the literature. This complex, impact evaluation and analysis should be of interest to HP-DP graduate students for discussion in class about the application of a TSD in real-world situation.

### Establishing a Non-Randomized Comparison (C) Group

A non-randomized comparison (C) group may represent the only feasible alternative if an agency establishes a policy to deliver the HP-DP program to all participants at all sites. The Design #2 example provides one method to create a (C) group. In using a (C) group, an evaluator is attempting to replicate an experimental study in every way, with the exception of randomization. An evaluator has the challenge of identifying candidate participants or units/sites, and selecting a (C) group from among these options. In identifying a (C) group, considerable attention must be given to selecting individuals or groups who are as similar to the E group as possible. An evaluation must document at baseline, however, the similarities and differences between the (C) group and E groups.

The rationale and methods to identify individuals, units, or groups to serve as a (C) group must be well defined. The (C) groups selected will either be a historical group (Design #1), or another group that is not exposed to the new intervention (Design #2). This will always be a complex task. *Evaluation study results and conclusions are always diminished, and in almost all cases internal validity is lost, when a quasi-experimental design is unsuccessfully implemented.*

An evaluation may attempt to match program data at individual sites (E group) to program data at a site or comparable area (C) group where the new intervention will not be introduced. This design is not feasible, however, unless a uniform database exists or can be introduced at all comparison locations, for example, clinics, hospitals, or schools. In identifying site/subjects to serve in a (C) group, approximately the same numbers of individuals per site as in the E group are needed. If the candidate (C) sites have a monitoring system, an evaluation may identify a number of units whose participants may have comparable baseline demographics to the E group. A major barrier to using this method is gaining the cooperation of intact comparison groups or sites (C) at other locations.

### Quasi-Experimental Designs and Bias

A quasi-experimental design, by definition, will exert variable control over the major biases to internal validity. Thus, caution is advised in interpreting results from a quasi-experimental study. Selection and historical bias will always be the initial, major biases to examine when a quasi-experimental design is used. After matching on one or two baseline variables, it usually becomes impossible, in most cases, to match on a third major population baseline characteristic. *The initial, pre-treatment differences from known, and especially numerous unknown, selection biases make all E and (C) group adjusted post-test comparisons challenging.*

There is a lack of consensus in the literature about what analytical technique is the most appropriate for results produced by non-randomized comparison group designs. This issue has been discussed in the social and behavioral science literature for 35 years, for example, see Cook and Campbell (1979) and Kenny (1979). Statistical adjustment methods cannot fully adjust for known, and cannot adjust for multiple unknown, selection characteristics of participants or matched groups/sites. Grossman and Tierney (1993) in "The Fallibility of Comparison Groups," provided an excellent methodological and analytical discussions about the use of a (C) group and quasi-experimental designs. They noted: "despite using a comparison group explicitly designed to overcome many self-selection issues endemic to quasi-experimental methods and using a variety of statistical methods to control for selection bias, quasi-experimental designs are still subject to the threat that the comparison group did not adequately represent a non-treatment state."

## Design #4: Randomized Pre-Test and Post-Test Design

An experimental design typically enables the evaluator to establish by randomization of individuals (or sites), two (or more) groups not significantly different at baseline for all (or almost all) independent or dependent predictors of impact. There are several methods to plan and conduct an experimental study. A common approach is to evaluate an existing program with the usual intervention (X1) provided to C group participants and comparing this group to an E group exposed to a hypothetically more effective program with additional intervention procedures (X1 + X2 + X3 + X4). Standardized baseline (O1) and follow-up assessments (O2 + O3) are conducted for all C and E group participants during specific observation periods. If a large number of participants (400–1,000) are needed in the evaluation, individuals can be randomly assigned (R) at each program site to the E or C group to control for inter-site selection biases.

Random assignment may be conducted daily if participants enter the program on the same day, or participants may sign up every week when they enter the program over a defined period of time. This design should produce excellent control over the three major biases to internal validity, assuming no major implementation problems. Confirmation that the randomization process has been established with equivalent groups at each site and overall is essential. Case studies 5, 6, 7 in this chapter (and case studies in Chapter 6) are examples of Design #4. Case study 7 is also an excellent example of a group randomized design in a low-income country: Nepal. The Nepal case study and many comparable examples demonstrate the complexity of a GRCT. It also confirms that this design can be successfully implemented not only in high-income, but also in low-income countries.

### Establishing a Control (C) Group

A randomized design will typically assert control over independent variables and minimize **M-S-H** biases by equally distributing, between the E and C group, participants with variable baseline characteristics. Each variable may have an independent or interactive effect, explaining part of an observed impact rate. The key question in establishing a C group is, Does it adequately control for independent predictors of change in the impact and outcome rates? Baseline equivalence of an E and C group needs to be documented: randomization does not always produce equivalent groups at baseline. Ideally, E and C baseline data confirm that they are almost identical for all dependent impact or outcome variables, and independent variables.

An issue, which at times has been a common barrier to C group establishment, is that program staff may not want to withhold the new treatment methods (X1 + X2 + X3 + X ... ) from participants. This may seem to be a serious barrier at first glance; it should not be in practice. *Remember*: an evaluation is being planned to confirm intervention efficacy or effectiveness. Valid impact data from a sufficient number of completed evaluations supporting the internal validity of an existing program or new program for your population or setting may not be available. Although the standard or minimum program (X1) should be delivered to all participants, the intensity and duration of methods and materials or the frequency of program procedures can be varied to document what is most effective. The C group, the standard program (X1) can be compared to a "best practice" program (X1 + X2 + X3 + X4) among an E group, where X2 is a brief, face-to-face reinforcement, X3 is follow-up telephone counseling, and X4 is systematic family reinforcement.

An evaluation should be designed to answer important practical questions about the feasibility of delivery, impact, cost, and cost-effectiveness of an HP-DP program for a public health agency or primary care organization. How effective is the existing program, and what new, best practices methods could be feasibly applied in all practice settings that might significantly increase the current level of behavior change and improve health? *This type of evaluation may be described by some researchers as* "Comparative Effectiveness Research" (IOM, 2009).

## Random Assignment and Group Comparability

Randomization of participants into E and C groups is the best method for establishing equivalent groups for evaluation purposes and to control for the primary biases to internal validity. Multiple computer programs are readily available to generate a random assignment list for participant each site. If participants are randomly assigned as they are recruited, assignment may take a number of forms. If the numbers of participants is 100+/site, then simple random assignment at each site may be adequate to establish equivalent E and C groups, overall and at each evaluation site.

A program planner, however, may choose a stratified system of randomization to achieve greater precision. Participants are grouped at the baseline assessment into clusters by demographic characteristic predictive of the impact rate, for example, age-gender-race, with other participants with similar characteristics. If the site is used as the unit of treatment and analysis, sites can be matched into dyads by major predictors. Individuals can be randomly assigned within a site or from dyads to an E or C group. Establishing comparability of the E and C or (C) groups at baseline for predictors of an impact rate is an essential evaluation task.

Data in Table 3.6 document the comparability of the E and C group and patients lost to follow-up (LTF), E-LTF + C-LTF, in a large randomized clinical trial (SCRIPT Trial III). The aim of Trial III was to determine the effectiveness of counseling methods for pregnant smokers enrolled at 10 prenatal clinics from eight randomly selected counties in Alabama. These counties and patients were a representative sample (15%) of the annual Medicaid-supported population of Alabama.

During Trial III, over 30 months, 28 regular nursing and social work staff screened 6,514 patients at the first visit: 1,736 (26.7%) were smokers. Of the 1,736, 1,340 (77%) gave consent. After randomization at each clinic, of the 1,340 in the C or E group, 247 patients (18%) from two counties became ineligible. The Medicaid contracts were rebid in years 3 and 4, and 247 randomized patients moved to other care sites. Thus, regular staff recruited 73% (1,736–247/1,093) of eligible patients. *Analysis of the baseline characteristics, age, race, education, and parity of patients who left care confirmed no statistically significant differences on entry into care.* The data indicated that **selection bias** was very small. The data and the original random selection process to identify the eight counties provided strong evidence for the representativeness of the Trial III sample and evidence of the external validity of results to the Medicaid population of the state of Alabama.

TABLE 3.6 Baseline Comparability of Trial III Patients

| VARIABLES | C GROUP | C-LTF | E GROUP | E-LTF | SIG. |
|---|---|---|---|---|---|
| Mean Age | 22.4 yr. | 24.0 yr. | 22.2 yr. | 23.0 yr | Ns |
| Black | 15.7% | 19.6% | 15.4% | 14.7% | Ns |
| CPD | 9.8 | 10.3 | 10.4 | 12.0 | Ns |
| Lives w/Smoker | 69.8% | 75.3% | 73.7% | 66.0% | Ns |
| Mean Cotinine | 163 ng/ml | 181 ng/ml | 181 ng/ml | 178 ng/ml | Ns |
| EGA | 10.0 wk | 9.2 wk | 9.2 wk | 9.6 wk | Ns |
| | N = 449 | N = 97 | N = 452 | N = 95 | Total = 1093 |

CPD = cigarettes per day; EGA = estimated gestational age; LTF = lost to follow-up

## Case Study 1: A Group Randomized Design for School-Based Evaluation

R. Windsor, S. Middlestadt, and A. Radosh, "Evaluation of Secondary School HIV/STD Prevention Education Programs: Methodological and Design Issues to Improve the Science Base," Project Report of the Academy for Educational Development (AED), to the CDC, Division of Adolescent and School Health (CDC, DASH, 1997).

The following discussion is a synthesis of a report describing the methods used to plan and implement a group randomized clinical trial (GRCT) funded by the CDC for three cities in New Jersey. The author (Co-Principal Investigator Windsor) and contributing authors (Co-Principal Investigators Middlestad and Radosh) were colleagues at the Academy for Educational Development (AED), responsible for the CDC evaluation contract. Although middle schools were the unit of random assignment, treatment, and analysis, the methods described are applicable to any defined unit of a target group being considered by an evaluation. In this example, students in the seventh- and eighth grade classes were the unit of matching, randomization, treatment, and impact analyses.

### Introduction

A meta-evaluation of 23 published studies to determine the efficacy of school-based HIV/AIDS education programs to significantly reduce adolescent sexual behavior noted multiple, serious methodological problems. The review noted that the ability to reach definitive conclusions was limited by the few rigorous studies of individual programs, and by methodological limitation of individual studies. Additional research needs to employ more valid and statistically powerful methods. Multiple reviews during this period identified and discussed the same issues.

In 1993 the CDC funded an evaluation of a new HIV/AIDS prevention program in New Jersey: Healthy & Alive (HA). This skills-based curriculum was designed to change social norms and behaviors of seventh and eighth grade students through (1) modification of risk-related attitudes, intention, and behaviors, (2) improvement of communication and refusal skills, and (3) strengthening self-efficacy to avoid sex or to use prevention methods. It was developed for implementation at three multi-racial and multi-ethnic cities in New Jersey where sexually transmitted prevalence rates were high. The three urban school districts ranged in size from

18,829 to 32,196 students. The evaluation of HA was conducted from 1994 to 1997 as a collaborative effort of colleagues at the Academy for Education Development (AED) and the CDC.

Case material from the Healthy and Alive evaluation (1994–1997) illustrates how serious methodological problems noted in our meta-evaluation of completed studies, such as weak evaluation research designs, insufficient sample size (number of schools), and low statistical power, can be addressed. It demonstrates how stratification within school districts of multi-ethnic sites on one or two salient baseline predictor variables, and matching the sites (schools) into dyads in the same district for randomization, can be used to create very comparable E and C groups for an evaluation of the impact of an HP-DP program for students in schools.

## Evaluation Design: Controlling for Biases to Internal Validity

School-based evaluation studies need to be especially concerned about two major sources of bias: (1) selection biases caused by E versus C school/class/student differences and participation rates at baseline; and (2) selection biases caused by non-random E versus C school/class/student attrition rates at follow-up. In an evaluation where the number of units of treatment and analysis, for example, schools or clinics, available to randomize to the E group is < 10 or C group is < 10, the need to balance independent predictors of student behavior is compelling. Potential, large selection biases in a multi-school evaluation may be addressed by applying a stratified, matched GRCT.

If school-student heterogeneity within and between districts is large, as was apparent in this evaluation, simple random assignment of schools would not achieve E group and C group baseline equivalence. Stratification within each district, matching of dyads, and randomization of a large number of schools could significantly increase control over the large number of known and especially unknown independent characteristics that predict student behavior. Stratification and matching before randomization, if a sufficient number of schools are available, should substantially increase the probability of E group and C group equivalence and should increase statistical power.

Conversely, a quasi-experimental design, for example, matching only (Design #2), would introduce multiple, serious methodological problems. Matching, without randomization, particularly if the total number of units is 8–10, and only 4 or 5 E and C sites are available, will not have sufficient statistical power and will not provide sufficient control for large selection biases in participation and attrition rates. It will not create baseline equivalence for school/teachers/students. *The stratification and matching methods and group randomized design used to evaluate Healthy and Alive had not been previously used in school-based HIV/AIDS evaluation studies.*

## Stratification and Matching of Schools Within a District

The group randomized design applied in the HA evaluation is diagrammed in Table 3.7.

A major challenge in the application of the matched group randomized design in this evaluation and other school-based evaluations is having the opportunity to randomize schools. The design was presented and discussed by all key stakeholders in the leadership group, including senior CDC and AED staff, and senior representatives from the school districts. The presentation educated and convinced the school leadership in New Jersey of the serious weaknesses associated with the use of a quasi-experimental design. Fortunately, the superintendents in each city and the principals agreed to participate and have their schools randomized to an E or C Group. This decision resulted in the matching and random assignment of all 57 schools in the three cities.

In this example, school District #1, #2 and #3 were stratified into three demographically homogenous groups by the first author, using the sixth grade student census: School Group #1: majority black (> 50%), School Group #2: majority Hispanic (> 50%), and School Group #3: mixed ethnicity (> 50%) black and (< 50%) Hispanic. Schools within districts were then rank ordered within these three groups. Using the actual percent ethnicity as the first matching variable, contiguous dyads of schools were identified. Wherever possible, the sixth grade census was also used as a second matching variable in many dyads. Dyads for some schools were less similar than dyads in other districts. In District #1, with six demographically dissimilar schools, meaningful dyads could not be formed by race or ethnicity. Only class size was used to match District #1 schools. These methods produced an approximately equal number of students in the E and C group schools.

TABLE 3.7 Matching and Group Randomized Design

| GROUP | T1 | T2 | T3 | T4 | T5 |
|-------|-----|--------|-----|---------|-----|
| MR > E | O1 | X1... 12 | O2 | X13... 12 | O3 |
| MR > C | O1 | | O2 | | O3 |

T = Years; M = Matching; R = Randomization; O = Observation-survey
X1... 12 = 12 Sessions > 7th Grade + X13... 24 = 12 Sessions > 8th Grade

Three dyads for six schools were created in District #1. Six dyads plus one extra school were created in District #2 with 13 schools, and 19 dyads were created in District #3 with 38 schools. One school in each dyad was randomly assigned to the E group or to the C group. The final number was 29 E group schools with 1,573 students and 28 C group schools with 1,345 students.

## Measurement

In the fall of 1994, all seventh and eighth grade students at the 57 schools were assessed by a standardized, written, self-administered survey form adapted from the Youth Risk Behavior Survey (YRBS) developed by the CDC's Division of Adolescent and School Health (DASH). An 88% response rate was documented. School/students were surveyed again in the spring of 1995 and spring of 1996. Although 57 schools were matched and randomly assigned, 46 schools (25 E and 21 C group schools) completed the baseline assessment. Four E group schools and seven C group schools withdrew in the summer of 1995 after the baseline survey. Teachers were not available to be trained to deliver the curriculum, and/or staff were not available to conduct student follow-up surveys.

*Note*: This substantial, adverse historical event, the loss of 11 schools, produced significant selection biases to the final HA impact analysis and results. It compromised the statistical power of the evaluation and compromised the final results. Neither the CDC nor AED had any control over the loss of schools. No resources were available to modify the design and select new school districts, or to add at least 10–12 replacement schools. The following discussion, however, confirms that the methods to plan the GRCT were very successful in creating equivalent E and C groups of schools.

## E and C Group Baseline Comparability

The first steps in the evaluation after baseline measurement were to document E versus C group baseline comparability. Data presented in Tables 3.7, 3.8, and 3.9, confirm E and C group equivalence for multiple demographic, psychosocial, and behavioral predictors of future adolescent sexual behavior. The difference in sample size (200+) between the E and C group was attributable to having one more E group school. Data in Tables 3.7, 3.8, and 3.9, confirmed that stratification, matching, and the random assignment process were very successful. As indicated in Table 3.10, the only variable for which there was a significant baseline

TABLE 3.8  E and C Group Baseline Demographic Characteristics*

| STUDENT CHARACTERISTICS | E (1,573) | C (1,345) |
|---|---|---|
| Age: 11 | 5% | 6% |
| 12 | 54% | 54% |
| 13 | 30% | 29% |
| 14 or Older | 11% | 10% |
| Gender: Male | 51% | 53% |
| Female | 49% | 47% |
| Race/Ethnicity: Black Non-Hispanic | 50% | 49% |
| Hispanic | 30% | 32% |
| White-Non-Hispanic | 9% | 10% |
| Asian/Pacific Islander | 3% | 3% |
| Education: Mother—H.S. Graduate | 86% | 86% |
| Father—H.S. Graduate | 90% | 91% |
| Usual Grades—As & Bs | 31% | 31% |
| Language home—English only | 53% | 53% |

* 57 Schools + 88% Student response rate.

TABLE 3.9  E + C Group Baseline Psycho-Social Characteristics

| CHARACTERISTICS* | SCALE RANGE | CRONBACH ALPHA | SCALE MEANS | |
|---|---|---|---|---|
| | | | E GROUP | C GROUP |
| STD/Condom Knowledge | 0–8 | 0.54 | 2.6 | 2.4 |
| Sexual Beliefs: Peer | 0–6 | 0.65 | 4.4 | 4.4 |
| Sexual Beliefs: Personal | 0–6 | 0.63 | 5.2 | 5.1 |
| Beliefs: Combined | 0–12 | 0.75 | 9.6 | 9.5 |
| Adolescent-Adult Communication | 0–10 | 0.82 | 3.9 | 4.0 |
| Condom Use: Self-Efficacy | 0–11 | 0.75 | 6.2 | 6.2 |
| General Self-Efficacy | 0–16 | 0.86 | 11.6 | 11.6 |

* Standardized CDC Instrument and Scale

difference was the percent of adolescents who reported having sex in the last three months. This difference was primarily caused by the very diverse demographic characteristics of the six middle schools and students in District #1.

*A post-hoc application of alternative assignment methods was conducted, using five demographic and three behavioral variables from baseline data. Six assignment options were applied. Two completely unstratified and unmatched samples of schools were also randomly selected. The stratification, matching, and random assignment process used in the study was the most successful method to control for potential selection biases.*

TABLE 3.10  E and C Group Baseline Behavioral
Characteristics

| BEHAVIORAL CHARACTERISTICS | E GROUP | C GROUP |
|---|---|---|
| Ever had sex | 397 (26%) | 348 (27%) |
| Sex first time: 10 or younger | 131 (36%) | 115 (34%) |
| Used condom: first sex | 206 (55%) | 185 (55%) |
| Always used condom | 225 (62%) | 197 (62%) |
| Used condom last sex | 141 (40%) | 133 (41%) |
| Used condom and pill, last sex | 67 (19%) | 62 (19%) |
| Had sex: past 3 months | 194 (52%)* | 189 (57%)* |
| Number of partners: 1 | 80 (45%) | 78 (44%) |
| 2 | 34 (19%) | 48 (27%) |
| 3 | 17 (10%) | 19 (11%) |
| > 4 | 47 (26%) | 32 (18%) |

* Significant at the 0.05 level

## Statistical Power

Meta-evaluations of school-based intervention programs cited in the introduction of this case study indicated that the issues of statistical power and sample size estimation were rarely addressed by previous evaluation research. Most school-based HIV/STD intervention studies prior to and during this period had failed to have an adequate number of equivalent units, and had inadequate power for an impact analysis. The stratification, matching, and randomization of the 57 schools were designed to reduce the variance among schools and increase power. Thus, the number of schools ($N = 57$) was perceived by the CDC and the evaluation team to be adequate for year 3 impact analyses.

This case study illustrated the complexity of using the school as the unit of randomization, treatment, and impact analysis. It described one successful example of a process to establish equivalent units and how to increase the internal validity of results from a school-based evaluation of an HP-DP program. Murray (1998) in *Design and Analysis of Group Randomized Trials.* provides a comprehensive discussion of the methods and analytical issues discussed in this section.

## Determining the Sample Size for the E and C Groups

*One of the most frequently asked questions in planning an evaluation is probably this: How many participants should be in the C or (C) and E groups?*

The next section presents a discussion of methods that all evaluations need to apply: how to estimate the group sample sizes. As noted in previous discussions of meta-evaluations, evaluation design, and validity of measurement, the adequacy of sample size–statistical power is one of the three fundamental issues that an evaluation must address. The sample size and minimum number of participants or sites/units to be recruited in each group must be estimated in all evaluation plans and/or proposals to funding agencies.

Knowledge of what the sample size needs to be for the E and C groups is necessary to ensure sufficient statistical power in data analysis and interpretation. It is also essential to determine how long the evaluation will take, to estimate staffing needs, and to define how many participants or sites (minimum number) will be needed by the evaluation. This information is critical to prepare a budget describing how much it will cost to conduct the HP-DP program evaluation and to prepare a time/task-line for implementation. Grant proposals to conduct impact evaluations to almost all agencies require a detailed discussion and justification of sample size and statistical power. A meta-evaluation will define the level and range of behavioral impact of completed evaluation studies. A meta-evaluation and a formative evaluation (Design #1) are essential to provide sufficient empirical data and information to document current levels of behavior and to estimate effect sizes and sample size needs from each and all evaluation sites.

Two types of error need to be considered in planning an evaluation: Type I and Type II.

*A Type I error is the probability of rejecting a null hypothesis (H0) when it is true, and a Type II error is accepting the hypothesis when it is false.* A null hypothesis is a statement of no significant differences between the E and C groups. Because the objective of a program is to have a significant impact (**reject the $H_0$**), large enough E and C groups at follow-up need to be established to control for Type 1 and 2 errors. Regardless of the total number in each group, the sample size and number of sites of each study group should also be approximately the same.

Four statistics must be available to estimate the most efficient sample size for E and C group comparisons. An accepted convention for statistical significance to be used by a PHASE 1 and 2 Evaluation is $\mu = 0.05$ with a two-tailed test. *Note*: The primary aims of a PHASE 3 and 4 Evaluation is to document the level of delivery and acceptability by regular staff and clients of the program and to document effect size/level of behavioral impact. *In a PHASE 3 and 4 Evaluation, a one-tailed test may be used to test statistical significance and to estimate sample size. The use of a one-tailed test may be justified, if there are no safety or harm concerns. This decision also has a practical value. It reduces the number of sites and total sample size needed for each evaluation study group (E + C) and reduces the time and cost of the evaluation.*

Having specified the $\mu$ level, selecting a "Power" level is required. A power = 0.80 is an accepted standard for behavioral impact evaluations (Cohen & Cohen, 1975; Fleiss, 1981). In a health outcome evaluation, where the level of potential harm or risks associated with an evaluation of treatment methods may be higher, a higher level of Power = 0.90 and alpha = 0.01 is often selected. These levels will substantially increase (two to three times) the sample size of each evaluation.

Expected behavioral impact levels need to be estimated for the C and E groups. An ME or MA and a rigorous formative evaluation (Design #1) will help to define the current base rate of change. An estimate of the current level of program (X1) impact (effect size; ES) being produced is essential. The process of estimating ES is described in the following example. A meta-evaluation and formative evaluation may indicate that the cessation rate ($P_1$ = Probability of Effect) annually for one year among pregnant smokers receiving care and routine counseling (X1) at your 10 primary care clinics is 5%: P1 = 0.05. The methods described in the Design #1 example need to be used by *all* HP-DP programs to document a $P_1$. Valid and representative data of the target population behavior from all evaluation sites are essential to compute sample size.

A formative evaluation and meta-evaluation would confirm that a reasonable expectation of impact for a "best practices" program (X1 + X2 + X3 + X4) for pregnant smokers in a primary care setting at a third trimester follow-up is a 15% cessation rate: P2 = 0.15. With these four parameters, $\mu = 0.05$, Power = 0.80, P1= 0.05, P2 = 0.15, a standard sample size table can be used to estimate how many participants an evaluation must have in both E and C groups at O1 and O2 to test the significance of a difference in rates. If the difference in impact was 5%, the sample size for each group at follow-up would need to be 474 per E and C groups. The Epi-Info, statcalc module: sample size and Power, a free web service of the CDC (cdc.gov), or a hand calculator can be used to estimate samples sizes/group. Using the four parameters, standard statistical formulae are available to estimate sample sizes for a comparison of impact rates.

Data presented in Table 3.11 for a two-tailed test of proportions specify the sample sizes needed for an E and C group for alpha/$\mu$, power = 0.80, P1, and P2 statistics. Using the statistics from the cessation example, data in Table 3.11 indicate that the program would need

TABLE 3.11 Sample Size Per Group: Two-Tailed Test

| P 2 | P1 = 0.05 = C GROUP RATE | |
| --- | --- | --- |
| | POWER | |
| | 0.90 | 0.80 |
| 0.10 | | |
| 0.01 | 760 | 686 |
| 0.05 | 621 | 474 |
| **E Group Rate = 0.15** | | |
| 0.01 | 285 | 228 |
| 0.05 | 207 | 160 |
| 0.20 | | |
| 0.01 | 155 | 125 |
| 0.05 | 113 | 88 |

160 participants *per group* at follow-up (O2) to confirm as statistically different the hypothesized difference between P1 (C group) and P2 (E group). These data refute the common statement: > 100 per group is an adequate number. There is no chance of finding a statistically significant E versus C group difference with sample sizes of N = 100 each, when P1 = 0.05 and P2 = 0.15.

It is also critical to note that the sample size and power estimates are based on the number of follow-up observations (O2) for each sample of E + C group participants. Thus, it is prudent to randomize an extra 15% or 20% per group to ensure an adequate number of O2 or O3 observations. For example, an evaluation with a P1 = 0.05 and P2 = 0.15 should randomize > 380 participants. This method also defines how many participants need to be recruited each week-month-year at each evaluation site. These are essential data to prepare a time- and task-line and evaluation budget. The methods presented in this section represent critical methods that must be applied in future evaluations to improve the quality of the HP-DP science and practice base.

## Sample Size Estimates for Group Randomized Design

The information needed for a sample size calculation for group random-ized trials (GRT) is similar to that needed for a randomized clinical trial (RCT). A GRCT may be more appropriate than an RCT, because the E group program has to be implemented at a group level (e.g., health educa-tion for all students in a school, or adult patients in a primary care clinic), or the behavioral impact or health outcome is confirmed at the group level, for example, reduction in infant morbidity or mortality cases in villages. As noted in the Healthy and Alive evaluation, in a GRCT the unit of analysis, treatment, and randomization is by group, or cluster, of participants: students in schools, a specific cohort of patients in hospitals, users at healthcare practice site, or adults in communities. Baseline observations are made on all eligible individuals in a group at each evaluation site.

Some advantages of GRT are that, unlike the RCT, one need not enumerate the entire study population in advance, but just groups to be randomized. Within-group interaction exposure and "treatment contamination" biases are minimized: the GRCT may be more economical. The trade-off is that elements in the same group are expected to be more similar to one another (within-group homogeneity), which causes higher variance–standard errors. The individual elements, when groups are the unit of analysis, violate the assumption of independence. This must be accounted for in sample size calculations and analysis of a GRCT.

The intra-class correlation coefficient (ICC), called *rho*, or $\rho$, is a measure of the association among units within a group and varies from 0 to 1. If $\rho = 0$, then there is no correlation within cluster elements. This is equivalent to independence, and is observed through simple random sampling. If $\rho = 1$, then there is perfect positive correlation among group elements. For almost all impact rates, there is some degree of correlation: *rho* typically varies between 0.01 and 0.04. Quantifying the ICC is a standard practice in GRCT. Estimates are essential for the most accurate sample size estimation. ICCs tend to be larger for smaller clusters, for example, $0.05 > 0.12$ for spouse pairs, $0.0016 > 0.0126$ for MD practices, and $0.0005 > 0.0085$ for counties (Murray et al., 2004).

As *rho* increases, the number of groups/sample size increases. More groups with fewer members will have much greater power than a few sites with a large number of eligible participants. For GRCT, sample size estimates and power analyses utilize similar information needed for an RCT, with the addition of the ICC (Friedman et al., 1998) to adjust the sample size estimate from an RCT to reflect the magnitude of the ICC. Evaluators may also use, as an alternative, the coefficient of variation, k, (SD/mean) of the true rates (proportions or means) within each group.

An additional factor to consider is the use of pair-matched groups to improve the baseline comparability of groups that may be compromised from randomization of a relatively smaller number of groups, rather than a larger number of individuals, as in an RCT. Other assumptions for sample size estimation are **a** level, typically 0.05, and Power (1-b) = 80% or greater, to examine the a priori specified two-tailed test differences between groups. If determining sample size and selecting analysis methods are especially complex, for example, a group randomized design, statistical consultation should be sought.

## Determining Sample Size for Pair-matched GRCT Using a Coefficient of Variation

A GRCT is presented in this chapter describing an evaluation of the effectiveness of a health education–community participatory intervention on infant birth outcomes in Nepal (Manandhar et al., *Lancet*, 2004). This evaluation had estimates of *rho* for neonatal mortality and *km*, the cluster coefficient of variation for the expected neonatal mortality rate. It utilized the *km* to estimate the minimum number of clusters needed to achieve a reduction in neonatal death rate of > 25%. There were 43 eligible districts, and to minimize contamination, the investigators created 21 pair-matched districts based on similarities of topography, ethnicity, and population density. One district in each pair was randomly allocated to the E or C group.

Mortality data were not available at the group level so the expected neonatal mortality of the country, 60 per 1,000 live births, was used to estimate outcome levels. A 25% reduction provides an expected neonatal mortality in the intervention groups to 37– 44 per 1,000 live births. The coefficient of variation was estimated to range from 0.15–0.30 between clusters with matched-pairs. Approximately 300 births over the study period were expected per cluster. If 80% power was required ($z = 0.84$) for a significant difference at $p < .05$ ($z = 1.95$) then the number of pairs, c, required in the intervention and control arm was estimated by:

$$c = 2 + (1.96 + 0.84)^2 \left[ \left( (0.06 * 0.94) / 300 \right) + \left( (0.044 * 0.956) / 300 \right) \right.$$
$$\left. + 0.15^2 \left( 0.06^2 + 0.044^2 \right) \right] / (.044 - 0.06)^2$$

c = 12 cluster pairs, or 24 of the eligible cluster were selected.

Ignoring clustering and applying the standard sample size calculation equation with the same parameters, the study required > 3,500 pregnancies/year: the number observed in the Nepal evaluation.

# Evaluation Design Case Studies: Translating Population Health Science to HP-DP Practice

Detailed discussions from seven case studies are presented to illustrate the strengths and weaknesses and the validity of evaluation results for Designs #1, #2, #3, and #4. They have been selected because they are part of the published literature and represent evaluations of different interventions for different problems, populations, and HP-DP program delivery settings, for example, schools, worksites, communities, or health clinic settings.

## Case Study 2: A One Group Pre-Test + Post-Test Design for a Public Health Policy

J. Pearson, R. Windsor, A. El-Mohandes, and D. Perry, "A Formative Evaluation of the Immediate Impact of the Washington, D.C. Smoke-Free Indoor Air Policy on Bar Employee ETS Exposure," *Public Health Reports* (August 2009) (see publication for references).

### Introduction

According to the 2006 Surgeon General's report, even small levels of environmental tobacco smoke (ETS) exposure produce increased risks of coronary heart disease, lung cancer, stroke, and respiratory symptoms. Over the last decade, a large number of communities, states, and countries have passed smoking bans in restaurants and bars to protect employees. Impact evaluations of these laws have consistently reported significant reductions of ETS and improvements in employee health. In April 2006, the Washington, D.C., City Council passed a Smoke-Free Indoor Air Law. On January 2, 2007, the indoor smoking ban was initiated in bars, restaurants, and pool halls. *The passage of this new law presented a unique opportunity to evaluate its immediate impact. This formative evaluation tested the hypothesis that the law significantly reduced cotinine-confirmed levels of ETS exposure by bartenders > 50%.*

### Methods

#### Study Population Selection

This evaluation focused only on workers in establishments defined by the D.C. Official Code as a "club," "brew pub," "nightclub," or "tavern." In May 2005 a Yellow Pages search with these descriptors identified 273 sites, and 1,950 bartenders. We excluded 11 bars that had enforced restricted smoking policies prior to the ban, or that were exempt. One hundred eighty-four (71%) of the 262 eligible sites from six high-density areas where adult customers congregated seven days a week were selected. Because of time and resource restraints, we could not include 78 small neighborhood bars distributed throughout the city. Using a Power = 0.80, alpha = 0.05, a one-tailed test, and effect size of > 50% in cotinine levels based on employee ETS research, we needed ≥ 35 sites/employee pre-ban and post-ban assessments. We randomly selected 41 bars.

### Site and Employee Recruitment

Letters were sent and calls made to the randomly selected sites to describe the study and to seek permission of managers to approach employees. These were ineffective. We then trained 12 volunteer staff (MPH students) to approach managers from December 2 to December 21, 2006, to seek permission to conduct the study and recruit employees prior to the ban (O1). Participants had to be (1) a nonsmoker, (2) not using other forms of tobacco, (3) did not live with a smoker, or the smoker did not smoke indoors, and (4) employed > 20 hours/week at the site.

Fifty-two (78%) employees identified themselves as bartenders. Other staff categories, 6 servers, 3 barbacks, 3 managers, one owner, and one host, were recruited who met all screening criteria and served customers. After consent, staff collected baseline information, saliva samples, ETS exposure, and respiratory and sensory symptom reports, and attitudes on the ban (O1). Employee assessment procedures (O2) were replicated from February 1 to February 21, 2007, after the ban.

### Impact Measurement: Salivary Cotinine

Our primary impact measure was employee cotinine levels: the major proximal metabolite of nicotine present in a person's body fluids. A cotinine half-life of 18 hours makes it a valid measure for ETS exposure. This study used a recommended < 10 ng/mL cutoff for nonsmoking self-reports. Saliva samples were collected using a Salivette sample vial and frozen < 3 hours. In < 7 days after assessment, samples were thawed, centrifuged and shipped in dry ice to the Pharmacology Laboratory at San Francisco General Hospital/Univeristy of California, San Francisco, for analysis. Saliva cotinine was measured using tandem liquid chromatography–mass spectrometry (LC-MS/MS). This analysis has a minimum detectable level = 0.05 ng/mL, is the most sensitive type of cotinine measurement, and has "excellent" specificity.

### Self-reported Symptoms

After screening, a questionnaire elicited descriptive information, respiratory and sensory symptoms, and smoking ban attitudes. Respiratory symptoms questions in the past four weeks were from a validated form used in comparable hospitality-bar employee assessment studies: International Union Against Tuberculosis and Lung Disease (IUATLD) Bronchial Symptoms Questionnaire.

### Statistical Analysis

Analyses of changes were restricted to employees with O1 and O2 assessments, who were cotinine-confirmed nonsmokers, and were employed at the same bar during both collection periods. Salivary cotinine levels and symptom data were analyzed by computing O1 and O2 difference. Respiratory and sensory symptoms were analyzed by change in the number of symptoms. Analyses were completed with the SAS System 8.02.

### Results

Of the 102 employees approached at the 41 bars, one did not understand enough English to give consent. One worked in a bar with ETS restrictions. Of the 100 remaining, 17 (17%) were smokers: 17 nonsmoking employees (17%) refused to participate. Between December 2, 2006, and December 21, 2006, staff recruited 66 eligible employees who had worked at least two hours at the time (> 8:00 p.m.) of baseline data collection. Of the 66 assessed, 16 were not eligible for follow-up. Two reported smoking, and 14 were ineligible due to a change of job (6), bar closing (6), bar exemption (1), or death (1). This left 50 eligible participants. Only three eligible participants were lost to follow-up, unreachable at work or by phone. Only one employee refused the O2 assessment. Thus, follow-up data were collected on 46 of 50 (94%) eligible employees

### Analyses

Two employee samples at O2 were below levels of laboratory quantification. We imputed O2 cotinine levels to be 0.05 ng/mL. Six samples did not have sufficient volume for analysis at either O1 or O2. We imputed their cotinine values, assuming, conservatively, no O1 or O2 changes.

TABLE 3.12 ETS Exposure at Baseline and Follow-up of Bar Employees

| MEASUREMENT | BASELINE MEAN | FOLLOW-UP MEAN | P VALUE | DIFFERENCE |
|---|---|---|---|---|
| Saliva Cotinine | 2.37 ng/mL | 0.49 ng/mL | < 0.0001 | < 79.3% |
| # hrs at work: < week | 35 (25–40 hr.) | 35 (25–50 hr.) | 0.43 | n/a |
| # hrs ETS work: <week | 30 (18–40 hr.) | 0 (0–1 hr.) | < 0.0010 | < 100% |

**Cotinine levels**: As noted in Table 3.12, the cotinine levels of the 46 employees declined significantly, by 79.3%: O1 = 2.37 ng/mL and O2 = 0.49 ng/mL.

**Self-reported ETS levels:** As noted in Table 3.12, the number of hours reported working did not change significantly between O1 and O2, nor did reported hours of ETS exposure outside of work. The hours exposed to ETS at work declined from a median of 30hr/wk at O1 to 0hr/wk at O2.

## Discussion: Main Findings

This evaluation documented that the smoking ban in Washington, D.C., eliminated hospitality employees' reports of exposure to ETS at work. Follow-up salivary cotinine levels dropped by 79%, confirming employee ETS exposure reports. Respiratory and sensory symptoms were reduced by 83%. Attitudes toward the law, 9.0 at O1 and 10 at O2, did not significantly change.

## Comparison With Other ETS studies

Six studies, including two in the United States, evaluated the impact of bans on hospitality employees' exposure to ETS. Table 3.13 presents

TABLE 3.13 Cotinine-Confirmed Employee ETS Exposure Studies

| FIRST AUTHOR, SITE, YEAR CITED | N | COTININE TEST | $O_1$ NG/ML | $O_2$ NG/ML | DIFFERENCE (%) |
|---|---|---|---|---|---|
| Allwright et al., Ireland, 1998 | 158 | Saliva | 5.10 | 0.90 | < 82.3% |
| Farrelly et al., US, 2005 | 104 | Saliva | 3.60 | 0.80 | < 77.8% |
| Mulcahy et al., Ireland, 2005 | 35 | Saliva | 1.60 | 0.50 | < 68.8% |
| Abrams et al., US, 2006 | 107 | Urine | 4.93 | 0.30 | < 93.9% |
| Menzies et al., Scotland, 2006 | 105 | Serum | 5.15 | 2.93 | < 43.1% |
| Goodman et al., Ireland, 2007 | 65 | Saliva | 5.10 | 0.60 | < 81.0% |
| Pearson et al., US, 2007 | 46 | Saliva | 2.37 | 0.49 | < 79.3% |

a comparison *only* of the cotinine results of the six studies and the current study. All evaluations documented large, significant decreases in cotinine-confirmed self-reported ETS exposure levels. The average decrease in cotinine levels of the 620 employees from the seven studies was 77%: 4.41 ng/mL to 1.02 ng/mL. These data, and other employee ETS studies, confirmed the hypothesis: indoor air laws eliminate employee ETS exposure at work.

### Discussion of Internal and External Validity of Results

This evaluation used a one-group pre-ban and post-ban design (Design #1) with the subjects as their own controls. This design has three major threats to the internal validity of results: *measurement bias, selection bias, and historical bias.* Each bias was examined to determine if it and not the ETS law was a plausible explanation of reported results. These methodological issues and biases had not been adequately discussed in previous employee ETS evaluation reports.

In this study we used standardized laboratory methods to independently document employee baseline and follow-up cotinine levels and ETS exposure. We used the most highly recognized reference laboratories in the United States and the most sensitive method of measuring cotinine, tandem HPLC-mass spectrometry, to document employee ETS exposure. When we did not have an employee O1 or O2, we imputed a value of no change between O1 and O2. There was no inter-site variability in reported ETS exposure: employees reported 100% reduction in ETS exposure at O2. The magnitude of the observed impact on cotinine levels was consistent with other studies that used cotinine measures to evaluate ETS exposure.

We used a validated instrument used by multiple employee ETS exposure studies to assess respiratory and sensory reports. While the IUTALD instrument has confirmed validity, because employees could not be blinded to the aim of the city-wide ban and evaluation, the respiratory and sensory reports in this study (and results of all other studies), may have, in part, reflected socially desirable employee responses. *We concluded that the significant changes in employee ETS exposure and cotinine values were not attributable to measurement bias.*

Although our sampling frame of 184 sites included 71% of eligible sites, 78 smaller, older bars distributed in neighborhoods in the city were not included in the sampling and random selection of sites. If we had randomly sampled 20% of these sites, it would have added 16 sites/employees to the study. While the methodology applied suggested some degree of selection bias, an ETS study by Repace (2004) at a gambling casino in Delaware and the Surgeon General's Report (2006), however, documented that larger bars with more open space have significantly lower ETS concentrations of breathable particles and carcinogens than smaller bars. The majority of sites randomly selected in the evaluation were new, or recently renovated, large-capacity bars with high volumes of people in each area. Completed ETS research on bar size, ventilation, and structure suggested that if we had included a random sample of >15 neighborhood bars, employee reports of ETS exposure and baseline cotinine levels at these sites may have been higher than the levels documented. *Thus, exclusion of the smaller neighborhood sites may have produced a small underestimate of employee baseline saliva cotinine levels and reports of ETS exposure at work.*

Another strength of the study was that it defined the population of sites for a specific geographical area, and used a random selection process. The two studies conducted in the United States that used cotinine analyses to document bar employee ETS exposure, Farrelly et al., 2005 and Abrams et al., 2006 used posters, newspapers, and so on. Our random selection and sampling of sites, combined with the documentation of high employee baseline (82%) and follow-up rates (94%), enhanced the city-wide generalization of the results. *Selection bias was an implausible explanation of the results.*

The very short time span between the O1 assessments in December, implementation of the law in January, and O2 assessments in February, makes it very unlikely that an independent, external, city-wide public health or policy intervention (**historical biases**) may have influenced the validity of results. There were no other legislative actions or public health campaigns to eliminate employee ETS exposure in Washington, D.C., Maryland, or Virginia during the evaluation periods or calendar years 2006 and 2007. Because all assessments were conducted during the late fall and early winter months, and none of the bars had open areas during this period, *we concluded that seasonal variation in exposure was not an explanation for the impact documented.*

We *concluded that the ETS law and policy banning smoking in D.C. bars were the only plausible explanations for the significant positive changes in employee ETS exposure and cotinine levels.* Our methods and results should be useful to city councils, and public health law/policymakers in any defined geographic area that have yet to go smoke-free. Because of the random selection and high levels of participation of bars and bartenders, excellent measurement, and because the ban was city-wide, we concluded that the results had high internal and external validity. We concluded that the results were generalizable to Washington, D.C., bars/restaurants.

Although it would incur considerably higher costs, because the stability of baseline and follow-up impact rates have not been typically confirmed by previous evaluations, we recommend at least two employee pre-ban employee exposure and impact assessments at 6 months (O1) and 3 or 1 month (O2), and two post-ban assessments at 1 or 3 months (O3) and 12 months (O4). Future studies should also consider including site air monitoring of breathable and carcinogenic particles, air quality levels, LC-MS/MS saliva or urine cotinine analyses and appropriate pulmonary assessments. These methods will produce the most comprehensive and valid evidence of the immediate and long-term impact of a new ETS law on employee exposure and respiratory health.

## Case Study 3: A Non-Randomized Comparison (C) Group Design for a State-Wide Program

R. Clark Windsor, J. Cleary, et al., "Evaluation of the Effectiveness of AHRQ Recommended Practice Guidelines and the Smoking Cessation and Reduction In Pregnancy Treatment (SCRIPT) Program: A Science to Primary Care Practice Partnership," *Maternal and Child Health Journal* (2013) (see publication for references).

### Introduction

The IOM Report, *Crossing the Quality Chasm: A New Health System for the 21st Century*, indicated that achieving our National Objectives demands elimination of the gap between usual practice and "evidence-based practice." Although the need to disseminate evidenced-based methods by providers to pregnant smokers is established, limited evidence is available about the effectiveness of **Smoking Cessation and Reduction In Pregnancy Treatment (SCRIPT)** methods in state-wide systems of care. Only one evaluation of Tobacco Treatment Guidelines and SCRIPT methods delivered by regular staff to a large, representative sample of Medicaid-supported pregnant smokers in Alabama has been reported by Windsor et al. (2011). *This report presents the methods and results of the WV Right From The Start-SCRIPT Dissemination Project.*

### The West Virginia (WV) Right From The Start (RFTS) Program

The RFTS Program, based on ACOG Guidelines, was established in 1990 in the Office of Maternal, Child and Family Health (OMCFH), West

Virginia Bureau for Public Health. It is managed by the Perinatal Programs Director (J. Clark) and eight regional care coordinators (RCC), all nurses. After being informed of availability from their physician, clients who want to enroll in RFTS are contacted by a designated care coordinator (DCC) to schedule a home visit. After a 60 minute screening visit, follow-up visits are tailored to client risk and need. DCCs, RNs, and LSWs at 50 agencies provide RFTS care in all 55 West Virginia counties. Since 2004, the RFTS policy has been that each smoking client is assessed by a carbon monoxide (CO) monitor and counseled by her DCC.

In 2004–2005, in response to a high smoking rate among pregnant women in West Virginia (45%), program and practice leadership of the OMCFH and tobacco treatment and evaluation specialists at George Washington University established a partnership. The RFTS-SCRIPT Dissemination Project was created to address challenges in the Blueprint to Improve West Virginia Perinatal Health Report. The Dissemination Project was designed to achieve two aims: (1) to conduct a Process Evaluation to document DCC delivery of the SCRIPT Program and the RFTS-SCRIPT Adoption rate; and (2) to conduct a SCRIPT Effectiveness Evaluation.

## The SCRIPT Program

Meta-analysis of five SCRIPT evaluations of 2,700 Medicaid patients with biochemically confirmed self- reports combined with five SCRIPT evaluations of 1,800 patients from Australia, Canada, Norway, South Africa, and Sweden and the AHRQ meta-analyses, documented the SCRIPT effectiveness. The SCRIPT Program includes (1) assessment and biochemical confirmation of self-reports at the first visit and once during care; (2) a tailored Patient Manual with a fifth to sixth grade reading level, "A Pregnant Women's Guide to Quit Smoking"; (3) a tailored, 8-minute counseling video "Commit to Quit: During and After Pregnancy"; (4) a trained provider delivering SCRIPT methods during a regular prenatal visit and systematic reinforcement by all providers; (5) promotion of telephone/QUITLINE counseling sessions; and (6) encouragement of a nonsmoking home policy and partner/social support to reinforce quit attempts and cessation.

## The SCRIPT Dissemination Project

The lack of DCC cessation training, limited RFTS evaluation expertise, and inadequate staff/resources prevented RFTS from fully implementing SCRIPT in 2006–2008. The SCRIPT Dissemination Project was implemented in two Phases. In Phase 1, October 2007 to December 2008, we (1) expanded the

Dissemination Committee to include two DCCs and a Hospital Association, Tobacco Quit-line, Perinatal Advisory Committee, and March of Dimes representative; (2) improved the RFTS evaluation infrastructure; (3) prepared a SCRIPT Counseling Guidelines and Procedures Manual to standardize delivery by DCCs; and (4) introduced a DCC training program to increase knowledge, skills, and comfort in SCRIPT implementation.

During Phase 2, January 2009 to December 2010, we (1) introduced new client assessment Forms to document the baseline visit, SCRIPT visit, and follow-up visit Procedures ("Appendix": TeleForms); (2) provided DCCs with a "SCRIPT Tool Kit" with client materials, TeleForms, and a CO monitor; (3) implemented a standardized SCRIPT Process Evaluation to document the fidelity of DCC delivery; and (4) conducted an Effectiveness Evaluation.

## Methods

### DCC Performance Metrics and Process Evaluation Methods

Seven SCRIPT Procedures (Pn) delivered by each DCC were documented by a Process Evaluation Model using standardized Teleforms. DCC performance data were aggregated to compute an annual **RFTS-SCRIPT Program Implementation Index** (PII). A PII = 100% confirms that all DCC clients received SCRIPT Program Procedures (P1–P7). During Phase 1, the SCRIPT Program, and O1 and O2, assessments were inconsistently implemented by DCCs in all Regions.

A SCRIPT PII = 80% was the consensus implementation performance metric selected by the Dissemination Committee to reflect a very good level of RFTS success. Client behaviors in scheduling, changing, and missing appointments were barriers to DCCs and RFTS achieving a higher performance level. During Phase 1, DCCs received SCRIPT training. During Phase 2, new DCCs were trained using comparable methods, and retraining programs were available. DCCs in 2009–2010 with low levels of fidelity, a PII < 80%, were sent a performance report as part of the RFTS-SCRIPT Quality Improvement process. The DCC, her RCC, vand primary care agency supervisor were informed that a consultation and retraining were required < 30 days.

### Client Assessment Methods

In 2004, RFTS policy stipulated that DCCs should assess tobacco use at the screening and follow-up home visits by self-report, number of cigarettes smoked per day (CDP), and exhaled CO using a monitor. Although client questions remained the same, inconsistencies in SCRIPT implementation in

2006–2008 warranted modification of RFTS policies to require new tobacco assessment TeleForms at screening, the SCRIPT visit (14 days), and follow-up assessments at 30–60 days screening. The new policies and three TeleForms were pilot tested in 2008 and implemented state-wide on January 1, 2009.

Exhaled CO documented client cessation or significant reduction (SR), because non-disclosure rates of 25% have been confirmed among Medicaid patients at the first visit. SR was defined as 50% reduction from a O1 CO, with a minimum CO > 10 ppm. Data were collected using a dual client tracking system. Teleforms were faxed and de-identified at George Washington University using Teleform software. These data were concurrently entered into a RFTS database.

### Effectiveness Evaluation Methods

The SCRIPT evaluation encountered several barriers to implementing an experimental design, using the DCC as the unit of randomization and treatment. This evaluation had to address the reality of annual variations within and between eight RFTS Regions, and DCC staff turnover. Several agencies terminated RFTS participation, and the annual DCC turnover rates were 5%–20%. Because the RFTS population was homogeneous, self-reported prevalence was stable, and we had CO confirmation of smoking status from 2006–2010, a quasi-experimental design was selected for the evaluation. *In the application of a quasi-experimental design, measurement, selection, and historical biases are three major sources of bias to internal validity of results.*

The following is a description of how we implemented a **non-randomized, matched comparison (C) group design** to address salient sources of bias, especially client selection bias. All RFTS clients who reported smoking at screening, and were > 18 years old, and < 32 weeks estimated gestational age (EGA) were eligible for the evaluation. In 2009–2010, 1,303 clients met these criteria. However, because RFTS participation is voluntary, the program is home-based, and the population is transient, 622 of the smokers (48%) declined SCRIPT at screening. And 285 (22%) changed their mind about participation before the SCRIPT visit. *Only 21% (n = 273) of RFTS smokers in 2009–2010 who wanted to quit and provided CO at screening received a SCRIPT visit. A detailed discussion of why this low level of participation occurred is presented in the 'discussion section.*

The SCRIPT experimental (E) group consisted of the 259 clients in 2009–2010 who had a valid CO at screening, wanted to quit, and received a SCRIPT home visit. We divided the 259 E group clients into 10 strata, using a screening CO as the first step in the application of the quasi-experimental design. The RFTS matched historical comparison (C) group was derived from the 688 clients, 295 in 2006 and 393 in 2007, who met the same eligibility criteria, had the same CO assessment methods as E group clients, and who reported receiving smoking counseling at follow-up. The 688 were stratified by baseline CO into the same 10 matched strata as E group clients. We randomly selected the number of (C) group clients equal to the number of E group clients in each of the 10 strata. (C) and E group clients were matched on a baseline CO value, because it is the strongest predictor of smoking behavior during pregnancy. This methodology produced equal-sized, CO-matched smokers in the (C) group (2006–2007) and E group (2009–2010).

## Results

### Process Evaluation Results

A process evaluation of DCC implementation of the seven core SCRIPT procedures documented a modest state-wide improvement in the delivery of the SCRIPT Program. The SCRIPT Program Implementation Index (PII) improved from a PII = 65% in 2006 to PII = 76% in 2010. Since RFTS is a home-based program, and client-driven, cancellation of a visit, failure of a client to be home for a visit, or not allowing a DCC entry into the home for a scheduled visit had direct, negative effects on achieving the target SCRIPT PII.

### RFTS (C) Group and E Group Comparability at Screening

As noted in Table 3.14 the (C) and E groups were comparable at the O1 assessment.

TABLE 3.14  (C) Group and E Group Comparison at Screening

| VARIABLE | (C) GROUP N = 259 | E GROUP N = 259 | P VALUE |
|---|---|---|---|
| Baseline CO (ppm) | 13.1 | 13.6 | 0.60 |
| EGA (weeks) | 18.0 | 17.2 | 0.17 |
| Smokers in house (%) | 81.3 | 77.7 | 0.27 |
| Mean Maternal Age (yr) | 23.8 | 24.3 | 0.17 |
| Mean CPD | 9.7 | 8.8 | 0.13 |
| Perceived harm: Smoking to self* | 8.7 | 8.9 | 0.22 |
| Perceived harm: Smoking to baby* | 9.4 | 9.5 | 0.30 |

* 1–10: 10 = most harm.

No significant selection biases were documented for the same variables for all 1,365 self-reported smokers in 2006–2007 and 1,303 self-reported smokers in 2009–2010. The annual RFTS populations were very homogeneous and stable; clients were pregnant, Medicaid-eligible, and 98% white from 2006–2010. *The CO confirmed non-disclosure rates at the follow-up visit were also very low and not significantly different for any cohort: 3.4% in 2006–2007 and 2.3% in 2009–2010.*

We also compared the baseline characteristics of the 259 (C) group clients randomly selected from the 688 clients in 2006–2007 to the 429 clients not selected. This documented if the randomly selected (C) group was representative of RFTS clients for 2006–2007. No significant differences were documented. The randomly selected (C) group was representative of RFTS clients in 2006–2007, and comparable to the population of smokers of 2006–2010.

### Effectiveness Evaluation Results

Table 3.15 presents analyses for the impact categories for (C) and E groups. Significant increases in the cessation rates were documented for the E (9.3%) versus (C) group (p = 0.0001). The difference of 9.3% was comparable to the average 8.0% E versus C group rate differences reported in SCRIPT Trials I–II–III. A significant difference in SR rates was also confirmed for the E (4.3%) versus (C) group (p = 0.05). The SR results were not as large as, but were consistent with, Trial I–II–III results, which used saliva cotinine analysis for confirmation. The half-life of CO is 2–4 hr versus 18–24 hr for saliva cotinine. CO is not as sensitive a measure of daily exposure as saliva/urine cotinine.

Data in Table 3.16 confirmed substantial levels of CO reduction for the E and (C) groups. A reduction from a baseline CO = 20–25 ppm to a

TABLE 3.15 Behavioral Impact Rates by (C) and E Groups

| VARIABLE | (C) GROUP N = 259 | E GROUP N = 259 | % | P VALUE |
|---|---|---|---|---|
| Smoke-free homes (%) | 32.0 | 33.6 | + 0.05 | 0.709 |
| MD/RN advice to quit (%) | 86.0 | 90.0 | + 4.70 | 0.170 |
| CO-confirmed cessation (%) | 4.6 | 13.9 | + 9.30 | 0.000 |
| CO-confirmed sig. reduction (%)* | 6.9 | 11.2 | + 4.30 | 0.050 |

* 50% reduction: > 10 ppm at screening.

TABLE 3.16 (C) and E Group CO Values at Baseline and Follow-up

| BEHAVIOR | (C) GROUP | | | E GROUP | | |
|---|---|---|---|---|---|---|
| | BASELINE (PPM) | FOLLOW-UP | % < | BASELINE | FOLLOW-UP | % < |
| Smoking cessation | 7.2 | 0.6 | < 92% | 9.0 | 1.3 | < 86% |
| Significant reduction | 25.8 | 9.2 | < 64% | 21.9 | 6.3 | < 71% |
| No significant change | 12.4 | 15.6 | > 26% | 13.4 | 15.3 | + 14% |

follow-up CO = 6–9 ppm represents an estimated 68% reduction in fetal/newborn carboxy-hemoglobin levels.

### Discussion of the Internal and External Validity of Results

While the Dissemination Project experienced many implementation barriers, RFTS achieved its primary Behavioral Impact Aims and almost achieved (SCRIPT PII = 0.76) the RFTS Adoption Aim of a SCRIPT PII = 0.80 in 2010. Although the (C) and E groups were not randomized, comprehensive analyses of the homogeneity, comparability, and stability of characteristics of the RFTS population for 2006–2010 for all predictor variables provided strong and consistent evidence for **selection bias** being an implausible explanation for E versus (C) group impact rates differences.

Smoking status was assessed by the same DCC at a screening and follow-up visit by the same questions and CO monitoring equipment and procedures for both Groups. The 2–4 hr half-life of CO versus 18–24 hr for saliva cotinine was an issue discussed by the Dissemination Committee. The use of the CO test also dramatically improved the RFTS client non-disclosure (deception) rates. The CO-confirmed (C) group non-disclosure rate was 30% at screening and 3.6% at follow-up for 2006–2007. The CO-confirmed E group non-disclosure rate was 25% at screening and 2.6% at follow-up for 2009–2010. The CO test provided valid immediate, specific, and inter-pretable client and DCC feedback about smoking status for both the E and (C) group. *Thus, measurement bias was not a plausible explanation for the observed differences.*

Implementation of the Dissemination Project was also affected by a state-wide and national recession. Unemployment in West Virginia increased from 4.5% (2006) to 9.3% (2010). These **historical biases** to implementation, however, may have provided additional support for the validity of the results. The Project achieved its behavioral and adoption Aims, even under especially adverse social and economic trends in West Virginia. *When selection, measurement, and historical biases were analyzed, we concluded that the Dissemination Program was the most plausible reason for the significant changes documented.* The increase in the SCRIPT Program Implementation Index (PII), 63% in 2006–20207 to 76% in 2009–2010, further supported this conclusion. A comprehensive meta-analysis of the MCH literature indicated that these process and effectiveness evaluation results are new for a home-based SCRIPT program as part of state-wide "Healthy Start" services.

The SCRIPT Dissemination Project produced salient insights about barriers to reaching Medicaid pregnant smokers through home-based care coordination. Only 21% of RFTS clients (N = 273) who wanted to quit and provided a CO at screening received a SCRIPT visit. This percentage was substantially lower than the patient participation rates for SCRIPT Trials I–II–III, which was 77%, 93%, and 73%, respectively. These Trials, however, were conducted at prenatal care clinics. The following describes why RFTS rates were so much lower than the Trial rates.

RFTS enrollment is voluntary, and all clients were screened in their second trimester: the average EGA was 18 weeks. The client EGA for the SCRIPT visit was 22 weeks, versus 10–12 weeks for the SCRIPT Trials. All RFTS smokers would have had multiple opportunities to quit prior to RFTS enrollment: when their pregnancy was confirmed, at their first prenatal visit when they received advice to quit from their MD and RN, and at prenatal visits 2, 3, and 4. The percent of RFTS clients still motivated to quit would be substantially lower at 22 weeks versus 10–12 weeks. A detailed discussion of these issues is presented in the published article.

The WV SCRIPT evaluation and two Australian evaluations confirm that a wide science-to-practice gap remains. The methods and insights from the SCRIPT Dissemination Project should be useful to prepare evaluation plans by other systems of care and Healthy Start initiatives throughout the United States. The results of the SCRIPT evaluation are especially important in light of the recent CMS policy mandating evidenced-based smoking cessation counseling and reimbursement. This evaluation study is an excellent example of the application of quasi-experimental design and successful in implementation of a "Practice-Based Participatory Research Project (PBPR)" for a state-wide perinatal program. *Because of the homogeneity of the home-based population, almost all white pregnant smokers supported by Medicaid, these results may be generalizable to comparable demographic populations in other home-based Healthy Start programs.*

## Case Study 4: A Time Series Design for a Community-Based Participatory Evaluation

R. Windsor, G. Cutter, and J. Kronenfeld, et al., "Increasing Utilization of Rural Cervical Cancer Detection Program." *American Journal of Public Health* (June 1981), 641–643 (see publication for references).

### Background and Objectives

The Alabama Department of Public Health established a Cervical Cancer Screening Program (CSP), initially with NCI support, to remove barriers to service availability, accessibility, acceptability, and cost in local rural communities. The CSP was designed to increase service use by women who have never used the program. A "Practice and Community-Based Participatory Research" effort was begun with representatives from the University of Alabama-Birmingham (UAB) public health faculty, Alabama Health Department-CSP program, Cooperative Extension Service, and leadership of 36 women's groups This group planned and evaluated a rural, county-wide Cervical Cancer Screening and Communications Program.

Our objective was to significantly increase the number of women who had never had a Pap test using the Hale County CSP during the second (Intervention) quarter of year 2 and 3. Eligible CSP residents were predominantly black, poor, and rural, with available but limited access to primary care services. The Hale County program was selected as a demonstration site because it had a large pool of women > 35 years of age (3,500) who had not been screened, was similar to a number of counties in south central Alabama, and was operational for two years.

### Health Education Intervention Methods

A multiple-component intervention was developed because the literature and experience confirmed that no single source of exposure could be expected to have a significant impact. Multiple messages and channels, particularly interpersonal sources, were applied. Two health education programs were implemented in Hale County during the second quarter, April–June, year 2 and 3. Two principal messages were communicated during the three-month interventions. Women > 35 years who had never had a Pap smear were at higher risk for cervical cancer. Cervical cancer was highly curable if detected early. If a woman met the criteria, she should contact the CSP. As shown in Table 3.17, there were five principal components of the health education intervention.

TABLE 3.17 Elements, Channels, and Purposes of the Hale County Intervention

| ELEMENTS | COMMUNICATION CHANNELS | PURPOSES |
|---|---|---|
| 1. Community Organization ($X_1$) | Local lay and professional leaders | Increase acceptance, support, and credibility |
| 2. Mass Media ($X_2$) | Electronic and print media: radio, local newspaper, church and club newsletters, posters, and bulletin boards | Increase awareness/interest in program messages<br>Reinforce program message |
| 3. Lay Leadership ($X_3$) | Leadership training: standardized package | Increase assumption of responsibility by locals Decrease misinformation<br>Increase program acceptance by peer groups |
| 4. Interpersonal Group Sessions ($X_4$) | Group process: 1- to 2-hour standardized cancer education program session | Increase efficiency of networking<br>Increase adaptability to personal evaluation and responsibility<br>Increase motivation and social support<br>Increase personalization of messages<br>Increase legitimacy of at-risk role |
| 5. Interpersonal ($X_5$) | Individual word-of-mouth<br>Individual sessions | Increase persuasion-diffusion-salience of messages<br>Increase trial and adoption |

Program planning, organizational development, leadership training activities, and evaluation methods were completed in year 1. Cancer communication intervention elements noted in Table 3.14were applied in the second quarter of year 2. This community organization effort recruited and trained 39 female lay leaders, 21 white and 18 black, from existing community groups to conduct programs to their women's group. They held 45 meetings with 15 to 20 participants at each session. Approximately 750 women were documented as having been directly exposed to the program. Considerable emphasis was placed on word-of-mouth diffusion by participants to female friends and family > 35 years of age. The second intervention applied solely by the local public health and community leadership in the second quarter of year 3 was a replication of the year 2 intervention.

Evaluation Design and Measurement

A time series design (TSD) with a repeated treatment was applied to evaluate the impact of the Cancer Communications Program (CCP). The computerized data system of the CSP of the Alabama Department of Health was used to confirm the monthly and quarterly pattern of new users. In applying a TSD, this project (1) established the periodicity of the pattern of behavior being examined, (2) collected impact data unobtrusively, (3) confirmed multiple data points one year prior to and one year following the CCP, and (4) applied and withdrew the intervention during a specific time. A TSD was used because it was the highest quality quasi-experimental design for the CCP.

## Program Impact

Figure 3.1 illustrates the frequency of new users by quarter and year. The pattern in Figure 3.1 for the three-year period suggests a significant difference in CSP use during the two CCP periods. The frequency of new users for five baseline quarters prior to intervention 1 was stable, although the increase in the frequency of new users in the second quarter of year 1 suggested a seasonal variation. An increase of 345% in new users, 20 > 89, was observed for the second quarter of year 2, the CCP quarter. In other words, 89 new clients used the service during this period, compared with an average of 15 in year 1, and a maximum of 20 for the second quarter baseline in year 1.

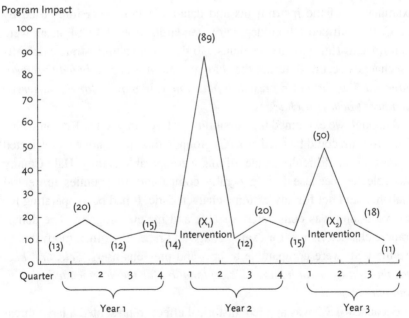

FIGURE 3.1 Frequencies of New CSP Users by Quarter and Year.

Another increase in client use, from 20 > 50 (approximately 150%), was observed during the second intervention period. In the aggregate, an estimated 100 more new users were motivated to use the CSP than would be expected from the pattern observed during the non-intervention periods in year 2 and 3. An analysis of the new-user increase using a linear regression model found that the observed frequencies for the intervention quarters were significantly higher (P > 0.01) than the observed frequencies for the non-intervention quarters. Throughout the three-year period, the demographic characteristics of the new users remained very stable. Analyses of utilization data from a contiguous, matched county revealed no changes in CSP use by new users of the magnitude noted in Hale County. *We concluded: the increases in 100 new CSP users during the two second quarters were primarily due to interventions X and Y.*

### Discussion of Internal and External Validity of Results

Evaluators of public health programs need to consider the plausibility that factors, other than the intervention, produced the observed impact. The TSD controlled for the effects of multiple observations by using unobtrusive measurement. Because the data observed were unobtrusive measures of behavioral impact (CSP use), this factor could not be a plausible explanation for the observed change during the intervention periods. An examination of the instruments and data-collection procedures used by the CSP confirmed a high degree of standardization. All CSP users were confirmed as Hale County residents. No significant administrative or staffing changes occurred during the study period. *It was concluded that measurement bias did not represent a plausible explanation for the observed significant behavior changes.*

Although we examined the possibility that a county in the Region with a CSP program could be used as a (C) group in this study, none was selected because of the difficulty in identifying a comparable county. Hale County was selected because it is generally comparable to counties in central Alabama, and not for any extreme characteristic. It had been operating for two years and was considered a stable and mature program. The demographic characteristics, for example, age and race, of women motivated to use the CSP were comparable to new and previous users. *Selection bias was thought to be an implausible explanation for the documented, significant impact.*

Because a TSD was applied, historical effects represented a large threat to the internal validity of the results. In examining the possibility that historical events caused the observed increase, the evaluators found that no local, countywide, area, state, or national cancer communication program or event had occurred during the three-year demonstration period. Local organizations that might have had an independent effect on CSP use were collaborators with or supporters of the project. No changes in CSP use of the magnitude noted in Hale County were evident in adjacent counties. It was concluded from the evidence and statistical analyses that a **historical bias** represented an implausible explanation for CSP increases in Hale County.

### External Validity in Alabama and the Utility of Community-Based Participatory Research

Our assessment of threats to internal validity confirmed that the most likely explanation for the observed changes in CSP use was the CCP applied in the spring of year 2 and 3. This conclusion was strengthened by the replication of the program by local colleagues in the year 3 evaluation. The observed increases were statistically and programmatically important in that the methods and issues examined were useful to community health education efforts. It was also concluded that the CCP Evaluation produced evidence generalizable to the large number of comparable counties in Central and South Alabama. *This project, conducted through the collaborative effort of existing programs, personnel, and funding sources, also demonstrated that a valid evaluation of an ongoing program can be conducted without the infusion of large budgetary funds. It was a successful example of the implementation of the CBPR methodology.*

## Case Study 5: A Time Series Design for a National Occupational Health Policy-Program

C. Montforton and R. Windsor, "An Impact Evaluation of Federal Mine Safety Training Regulation and Policies on Fatality and Injury Rates Among U.S. Stone, Sand and Gravel Workers: An Interrupted Time-Series Analysis," *American Journal of Public Health* (August 2010) (see publication for references).

### Introduction

When the public thinks of dangerous occupations, mining is typically first on the list because of high-profile news reports of entrapments involving underground coal miners. Workers in surface mining operations, however, face even higher risks of injury and disability than their counterparts in underground coal mines. The occupational injury incidence rate was 5.0/100 full-time workers in 2006 at surface dimension stone quarries: > twice the rate for surface bituminous coal miners.

The Mine Safety and Health Administration (MSHA) was established by the Federal Mine Safety and Health Act of 1977 to address hazards and prevent injuries and illnesses among US mine workers. In 1979, the agency issued mandatory safety and health training for any mine worker, including provisions requiring all new miners to receive at least 24 hours of safety training. All experienced miners must receive > 8 hours annually of refresher safety and health training.

While the increased risk and dangers of surface mining are well documented, the effectiveness of occupational safety and health regulations from the MSHA to prevent work-related injuries, illnesses, and fatalities among US workers continues to be debated. Although injury incidents rates have gradually declined over the decades since the OSHA and MSHA were established in 1977, there are very few well-designed evaluations measuring the effectiveness of interventions of mine safety training and policy interventions. *This evaluation was designed to assess the impact on injury and fatality rates at US surface mining operations of the mandatory worker safety policy and training regulations issued in September 1999 by the MSHA.*

## Methods

### MSHA Intervention

A multi-year spike in miner fatalities and a front-page story in *USA Today* about deaths at these operations created an opportunity for MSHA's assistant secretary, congressional appropriators, and representatives of the "exempt" mines to negotiate a plan to remove the long-standing rider. By congressional directive, the new training rules had to be issued by September 30, 1999. Mine operators were given one year to be in compliance. These new mandatory safety and health training regulations, known as Part 46, took affect on October 1, 2000.

### Injury Measurement of Population at Risk

The MSHA regulations require surface mine operators to file a quarterly report with employment hours. If an accident, injury, or illness occurs, the operator must report the event to MSHA < 10 working days. Data for 12 years of interest in this study, 1995–2006, were imported into SAS® version 8.2. The pre-intervention evaluation-analysis period was defined as January 1995 to September 2000. The post-intervention evaluation-analysis period was October 2000 to December 2006. MSHA regulations applied to about 10,000 mines and an estimated 110,000 workers. The mine sites in this evaluation met the following criteria: operational from January 1, 1995, to December 31, 2006; and had employees at the mine for at least eight quarters in *both* the pre-intervention and post-intervention periods. Of the 10,000, 7,998 (80%) sites met the inclusion criteria: 85% reported employee hours in at least 16 quarters in the intervention periods: 42.5% reporting employee hours in all 48 quarters. Nearly 55% of the eligible mines were intermittent operations: mines with at least one quarter/year with no reported employee hours.

### Evaluation Design and Analysis

An interrupted time series design (TSD) and analyses, based on models for sequential observations over time, evaluated the impact of the MSHA policy. With time-series data, analyses account for the correlation between proximal observations.

### Results

### Quarterly Fatality Rates

During January 1, 1995, to December 31, 2006, there were 259 fatalities at the study mine population: 160 in the pre-intervention period (O1) and 99 in the post-intervention period (O2). In the 23 quarters in the O1 period, the fatality rate was 0.025 per 200,000 employee hours. In the 25-quarter O2 period, the fatality rate was 0.017, a decline of 33% from the pre-evaluation period. The main intervention effect on the quarterly and semi-annual fatality rates of the MSHA was not statistically significant: (chi-square = 1.12; $p = 0.290$) and (chi-square = 2.39; $p = 0.122$). *The decline in fatality rates could not be attributed to implementation of MSHA's Part 46 training regulation.*

### Serious Injury Rates by Aggregate Type, Ownership, and Production Trends

Data for the 7,998 mines were stratified by relevant BLS codes, by year-round versus intermittent mining operations, and ownership, because 10 large firms were responsible for 50% of annual US surface mine production. Figure 3.2 presents the data comparing serious injury rates at mines, stratified by SIC codes. The period in which MSHA training regulation

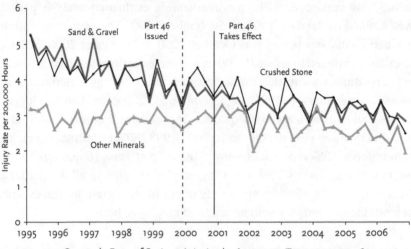

FIGURE 3.2 Quarterly Rate of Serious Injuries by Aggregate Type: 1995–2006

was issued is marked with a dashed vertical line. The effective date of the rule, September 30, 1999, is marked with the solid vertical line. Over the 12-year period, the overall rate of serious injuries declined by 52.6% at crushed stone operations, 46.2% at sand and gravel operations, and 38% at other surface mineral mines. *The time series analyses and model identification techniques provided no evidence that the large percent of change documented in serious injury rates in the post-intervention period could be attributed to implementation of the Part 46 training regulation.*

### Injury Severity

Nearly 96,000 injuries of varying severity, lost time (39%), medical treatment only (36%), and restricted duty (28%), were reported over the 12-year period. Figure 3.3 presents the quarterly rates by injury categories. *Over the 12-year period they declined by 56.4% and 60.3%.*

### Permanently Disabling Injury (PDI) Rates

The quarterly rate of permanently disabling injuries also declined by 54% (see Figure 3.4). *Analyses of the quarterly rates of injuries for lost time, restricted duty, and medical treatment injuries did not support the hypothesis that the rate changes from 1995 to 2006 were attributable to MSHA's Part 46 training regulation implementation. The analysis of main effects revealed a statistically significant difference in the time-series trend in the pre- and post-Part 46 periods (chi-square = 10.17; p-value = 0.0014) for permanently*

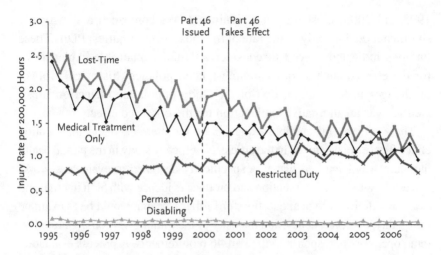

FIGURE 3.3 Quarterly Rate of Injuries by Severity: 1995–2006

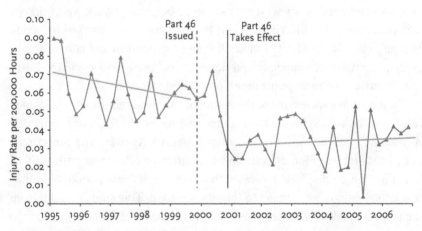

FIGURE 3.4 Quarterly Rate of Permanently Disabling Injuries: 1995–2006

*disabling injuries (PDI)*. A risk ratio estimate quantified the change in the population risk of experiencing a PDI in the two periods; the estimate was 0.59 (95% CI = 0.529–0.661). Miners employed after the MSHA's safety training regulation had a 41% less risk of suffering a PDI than workers employed in the period before the regulation and training intervention.

### Discussion of Internal Validity and External Validity of Results

Our time-series and regression analyses offer mixed results on the impact of MSHA's regulation on injury and fatality rates. Although large reductions in many injury-severity categories were documented between

1995 and 2006, most were not significant. We confirmed a statistically significant decline only in the rate of the most severe injuries: PDIs. These findings indicated a need to consider alternative plausible explanations for the effects, such as other mining-related policies (**historical Bbias**), or changes in the composition of the study population (**selection bias**). Neither was an alternative explanation for the observed effects.

There are several credible explanations for the lack of an intervention effect. These are discussed in the article. No efficacy study in the public health literature was identified that was specifically designed to evaluate a workplace safety-training intervention and produce evidence with high internal and external validity. A logical question for further research would be to examine the quality, time, frequency, and intensity of the training sessions instituted by mine operators in response to the Part 46 requirements. A process evaluation documenting these characteristics and confirming the degree of fidelity of program implementation might provide evidence and insight to explore hypotheses about *why* and *how* interventions worked or failed to work with workers. It is plausible that MSHA regulations failed to result in a marked reduction in injury rates at the affected mines because the political and administrative goals of compliance simplicity and flexibility eclipsed goals related to learning objectives and measurable injury prevention outcomes.

On the tenth anniversary of the National Occupational Research Agenda (NORA), the NIOSH issued *The Team Document: 10 Years of Leadership Advancing the National Occupational Research Agenda*. The report reiterated that intervention effectiveness research was "an underutilized tool when NORA began," and indicated that over the 10-year period, only limited contributions were made to the science base. This study's findings on the impact of MSHA's regulations illuminate the need for policymakers to consider the opportunities (or obstacles) to evaluating a regulation's impact prior to its creation and once it is in place. This Health Policy Outcome Evaluation is one good example of why agency officials need to consider the evidence base about how to improve injury rates and how the intervention will be evaluated. Specific process evaluation and implementation methods and data are essential to document delivery of intervention components and to conduct a rigorous (defensible) impact or outcome evaluation.

## Case Study 6: An Experimental Design of a Community-Based HP-DP Program

R. DiClemente, G. Wingood, K. Harrington, et al., "Efficacy of an HIV Prevention Intervention for African American Adolescent

Girls: A Randomized Clinical Trial Design," *Journal of the American Medical Association* (2004), 171–179 (see publication for references).

### Background and Objectives

While African American (AA) girls are at increased risk for HIV/ STD, very few sound evaluations of interventions to reduce associated risk behaviors had been reported prior to this study. This was a PHASE II Efficacy Evaluation designed to document the impact of four consecutive weekly, four-hour health education sessions (X1 + X2 + X3 + X4) among experimental group participants. The intervention was delivered to E group girls on Saturdays at a Family Medicine Clinic. Control group participants were randomly assigned to receive a general health promotion program also delivered as four four-hour sessions (Y1 + Y2 +Y3 + Y4) on consecutive Saturdays. The control condition emphasized exercise and nutrition.

After informed consent and baseline assessment, participants were randomly assigned to the E or C group. The evaluation design and sample size for each group at baseline and at the 6- and 12-month follow-up are diagrammed in Table 3.18. Effect size and sample size estimates were presented. With a base rate of 25% consistent condom use, a 50% increase in consistent use, a 20% attrition at the 12-month follow-up, and an alpha = 0.05 and Power = 0.80, the evaluation was designed to have > 250 per condition for a two-tailed analysis of impact.

### Intervention Methods

The intervention methods were developed collaboratively with AA girls in the community. Each of the four sessions of 10–12 participants was moderated by a trained AA peer educator. A central principle in the delivery of the program by the peer educators was "modeling skills" and "creating social norms" supportive of reducing their risks. Social Cognitive Theory and Gender Empowerment Theory were used to guide the development of intervention processes and content. Both the E and C group interventions were field tested prior to implementation.

TABLE 3.18 Evaluation Research Design

| BASELINE | GROUP | INTERVENTIONS | FOLLOW-UP 6-MONTH | FOLLOW-UP 12-MONTH |
|---|---|---|---|---|
| $O_1$ (N = 251) | R E | X1 + X2 + X3 + X4 | $O_2$ (N = 226) | $O_3$ (N = 219) |
| $O_1$ (N = 271) | R C | Y1 + Y2 + Y3 + Y4 | $O_2$ (N = 243) | $O_3$ (N = 241) |

### Measurement Methods

Multiple methods and measures were used to assess participants at baseline, and at 6 and 12 months. A total of 522 participants completed a self-administered instrument to document demographic and psycho-social characteristics, and were interviewed by a trained AA professional to document sexual behaviors. Interviewers assessed the skill of the AA adolescent to use a condom correctly. Participants also provided two self-collected vaginal swabs to be analyzed for STDs. The number of individuals assessed and lost to follow-up is presented in Table 3.18. A variety of psycho-social mediators were measured. Psychometric analyses confirmed reliability values: r = 0.68, 0.82, 0.68, 0.80, and 0.88. A detailed statistical analysis plan was presented.

### Results: Process Evaluation

All E group and C group sessions were monitored by trained staff who rated implementation fidelity: 98% of the activities planned for each of the four sessions were provided. Participant attendance was excellent for both groups: 95.2% of the E group completed all four sessions, and 94.5% of the C group completed four sessions. Both interventions were confidently rated on a scale of 1 to 5. Both received very high ratings: the E group rating was 4.82, and the C group rating was 4.76. Data in Table 3.19 confirmed that the random assignment process was successful.

### Results: Behavioral Impact Analysis

A detailed analysis of the effectiveness of the HIV/STD Prevention Intervention is presented in the publication. A synopsis of the Trial impact is presented in Table 3.20.

The following is a synopsis of several of the most salient results. The E group exhibited at both the 6-month (84.9% + 82.3%) and 12-month

TABLE 3.19  E Group vs. C Group Baseline Comparability

| VARIABLE | E GROUP | C GROUP |
| --- | --- | --- |
| Age | 15.99 yr | 15.97 yr |
| Public assistance | 45.8% | 48.7% |
| Has children | 23.9% | 23.2% |
| Condom use: Efficacy | 30.7% | 30.5% |
| % Condom use: 30 days | 79.2% | 77.5% |
| Positive gonorrhea test | 5.6% | 4.8% |
| Not in school | 10.0% | 8.9% |
| Age of first sex | 13.3 yr | 13.7 yr |

TABLE 3.20  E Group vs. C Group Impact Analyses

| IMPACT RATE | E GROUP | | C GROUP | | P VALUES | |
|---|---|---|---|---|---|---|
| | 6 MO. | 12 MO. | 6 MO. | 12 MO. | 6 MO. | 12 MO. |
| Consistent C. use: 30 days | 84.9% | 80.0% | 65.1% | 62.8% | < 0.001 | < 0.001 |
| Consistent C. use: 6 mo. | 82.3% | 73.5% | 61.7% | 57.6% | < 0.001 | < 0.001 |
| Unprotected sex: 6 mo. | 3.8 | 5.8 | 9.24 | 10.3 | < 0.008 | < 0.020 |
| New vaginal partner: 30 days | 2.7 | 3.6 | 7.4 | 5.6 | < 0.010 | < 0.010 |
| Self-reported pregnancy | 3.6 | 6.0 | 7.0 | 8.5 | < 0.040 | < 0.060 |

follow-ups (80.0% + 73.5%) significantly higher, adjusted rates of "consistent condom use in > 30 days and 6 months" compared to the C group 6-month rates (65.1% + 61.7%) and 12-month rates (62.8% + 57.6%). The E group reported significantly lower average number (3.77 + 5.77) of "unprotected vaginal sex in last 6 and 12 months" when compared to the C group (9.24 + 10.25). E versus C comparisons of a wide range of psycho-social constructs confirmed significantly higher, positive impacts for E group participants.

### Discussion of Internal and External Validity of Results

An examination of the primary threats to internal validity reveals that this efficacy evaluation asserted excellent control over each threat. The measurement of the impact rates used the most current methods to determine participant behavior. Bias of self-reported behavior was acknowledged. Because randomization of participants was successful, error that existed was not large and was equally distributed to each study group. The internal consistency assessments of knowledge and multiple psycho-social multiple constructs (r = 0.68, 0.82, 0.68, 0.80, and 0.88) ranged from borderline (< 0.70) to very good to excellent (> 0.80–0.88). The addition of biomarkers for STDs at baseline and 6–12 months added support for a limited **measurement bias**.

*The experimental design and qualitative evaluations provide excellent documentation that the significant E versus C group differences were not attributable to selection biases.* Figure 1 in the publication presents an excellent diagram and specific data that enumerate the flow and degree of participation and drop-outs for the E and C group. An 87% E group and 89% C group 12-month follow-up rate confirm a very small and equivalent level of selection bias. The evaluation recruited and randomized 86%

(522/609) of the eligible participants, an excellent accrual rate. Combined with an 88% retention rate, it provided very strong support for the internal validity of these results.

*The process evaluation and standardization of exposure levels for the E and C groups confirmed strong support for the absence of an internal (program) historical bias.* There is no indication that external historical events occurred in the United States or Alabama during the evaluation. Because of its methodological quality, it represents, with several small changes (most noted in the article and this review), a prototype for future STD/Pregnancy Prevention Program evaluations.

## Case Study 7: An Experimental Design for a State-Wide Primary Care-MCH Clinics—A Practice-Based Evaluation

R. Windsor, L. Woodby, T. Miller, et al., "Effectiveness of AHCPR Clinical Practice Guideline and Patient Education Methods for Pregnant Smokers in Medicaid Maternity Care," *American Journal of Obstetricians and Gynecologists* (2000), 68–75 (see publication for references).

### Background

Exposure to tobacco smoke during pregnancy is the most salient cause of infant morbidity and mortality in the United States. The need to disseminate and evaluate the level of adoption by regular staff and the effectiveness and cost-effectiveness of evidence based methods is well recognized. The objectives of Trial III, a PHASE 3 Effectiveness Evaluation, was to confirm the fidelity of delivery of counseling methods by regular staff and to evaluate the *effectiveness* of the methods among clinics and patients representative of a state Medicaid population.

### Methods

This Trial was a five-year, two-phase collaborative study between the University of Alabama at Birmingham (UAB) and Alabama Department of Public Health (ADPH). During Phase 1, organizational development and site selection were completed and a pre-Trial, non-experimental smoking history study was conducted to confirm normal rates of behavior change before training. After the smoking history study was completed, regular staff was trained to implement SCRIPT procedures, and a formative evaluation was conducted.

## Organizational Development and Site Selection: A Practice-Based Participatory Evaluation

Involvement of public health program leadership and clinic staff in planning and policymaking processes in the introduction and evaluation of new health education methods for routine clinical practice is essential. A science-management-practice partnership of senior investigators and Bureau of Family Health Services (BFHS) program directors, the SCRIPT Policy and Management Committee (PMC), was established to develop the proposal and direct the project. A Practice Advisory Committee (one staff member/clinic) ensured practice input.

A site selection process was designed to yield a representative sample of the state's Medicaid population. Eligible sites were identified in the 67 counties using self-reported smoking rates from annual vital statistics. Because a county needed > 50 pregnant smokers/year to participate (>1 smoker/week), 50 counties were ineligible. After stratification of the 16 eligible counties by number of smokers and percent black and white, eight matched dyads were created. One county per dyad was randomly selected. A comparison of annual statistics for the year prior to Trial III confirmed the representativeness of the eight SCRIPT counties randomly selected.

Staff orientation sessions and patient flow assessments (PFA) were conducted at all clinics within the first six months of the project. The SCRIPT procedures were introduced during training as a collaborative partnership (3 hours), reflecting a continuous quality improvement philosophy.

### Program Evaluation Design

During Phase 1, a representative sample of all new smokers and non-smokers for one month at all 10 sites, *a non-randomized historical comparison (C) group*, was assessed at their first visit and > 60 days. This study documented the "normal" self-reported and cotinine-confirmed prevalence and non-disclosure (deception) rates at the first visit. It also confirmed the "normal" cessation and significant reduction rates during care attributable to the health education methods routinely provided by regular staff to pregnant smokers at each clinic. It was conducted *before* SCRIPT staff training and *before* the intervention was introduced during the formative evaluation.

Following completion of the smoking history study and on-site SCRIPT training program, patients were recruited and randomized using a 3 to 1 ratio: 3 patients to the E group and 1 patient to the C group at each clinic.

This staged experimental design facilitated the routine delivery of the new SCRIPT methods by regular staff. Because they were all pregnant smokers from the same clinics and were assessed using the same procedures by the same staff, the C group patients randomized during this period were combined with the comparison (C) cohort of smoking history patients in Phase 1. This produced an E group of 139 smokers and a C group of 126 smokers.

### SCRIPT Procedures

The E and C Group received **Ask-Advise-Assess-Arrange** Procedures. E Group patients also received **Assist** Procedures: A "Commit to Quit Smoking During and After Pregnancy" Video, A Pregnant Woman's Guide to Quit Smoking, and a ≤ 10-minute counseling session. After an introduction, the Guide was given to patients to review while watching the 14-minute video (edited to 8 minutes post-Trial). The intervention process and content were derived from meta-evaluations, AHCPR Guidelines, patient flow analyses, and patient/staff interviews.

### Measurement Procedures

All patients completed a consent, a 12-question baseline form, and provided a saliva sample for cotinine analysis. Follow-up assessments were performed during a visit at > 60 days after the first visit, and < 90 days postpartum. Patients lost to follow-up (LTF) were counted as smokers. Assessment forms were faxed daily to the UAB Data Coordinator. In the SCRIPT Trial II, a significant reduction (SR) was defined as a patient with a baseline saliva cotinine > 30 ng/mL and > 50% cotinine reduction at follow-up. In Trial III, a baseline saliva cotinine had to be > 50 ng/mL and follow-up < 50% lower than the baseline for an SR patient. The new definition of increased the validity of the biochemical estimate of SR rates. It eliminated patients with ultra-low baseline levels.

### Process Evaluation Results

Data in Table 3.21 confirm E and C group baseline comparability. Process evaluation data for all sites documented that only one E group patient did not view the video at the site.

All baseline assessment procedures were completed for all E and C group patients. Approximately > 90% of all follow-up assessment procedures were completed. The SCRIPT and assessment procedures were delivered with fidelity by regular staff as components of prenatal care.

TABLE 3.21 E and C Group Baseline Comparability

| BASELINE VARIABLES | E GROUP | C GROUP |
|---|---|---|
| Mean age | 23 yr | 23 yr |
| Race: Black | 18% | 14% |
| Gestational age | 2.2 months | 3.0 months |
| Readiness score* | 2.0 | 2.0 |
| CPD | 10 CPD | 10 CPD |
| > 1 smoker-home | 77% | 84% |
| Mean cotinine level | 204 ng/ml | 201 ng/ml |
| Sample | N = 139 | N = 126 |

*0 = no; 3= very high
CPD = cigarettes per day

TABLE 3.22 E and C Group Effectiveness Rates

| BEHAVIOR | E GROUP | C GROUP | Z SCORE | P VALUE + |
|---|---|---|---|---|
| Cessation | 17.3% | 8.8% | 1.94 | 0.024 |
| Sig. reduction | 21.7% | 15.8% | 1.00 | 0.159 |
| **Sample** | **N = 139** | **N = 126** | **E vs. C** | **+ one tail test** |

## Impact Evaluation Results

Data in Table 3.22 confirm that the E group cessation rates were significantly higher than the C group rate. The E versus C group significant reduction rates were not significantly different.

These data were the first empirical evidence to confirm the behavioral impact and feasibility of routine delivery of AHCPR-recommended evidence-based patient education methods to pregnant smokers by regular staff. The deception rate, patients who said they quit but had a saliva cotinine value > 20 ng/ml, was 10% for both groups. Data in Table 3.23 present the cotinine level changes for the E and C Group. The average baseline cotinine of the E group who quit was 97 ng/mL (moderate daily exposure), in contrast to the corresponding C group value of 40 ng/mL (very light daily exposure). As noted in Table 3.23, the average significant reduction in cotinine values was 66%: 233 ng/mL to 78 ng/mL. Thus, a large percentage of very heavy, daily smokers (> 200 ng/m) in both the E and C groups dramatically reduced their tobacco exposure.

## Discussion of Internal and External Validity of Results

This PHASE 3 Effectiveness Evaluation was successfully implemented in year 1 and 2. The delivery of the new SCRIPT methods by the 28 public health nurses, social workers, and nutritionists was achieved. The site

TABLE 3.23 E and C Group Cotinine Values at Baseline and Follow-up

| BEHAVIOR | E GROUP | | C GROUP | |
|---|---|---|---|---|
| | BASELINE | FOLLOW-UP | BASELINE | FOLLOW-UP |
| No change | 218 ng/ml | 188 ng/ml | 195 ng/ml | 183 ng/ml |
| Cessation | 97 ng/ml | 4 ng/ml | 40 ng/ml | 4 ng/ml |
| Sig. reduction | 228 ng | 77 ng/ml | 238 ng/ml | 79 ng/ml |

selection process yielded a representative sample of the state's Medicaid population. A comparison of annual statistics for the year prior to Trial III confirmed the comparability of the sites and patients. The recruitment of > 90% and retention of > 90% of the eligible E and C group participants confirmed little **selection bias**. The small numbers of LTF patients were not different on baseline characteristics than E and C group patients.

The use of the most sensitive measure, a saliva cotinine test, in combination with patient self-reports, produced valid measures of cessation and significant reduction rates. No **measurement biases** were evident. There were no significant **historical biases**-events that could have plausibly produced the documented significant impact. In the aggregate, these data and the randomized design confirmed that the SCRIPT methods were significantly more effective than the normal, brief counseling provided to the C group patients. The internal validity of the evaluation of SCRIPT methods was excellent. *The methodological rigor of Trial III supported the state-wide generalizability of the process and impact results to pregnant smokers and providers: external validity. The results may be generalizable to other state-wide programs for Medicaid patients.*

## Case Study 8: A Group Randomized Community Trial for Rural Health Communities

D. Manandhar, D. Orsin, B. Shrestha, and the MIRA Trial Team, "Effect of a Participatory Intervention With Women's Groups on Birth Outcomes in Nepal: Cluster-Randomized Controlled Trial,: *Lancet* (2004), 970–979 (see publication for reference).

### Introduction

While infant and child mortality rates have declined over the past few decades in low-income countries, rates are still very high in low-income, resource-poor countries such as Nepal. Neonatal deaths account for the majority of infant mortality and are primarily due to home births without trained health professionals. In this study, investigators used a health education–community participatory approach to plan and deliver an intervention to women in randomly selected communities. Literate local female facilitators nominated by community leaders convened women's groups each month to discuss methods to reduce infant mortality.

## Methods

### Site Selection

The unit of randomization, treatment, and analysis was the village and village development committee (VDC) in a rural mountainous area, Makwanpur district, of Nepal. All 42 VDCs in the district were eligible for randomization: one was excluded due to security reasons. Of the 42 pair-matched VDCs, 12 village pairs were randomly selected: 12 experimental and 12 control villages. The study population included all married women of reproductive age (15–49 years) who had the potential to become pregnant and provided consent. Eligible villages were pair-matched on topography, ethnicity, and population density. The average village cluster was ~7,000 people. One VDC in each pair was randomly assigned to an E or C group. Systematic surveillance of all pregnancies and related outcomes was implemented for 2.5 years. Data on 28,931 women and all pregnancy-related events were regularly collected.

### Intervention

A local facilitator conducted nine women's group meetings in all nine wards every month. One supervisor for three facilitators attended the meetings and assisted in implementation. The intervention consisted of a series of 10 meetings, one per month, for one year. Through basic health education and participatory learning techniques, women discussed the purposes of the study and the intervention, learned how to identify maternal and neonatal problems and strategies to identify and share more information in the community, and how to prioritize mother and child health problems. They discussed possible practical solutions to address their problems and how to involve other community members. Strategies within the communities included community-generated funds for maternal and infant care, stretcher and transportation plans, and production and distribution of clean delivery kits. A film and card game created locally were developed and delivered as part of the health education program to improve infant and maternal health.

Sub-district-level neonatal mortality rates were not available, so the expected neonatal mortality rate, 60/1,000 live births, was that of the district. Using a range of estimates for the coefficient of variation ($k_m$) in outcome between clusters within matched pairs = 0.15–0.3, an average of 480 births per cluster, and alpha set at $p < .05$. Investigators determined that to detect a reduction in neonatal morality of 27%–28% (to 37–44/1,000 live births in the intervention clusters) with 80% power would require a minimum of 12 cluster pairs.

## Results

As noted in Table 3.24, baseline data for the E and C clusters indicated that the number of households and the ages of participants who became pregnant were very similar in the two groups.

Some very small differences in literacy and poverty indicators slightly favored the intervention clusters. With respect to outcomes, miscarriage rates, loss to follow-up due to migration, voluntary withdrawal, or incomplete surveillance data were equivalent.

### Health Outcome Results

As indicated in Table 3.25, in 11 of the 12 cluster pairs the neonatal mortality rates were lower. A pooled estimate (OR = 0.70%–95%, CI 0.53–0.94) indicates a 30% reduction in neonatal mortality in the intervention clusters compared with the control clusters.

The maternal mortality ratio (MMR) in the E group clusters was 69 per 100,000 population and 341 for the C group clusters. This represents a 78% lower MMR in the intervention area. While the sample size was not adequate

TABLE 3.24 Comparability of Experimental and Control Clusters

| VARIABLE | E GROUP = 14,884 | C GROUP = 14,047 |
|---|---|---|
| Clock-Radio-Iron-Bicycle | 4,094 (30%) | 4,476 (37%) |
| Food sufficiency: < 8 months | 30% | 28% |
| Age: < 20 | 8% | 8% |
| 20–29 | 38% | 39% |
| 30–39 | 32% | 31% |
| > 40 | 22% | 22% |
| Education: None | 82% | 88% |
| Could not read | 66% | 79% |

TABLE 3.25 Mortality Rate Comparison of the E and C Clusters

| VARIABLE | E GROUP | C GROUP | ODDS RATIO |
|---|---|---|---|
| Live births | 2,899 | 3,228 | |
| Neonatal deaths | 76 | 119 | |
| Neonatal mortality | 26.2 | 36.9 | 0.70 (0.53–0.94) |
| Maternal deaths | 2 | 11 | |
| Maternal mortality | 69.0 | 341.0 | 0.22 (0.05–0.90) |

to evaluate the impact of the intervention on maternal mortality, the observation of this trend was encouraging. There were no significant differences in stillbirth rates or usual causes of neonatal deaths between groups.

A process evaluation confirmed the following. Women in the intervention group were more likely to have antenatal care (E = 55% vs. C = 30%), had taken iron and folic acid supplements (E = 49% vs. C = 27%), had visited a health facility for illness (E = 50% vs. C = 22%), gave birth in a health facility with a trained health professional (E = 9% vs. C 3%), used a clean home delivery kit (E = 19% vs. C = 5%), and used sanitary practices at birth (boiled blade: E = 54% vs. C = 26% + attendant washed hands: E = 68% vs. C = 33%). Mothers in the E group (24%) versus the C group (10%) were much more likely to take their infant to a health facility when their baby was sick.

### Discussion of Internal and External Validity of Results for a Group Randomized Evaluation

This is an excellent example of a GRCT conducted to assess the feasibility of delivering an intervention to reduce neonatal mortality rate through "Community-Based Participatory Research" methods in a very low-income, rural district in Nepal. The results indicated that women and infants in the E group villages experienced a 30% reduction in neonatal mortality compared with women and infants in the C group villages.

In the context of current sociopolitical situation in Nepal (a civil war), it was remarkable that the program and evaluation were successfully implemented. In fact, it is very likely that the presence of a war would usually compromise the fidelity of intervention delivery and results. While security problems forced postponement of some women's group meetings, it did not cause groups to ever disband. It is unlikely that these **historical biasing** events impacted the results. The results support the investigators' contention that interventions using health education and participatory communication techniques can be used in resource-poor and politically unsettled regions. The outcome differences were probably an underestimate of intervention effectiveness.

Because the study applied a group randomized design, two issues need to be examined: randomization at the group level does not assure the same level of minimization of confounders as individual randomization, and delivery of the intervention to groups rather than individuals does minimize threats of contamination. Slight differences in the E and C groups were observed, but do not explain the significant reduction in mortality. The villages were a representative sample of the eligible sites for the evaluation. Thus, **selection bias** was an implausible explanation for impact. Because it is very unlikely that the death of an infant or mother would not be counted, **measurement bias** was not perceived as a plausible explanation for the results.

These findings, and other studies like it, for example, Tripathy, Mair, Barnett, et al., "Effect of a Participatory Intervention With Women's Group," *Lancet* (March 2010), in Jharkhand and Orissa, India, provide strong and consistent evidence that maternal and infant health can be substantially improved at a very low cost. *The Millennium Development Goals for maternal and child mortality can only be achieved by disseminating these types of acceptable, effective, efficient, and sustainable health education, consensus building, and community-based interventions.*

## Summary

In evaluating the impact of HP-DP programs, there are many critical methodological issues to address. The time frame, resources, and capabilities of a program need to be considered prior to selecting a design or methods. While a number of designs exist, only a few are really useful for a program evaluation. Four designs were identified: a One-Group Pre-test and Post-test, a Non-Randomized Comparison Group, a Time Series, and a Randomized Pre-test and Post-test with Control Croup. In deciding what design to implement, an evaluation team needs to appreciate the strengths and weaknesses of each. *An evaluation team also needs to blend the application of CBPR and PBPR methods and philosophy in its planning and organizational development. As noted by multiple examples in this chapter, when CBPR and PBPR methods were applied successfully, the evidence produced for each specific problem and target groups can be translated into future HP-DP practices to "improve population health."*

There are a very small number of ways to establish a C or (C) group that are equivalent at a baseline observation. Although, at first glance, using a randomized design may seem impossible, careful thought about the key questions to be answered, combined with a consultation and literature review, may provide insight into the use of a (C) group instead of a C group in evaluating a program. Regardless of the design applied, the degree of comparability of study groups at baseline and at follow-up must be established. Because designs play a prominent role in increasing the probability of a demonstrable effect and in determining significant observations, it is essential to estimate effect sizes, and the needed sample size for each group during planning. This issue has critical implications for the budget and timeline of all evaluations. These issues and the quality and completeness of evaluation measures are of paramount importance. While all issues represent challenges that each evaluation faces, this chapter has described how each issue can be addressed. In summary, the theory and applications discussed in this chapter represent an essential body of information that program evaluation leadership and staff should know and should be able to apply to plan, manage, and evaluate any HP-DP program.

# 4 | Measurement and Analysis in Evaluation

Those who cannot remember the past
are condemned to repeat it.

—*George Santayana*

## Introduction

In Chapter 3 (Efficacy and Effectiveness Evaluation), *measurement, selection*, and *history* are identified as the first of three primary threats to the internal validity of evaluation results. *Measurement and confirmation of the validity, reliability, and representativeness of data are the most critical methodological issues every evaluation must address.* A major responsibility in planning a HP-DP program is identifying measures and instruments to document predictor, process, impact, and outcome rates. Evaluators need to select and apply methods to eliminate measurement error as a plausible explanation of observed significant differences. Evaluators need to be thoroughly knowledgeable about measurement science, reflecting well-defined global ("gold") standards and methods to establish data validity. Multiple basic issues need to be considered in selecting the type and frequency of evaluation measures. In this chapter we introduce salient principles of measurement, review data collection procedures, and introduce selected analysis methods and case studies to document impact data and scale validity and reliability.

# Measurement and Data Collection

## Concepts, Constructs, and Variables

Planning an evaluation of an intervention, especially **PHASE 1** and **2** evaluations, is best approached using a *conceptual framework*. Using a conceptual framework means that a theory or, at a less formal level, a planning model is selected to hypothetically explain how the program and its core intervention were designed to change behavior. The PRECEDE/ PROCEED Model by Green and Kreuter (2004) discussed in Chapter 2 is a good example. A conceptual framework provides logical steps and components to select salient measures and an intervention for an evaluation. A model will describe the types of variables that need to be measured and the types of data to be produced. A model is based on one or more theories that describe expected relationships between two or more variables. A theory or model should (1) identify a set of core variables unique to the theory that need to be measured, (2) explain/hypothesize how the variables selected are expected to be significantly associated with each other, and (3) explain how the major variables of the model should be predictive of a dependent impact or outcome rate. A **Theory-Based Evaluation** (TBE) should be conducted in PHASE 1 and 2 evaluations for a specific problem and population.

If the program is based on a theory or model, it should be evaluated against the underlying variables/constructs of the theory or model. Social cognitive theory (SCT; Bandura, 1986) is frequently used by health promotion and disease prevention programs, and has been tested for various problems and populations. If SCT, for example, is selected for use by an HP-DP project, the evaluation must include measurements of constructs such as self-efficacy. This is necessary because analyses may reveal that changes did not occur in one or more primary dependent variables, thereby decreasing the probability of behavior changes. Selecting a model is both an empirical and a creative process. A planning and evaluation team tries to design interventions that effectively translate underlying theoretical constructs (concepts) of behavioral science theory and measurement scales into professional practice.

Members of a planning and evaluation team may ask, why a theory or model is necessary. There are several reasons. A behavioral intervention program and evaluations should be based on what is known about theories of behavior for specific health problems, populations at risk, and practice settings. The primary purposes of social and behavioral science research are to conduct basic and applied surveys and evaluations to improve an understanding of behavior. If the science base for a problem is at least moderately well developed, a meta-evaluation and meta-analysis may provide this type of insight. Valid research should help a team to decide how specific behaviors might be positively changed among a target group. Behavioral science theory may also provide a framework in which results across evaluation studies can be synthesized to improve comprehension of how to change human behavior. A Theory-Based Evaluation (TBE) should provide a foundation for thinking and should give direction about what to measure, as well as defining steps to enhance reaching a final objective. It may document the cause(s) of behavior change: theory validation.

If a theoretical model is validated by basic laboratory and applied behavioral research, then a program should have more confidence that the theory applied is more likely to provide valid data and insights about plans to change behavior among its target population. HP-DP programs should have a higher probability of being effective, if they are based on the most valid theories and models of health behavior change. *It is also important, however, to understand that the validity of a behavior change model may be strong for a specific disease, behavior, or population at risk, but weak for other diseases, groups of people, or locations.* While adult females with high blood pressure in Chicago, St. Louis, and Detroit in the United States, or London, Manchester, and York in England, may have large similarities, they are also likely to have large baseline differences that predict behavior change. Direct evidence and data from a representative sample of a target population form the multiple evaluations that are needed to support the evaluation of a behavior change model.

In the majority of cases, a behavioral intervention program is typically based on a combination of theory, experience, judgment, and available resources. A common mistake identified in systematic reviews of the social and behavioral science literature, however, is the poor quality of measurement of major constructs of a model, and/or the erroneous use of a model or its instruments without appropriate psychometric and factor analyses of validity and reliability. *One behavioral model or instrument does not fit all health problems, risk factors, or populations.*

A number of constructs in HP-DP theories focus on psycho-social variables and their effect on changing behavior. The unique nature of behavioral interventions poses special challenges to measurement. For example, a core construct of social cognitive theory is self-efficacy: the perception of how confident a person feels about performing a specific activity. Such measures are much more difficult to measure compared to an observable behavior or a standardized biochemical test. Biochemical variables or the behavior, for example, blood pressure control or smoking status, can be directly measured. Psycho-social constructs, however, are likely to be pivotal in changing an individual's behavior, and are an essential part of measurement in a program evaluation. An evaluator has to decide which constructs to measure, how these constructs can be translated into a set of items, and identify valid and reliable tools to measure each construct.

A meta-evaluation related to an evaluation of a problem among a population may identify specific types of impact and outcome data that a project must collect to provide convincing evidence of an effect. A thorough literature review is essential to identify established predictor measures and scales, and their applicability to the problem and population of interest. Valid and complete data on each dependent and independent variable for all participants is needed to compute rates and levels of change, and to assess important relationships over time. An evaluation needs to differentiate between independent and dependent variables. Independent variables, such as self-efficacy, may be predictive measures of the impact or outcome rate(s). Dependent variables or rates from a sample of a population at risk are the impact measures that an intervention is trying to change. The dependent variable may be the behavior itself or a health status outcome or indicator that documents the level of health status of a person or a defined population.

As noted, SCT is an extensively applied model in the HP-DP literature to try to explain people's behavior. Consider, for example, a model that hypothesizes how adults with Type 2 diabetes can have very good control over this condition, increasing self-efficacy, by learning to lower calories from dietary fat or sugar, by losing weight, and by increasing their physical activity each week. The model diagrammed in Figure 4.1, based on SCT (Bandura, 1977), proposes that the probability that a person will reduce fat or sugar intake in a diet and walk more often is related to multiple variables: increasing self-efficacy or perceived self-confidence at being able to perform the behaviors; changing his or her preference and selection of low-fat and/or low-sugar foods; changing environmental-social support and reinforcements to not buy, consume, or serve specific foods; and becoming more physically active each week.

According to the SCT, a patient education program should be designed to increase patient preference, behavioral capability, and self-efficacy for fat-sugar reduction among the high-risk group. It should also increase support in the family and social group to select and purchase low-fat and

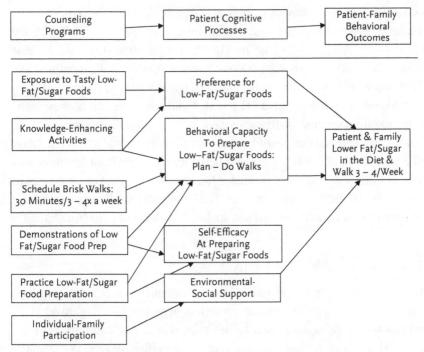

| Counseling Programs | → | Patient Cognitive Processes | → | Patient-Family Behavioral Outcomes |

FIGURE 4.1 Social Cognitive Theory (SCT) Diagram

low-sugar products and to schedule more physical activity each week. The SCT model hypothesizes relationships between four categories: (1) the basic concepts or building blocks for an intervention program; (2) types of variables to measure; (3) specific components of the intervention; and (4) specific directions for action.

The direct method to evaluate the impact of a program based on this model would be to measure dietary fat and sugar consumption by the target group, using a 24-hour food recall questionnaire, and physical activity, using a 7-day activity questionnaire. Although expensive, a variety of analyses of biological samples (blood or urine) could be applied to measure fat and sugars. The initial participant and family behavior would be to prepare and use a written list and menu of items to select and buy low-fat and low-sugar or no-fat and no-sugar products. Each patient would also be asked to prepare a weekly schedule and to complete a walking diary each week, documenting a 30–40 minute brisk walk/day, for three to four days per week. The evaluation would measure self-efficacy to determine its relationship to achieving changes in behavior.

The family would be involved in a discussion of how to routinely support the person with diabetes to gain control. If the study's objective is to know whether the behavior change was "predictive" of the hypothesized model, the group's preferences, behavioral capability, and self-efficacy for low-salt foods need to be measured at a baseline (O1) and at least three follow-ups at 3 months (O2), 6 months (O3), and 12 months (O4). A measure of hemoglobin A1C, the biological marker for diabetes control, would be documented at O1 to O4. Valid measurement of these variables requires specific instruments and methods to collect essential data. This is an explicit example of how to use a theory in evaluation planning. The evaluation not only focuses on behaviors and resulting health condition, but also measures and evaluates the change and level of predictors in psycho-social factors. This kind of TBE can validate the use of specific components of an intervention and its level of effect in behavior change.

## Instruments and Measurement

The word *instrument* is typically used to identify a method to produce a numerical measure of specific variables: demographic, cognitive, skill, psycho-social, behavioral, and health-related status or conditions. In the physical sciences, an instrument refers to a machine, device, or standardized method designed to produce and consistently reproduce very accurate and meaningful scores or numbers. Although at times an evaluation may use a machine as an instrument to measure behavior change, evaluations almost always have a sequence of questions, with numerical, pre-coded response alternatives, to measure a variety of types of participant characteristics. These sets of questions are also called *instruments*" Instruments are sometimes also referred to as *tools*. The questions in the instrument, or tool, are called *items*. A set of items is created to measure a construct or elements of a construct.

A *construct* (e.g., self-esteem) is a term used to identify a psycho-social variable composed of a set of basic elements that represents it. *A "construct" can also be called a "latent variable": it is not directly observable.* We infer a degree of quality or value-score from the responses to each specific question. It is *variable* because the response-score selected by each person will vary by the construct of interest, time, and by the target population. Through an iterative process, a *universe* of questions are drafted to define the elements. Psychometric analyses, including factor analyses and scale and item internal consistency and stability analyses, establish the basic validity and reliability of the items and elements of a construct. The application of these analytical methods need to be derived from assessments of > 100 eligible participants.

The numbers that come from applying the instrument to a person are called *measures*. Two or more instruments or items may produce or attempt to produce the same measure, for example, reports of smoking status, a urinary cotinine test, or an exhaled carbon monoxide test. The instrument includes not only the specific questions, but also instructions to the user or interviewer to ask the questions or probe initial responses. Procedures for eliciting responses and producing numbers to produce the measure are well defined and replicable. The terms *instrument* and *measure* are often used interchangeably in discussions of measurement categories. In this chapter, *instrument* will be used primarily to refer to a set of items and procedures that measure human characteristics.

The development of an instrument is a science and an art. Evaluators need to be well versed both in the core content of the area, for example, diabetes care, smoking cessation, child development, and so on, and in psychometric methods and analysis. Care and diligence should be involved in creating items for any psycho-social instrument, with a number of steps involving many experts both in the content area and in psychometrics. Windsor, Cleary, Ramiah, and Abroms, *Maternal and Child Journal* (2013), developed a scale, discussed later in this chapter, to measure the perceived attributes of routine use by regular nurses and social workers of an AHRQ evidence-based smoking cessation program for patients. A scale, **the Smoking Cessation and Reduction In Pregnancy Treatment (SCRIPT) Adoption Scale (SAS)**, was developed by a systematic review of the "Diffusion of Innovation" literature, item creation and review by expert panels, two surveys of the population of clinical users of the SAS, and factor and psychometric analyses of the data from the surveys.

In the application of the systematic process, the evaluation team established face and content validity. Two expert panels were used to develop the SAS instrument. The SAS development process, administration, and psychometric analysis will be a useful reference for "How to Develop a Theory-Based Scale." If a valid and reliable instrument for measuring variables of interest exists for a specific problem and population, it may be an excellent candidate scale to start the process. However, an evaluator should not use a developed instrument or measurement blindly without adaptation and pilot-testing.

An excellent meta-evaluation of psychometric methods and quality of 967 studies is presented by Barry, Chaney, Piazza-Gardner, and Chavarria, "Validity and Reliability Reporting Practices in the Field of Health Education and Behavior: A Review of Seven Journals,"

*Health Education and Behavior* (2013), 12–18. This article reviewed the application of standard psychometric methods for the seven professional journals for only a four-year period. It confirmed that only 25% of the studies presented data on the validity of their measures.

*This HEB review and many other reviews confirm the deplorable lack of scientific methods and inconsistent application of "gold standard" practices in health education, health promotion, and the social and behavioral sciences. The validity and reliability of all measures and existing scales must be re-evaluated for each new HP-DP program and population. Reader beware: Publication and peer review are not clear indicators of the quality and validity of data and/or results of an HP-DP evaluation.*

## Types of Variables

Multiple types or categories of variables can be measured to describe the characteristics of samples of a population at risk. The following categories of variables are the most commonly measured by HP-DP programs:

- Demographic
- Cognitive
- Skill
- Psycho-social
- Behavioral
- Environmental
- Health status
- Cost (discussed in Chapter 6).

### Demographic Variables

Demographic variables describe the social characteristics of populations, such as age, gender, race-ethnicity, occupation, and education level. These types of data and characteristics of people are usually not changeable, or at least not during an evaluation. Demographic variables, almost always classified as independent variables, separate people into common groups useful for assessing differences in program impact (efficacy) or to define the population to which an evaluation's results can be generalized (effectiveness). These data are essential to define who participated in your program, and who refused, and for comparison to similar groups in other programs, or to the population at risk. These data document to whom a program was delivered or not (potential selection biases). Demographic data document the representativeness of the evaluation study sample. The remaining categories of data, typically dependent variables, represent categories or types of data used to document changes in rates over time: process, impact, or outcome data.

### Cognitive Variables

Cognitive variables can be labeled *knowledge* variables. Measures of a person's health-disease-related knowledge assume a correct or incorrect answer. A knowledge score is derived for each participant based on multiple item responses: the higher the percentage of correct answers, the more knowledgeable the person. Health information data are commonly used to confirm levels of a target audience's awareness of a problem, program or activity, for example, the risks and harm of smoking and the benefits of cessation. Whether a percentage of people in your target area know that a problem or program exists is an essential type of data to design or refine a health communication and education campaign. Cognitive assessments may also measure the product of a mental process, for example, a person's ability to synthesize, analyze and/or apply knowledge related to a problem and solutions. The person synthesizes and interprets health information, processes its psycho-social and affective content, makes a conclusion, and/ or makes a positive or negative behavioral decision to take care of himself or herself, or a family member.

### Skill Variables

Skill or capacity variables represent a person's ability to perform a task; how well can a person perform a specific self-care behavior(s)? Like knowledge, there is a correct and incorrect answer, and a skill score is produced. Assessment of skill measures is important, because people cannot effectively perform the behavior or task daily/routinely at home unless they can demonstrate the skill in an assessment setting. For example, persons with Type 2 diabetes need to know how to and when to monitor glucose/sugar in their blood, how to respond to high or low levels and, if necessary, how to inject insulin. Persons with asthma need specific skills to use their inhaler, to manage and control their condition, and to respond to an asthma attack. Just because a person knows how to do it, however, does not necessarily mean that he or she will perform the task routinely. Does the person exhibit behavioral adherence to a self-care treatment?

## Psycho-Social Variables

This category measures psychological and sociological concepts, often called *constructs*, for example, adult health beliefs, self-efficacy, or social support. Attitude and belief variables or scales are developed to measure the feelings, opinions, and perceptions of people about specific health-related issues. Psycho-social constructs are not directly measured. Attitudes are considered to have three core components: (1) a strongly positive to strongly negative belief (scale 1 to 5) about a specific content or subject area, (2) a strongly positive to strongly negative value (scale 1 to 5) about the belief, and (3) a strongly positive to strongly negative predisposition (scale 1 to 5) to routinely act or behave. Psycho-social measures are collected using a representative series of questions related to the subject-content. A standardized scale of 1 to 5 or 1 to 10, positive to negative, attempts to assess the strength of these constructs among participants in an HP-DP evaluation.

## Behavioral Variables

All HP-DP programs are concerned with specific health-related behaviors: smoking cessation, drug treatment adherence, patient appointment keeping, or increasing weekly physical activity. Routine performance of a behavior reflects whether or not, or how frequently, one or more important behaviors are performed daily. Is the hypertensive patient regularly consuming fewer high-salt foods or taking her prescribed medications? Has the family with a new baby established a nonsmoking policy in a home? Is the diabetic's urine tested for blood sugar? Health screening or service utilization variables, a subcategory of behavioral measures, are used to describe behavioral patterns of clients in the use of health, medical or social services. What kinds of people use specific services, when are they using them, and how frequently?

## Environmental Variables

The physical or emotional environment in which an individual lives affects behavior and health. A wide range of environmental factors, for example, air, water, or other physical objects, may present major risks to individuals and communities. The social environment in which people live will also promote or inhibit exposure to positive or negative risks. For example, a safe neighborhood with access to bike trails, community activity/fitness centers, parks, and so on, enhances the physical activity of the community, whereas a community with a high crime rate, lack of a fitness center in close proximity, or lack of playgrounds and parks will hinder the physical activity of children in these communities. Other variables under this category include public policies, change in law, and so on. Some researchers refer to these categories as *ecological variables*. An evaluator may measure changes in the environment that are likely to predict or affect the behaviors or outcomes of interest.

### Health Status Indicators-Variables

Health (clinical or biological) variables may be used for multiple purposes: a health status outcome measure, or a change in the level of risk. Blood pressure control and reduction in elevated levels is a primary measure of the impact of a hypertension management program. High levels of high-density lipoprotein (HDL) cholesterol in blood protect against heart attacks and provide an estimate of the amount of regular exercise and physical activity. An evaluator may want to assess serum HDL cholesterol or triglycerides as a screen for whether a person should receive a counseling and exercise intervention. A saliva or urine cotinine analysis score confirms reports of smoking status.

### Variable Summary

There are an infinite number of variables to select for measurement by each evaluation. Each variable and measurement may have unique methods that must be known to the evaluation team. Each evaluation team must thoroughly understand the **measurement science** of each variable. Rather than focus on all possible variables, an evaluation should be very selective in choosing which to measure: high data quality, not quantity, should be the philosophy and objective of an evaluation. A thorough meta-analysis of the literature and expert consultation will define what variables are the **core** items that must be measured. As noted in Chapters 1 and 2, an HP-DP evaluation should define a very small number of high priority objectives and define the gold standard of measurement for each objective. **Ask:** Why are we collecting these types of data? How are we going to analyze the data on for each type of process, impact, or outcome variable? How can we achieve a 100% baseline and a > 90% follow-up assessment rate for core variables?

## Systematic and Random Error

There are two types of measurement errors: systematic and random. Bias and error reduces or destroys measurement validity. Bias is the distance between the true response and mean of the obtained responses. A good measurement tool should try to measure a variable as close to its *true* value. But it is almost impossible to measure the true value, even with biological values, because there is always some amount of error. An evaluator needs to plan, plot test, and implement methods to reduce the amount of error—both random and systematic error. Random error randomly affects measurement of the variable. But the positive interpretation about random error is that it does not have any consistent effects across the sample. In other words, the sum of all random error will be 0. Thus it does not change the conclusion of the study, but adds random (non-systematic) "noise" to the data and its values.

Systematic error is the major bias in measurement: values tend to be consistently positive or negative. A biased measure may lead an evaluation to make a different conclusion on a set of data for an impact rate than it would make if it had the true measure. Of course, evaluators do not usually know the true value, although it may sometimes be defined in the literature.

**Measurement bias** will always occur when not enough thought went into instrument development, if all measures and methods are not pilot tested, or the instrument was not used with care and attention to detail by assessors or participants. The assessment of the validity of an instrument is more difficult than the study of its reliability. Using the same instrument at two different times or with two observers (reliability) at the same time is relatively easy. Establishing validity requires an evaluation to obtain or to develop multiple measures of the dependent-impact-outcome variables and associated rates to determine which is the most accurate.

The assessment of salt in the diet provides an excellent example of potential, large measurement error. Because high salt intake is positively associated with high blood pressure (hypertension), a hypertensive control program may need instruments and methods to measure salt intake. A relatively accurate measure, not subject to self-report errors and biases, is an assessment of the sodium excreted in the urine. There is high day-to-day variability, however, in an individual's salt consumption because of the lag time between episodes of unusually high salt ingestion and a body's achievement of sodium balance. Several studies have estimated that an evaluator might need seven consecutive days of 24-hour urine samples to estimate regular salt consumption. Difficulties will arise in obtaining these samples. People do not want to carry urine sample bottles to work or to other activities because it is embarrassing and inconvenient. Multiple containers are needed to collect urine. They must be sterile, and urine must be collected at regular intervals. People will forget to provide every sample. The cost per individual would also be very expensive.

Multiple studies have been conducted to assess whether an overnight urine sample, testing for sodium and creatinine, can obtain similar information and replace the tedious and expensive 24-hour urine samples. Other investigators have used self-report measures of dietary consumption. In both cases, however, the seven consecutive days of 24-hour urine samples probably provides the criterion against which all measures of salt intake are assessed—"the gold standard"—because it was the more accurate and more valid measure of the variable desired.

## Validity

*Validity* is the degree to which an instrument measures what it is supposed to measure. Validity is also the extent of concordance between a measure and an underlying theoretical variable. Four types of validity, *face, content, criterion, and construct*, are presented in Table 4.1.

All evaluation must establish the validity (accuracy) and reliability (reproducibility) of data collected in measuring the eight categories of data noted in the introduction.

### Face Validity

Face validity, a dimension of content validity, describes the extent to which an instrument appears to measure what it is supposed to measure. Thus, the question, "How many minutes of exercise did you do today?" appears to measure one important component of aerobic activity for a particular day. This question may or may not produce good data for adults. This question would not be an accurate estimate of physical activity duration if young children were asked this question.

If an evaluation needs to assess aerobic activity that has cardiovascular benefit, a person must engage in aerobic activity for ≥ 20 minutes at a time (without stopping), for ≥ 3+ times every week. The activity must reach a certain intensity level, a heartbeat ≥ 60% of a maximum rate, calculated from commonly available tables for age and gender groups, to promote

TABLE 4.1 Definition of Types of Validity

| TYPE | DEFINITION |
|---|---|
| Face | The extent to which the instrument appears to measure what it is supposed to measure. |
| Content | The extent to which an instrument samples items from the full range of content. |
| Criterion | The extent to which a new instrument correlates with another more accurate (and usually more expensive) instrument (the criterion). |
| Concurrent | The extent to which the scores from two instruments or sub-scales are correlated. |
| Predictive | The extent to which an instrument administered during one time period can predict changes in a prospectively assessed criterion measure or rate. |
| Construct | The extent to which the measure of concern correlates with other measures in predicted ways, but no true criterion exists. |
| Convergent | The measure correlates with items with which it is predicted to correlate. |
| Discriminant | The measure does not correlate with items with which it is expected not to correlate. |

CVD fitness. Thus, it may be difficult to interpret an intensity response from the above.

Suppose the answer a person gives is "≥ 30 minutes." Was the activity sufficiently intense to merit the label "aerobic"? Did the person cover 4 miles (excellent CUD benefit) or 2 miles (modest CUD benefit) in 30 minutes? Were the 30 minutes in one block or two 15-minute segments? Each variation raises issues about whether the question elicits accurate data. You will need to create a self-report measure for adults to assess distance traveled, intensity (e.g., heart rate), and continuous duration of activity (segments in minutes). A measure, therefore, must be carefully written to assess impact. Face validity is a small first step toward overall validity of the instrument. As there is no quantitative measurement to face validity, experts are consulted.

## Content Validity

Most instruments measure multiple content domains. An instrument must sample items from each of the salient content areas to have content validity. Diabetes self-care and disease management is a complex activity requiring knowledge, skill, family support, and routine behavior in multiple content areas. Windsor and colleagues developed a standardized instrument to measure diabetic patients' self-care instruction, knowledge, skill, and daily self-care behavior. After an initial internal review of several drafts of an instrument by local, university diabetes care experts (MDs/RNs), this evaluation project used an external, expert panel of clinical diabetologists and behavioral scientists to validate the internal reviews of instrument content and items. The internal and external expert panels identified seven content areas for a diabetes self-care instruction and counseling program: (1) foot-skin care, (2) urine testing, (3) diet, (4) self-administration of insulin, (5) safety measures, (6) complications and use of medical services, and (7) self-care information.

Multiple knowledge and performance-skill questions/items were developed for each area. A sample of items within each major area of concern in diabetes self-care was written. Because of its completeness, as documented by a comprehensiveness literature review and internal expert panel review, this instrument has high content validity. If all of these content areas are positively associated, they would be documenting *concurrent validity*. If these measures of self-care are positively associated with reduced diabetes associated healthcare utilization, they would have *predictive validity*. As years pass, however, and more evidence is produced about diabetes, diabetic patients will be expected to do more or different things for themselves. The content validity of parts of an instrument may decrease. The instrument needs further development and refinement. Thus, the content, criterion, concurrent, and predictive validity of an instrument is time-limited. As a measurement science base matures, a disease-specific instrument needs updating.

For the SCRIPT Adoption Scale (SAS) in Table 4.6 below, 75 items were created using the five core adoption attribute domains defined by Rogers (1995): Relative Advantage, Compatibility, Complexity, Trialability, and Observability. After an internal expert panel review, 59 items were sent for an external expert panel review. This process documented SAS face and content validity. Following the second review by an internal expert panel, a 43-item SAS was administered to the target population of providers: 45 RNs and 40 LSWs. As presented in the case study in this chapter, factor analyses confirmed the construct validity of a five-factor, 28-item SAS instrument.

## Criterion Validity

There are instruments or measures that produce the most accurate data of a human characteristic. These measures use explicit methods and "criteria" to confirm the presence, absence, or degree of a variable. They are typically referred to as "the gold standard." Criterion validity may be assessed by using the two measures at the same time (*concurrent-criterion validity*) or by using a measure of a variable at one time to predict the measure of the variable using another measure at the second time (*predictive-criterion validity*). The process and analysis assessed in the development of the script adoption scale (SAS) documented concurrent validity.

Many variables have multiple methods of measurement with different levels of validity. If the correlation (validity coefficients) between values or scores that the two measures produces is high and produces an $r > 0.80$, the criterion validity of the second instrument or measure can be considered adequate. It can be used to assess groups of participants in an evaluation study. If the correlation is very high ($r \geq 0.95$), it may be used for individual assessments. Not all content areas, however, have "gold standard" measurements. In such scenarios, proxy measures could be used.

## Measures of the Validity of a Biological-Physical Test

There are four measures of validity to be considered for an existing or new physical measure: (1) sensitivity, (2) specificity, (3) predictive value (+), and (4) predictive value (-). Table 4.2 represents a sample of individuals who have been examined with a screening test for disease (rows) and a definitive diagnostic test (columns). A program can determine how well one test or measure performed in identifying individuals with or without a disease, risk factor, or behavior.

TABLE 4.2 Measuring the Validity of a Test or Measure

| TEST | PRESENT | ABSENT | TOTAL | PREDICTIVE VALIDITY |
|------|---------|--------|-------|---------------------|
| Positive | a = True Positives | b = False Positives | a + b | **Predictive Value (+)** $$\frac{a}{a+b}$$ |
| Negative | c = False Negatives | d = True Negatives | c + d | **Predictive Value (−)** $$\frac{d}{c+d}$$ |
| Total | a + c | b + d | Grand Total: a + b + c + d | |
| | **Sensitivity** $$\frac{a}{a+c}$$ | **Specificity** $$\frac{d}{b+d}$$ | | |

*Sensitivity* describes the accuracy of a test to identify correctly all screened individuals who actually have the disease or behavior. It is defined as the number of true positives divided by the sum of the true positives and false negatives. In Table 4.2, a total of a + c individuals are determined to have the condition, according to an established definitive measurement ("gold standard"). Suppose in a sample of 100, 12 had the disease. If the measure correctly identified all 12 cases, the sensitivity would be 100%. If the measure did not identify all individuals who exhibited the condition or behavior, then sensitivity would be less than 100%.

*Specificity* describes the ability of the test to identify only individuals who actually do not have the disease or condition. It is defined as the number of true negatives divided by the sum of false positives and true negatives. If a measure is not specific, individuals who do not actually have the condition or exhibit the behavior will be referred for additional assessment.

*Predictive value* (+) is the proportion of individuals screened positive by the measure who actually have the disease or condition. Predictive value (+) is the proportion a/(a + b) who actually have the condition as confirmed by the "gold standard" measure.

*Predictive value* (-) is an analogous measure for those screened negative by the measure; it is designated by the formula d/(c + d). It describes the proportion that does not have a condition, as confirmed by the "gold standard" measure. The only time these measures can be estimated is when the same group of individuals has been examined using the program measure-test and gold standard measure. The accuracy of a screening test is computed by the following formula: (a + d)/(a + b + c + d). Accuracy measures the degree of agreement between the program measure and "gold standard" measure. The same concept of sensitivity and specificity may be used in social and behavioral measurements in some situations.

## Validity Example

Multiple evaluation studies of smoking and pregnancy in the literature have documented the high levels of inaccuracy and bias from patient self-reports at their first obstetrical visit. Most studies have confirmed patient self-reports of smoking status by a urine or saliva cotinine test.

Hypothetical data in Tables 4.3 and 4.4 document the degree of accuracy of self-reports of smoking behavior by a sample of 400 pregnant women at their first prenatal care visit. A saliva cotinine (S-COT)

TABLE 4.3 Sensitivity-Specificity-Positive Predictive Value for Pregnant Women

| SALIVA COTININE TEST | BEHAVIOR PRESENT—YES | BEHAVIOR ABSENT—NO | TOTAL |
|---|---|---|---|
| > 20 ng/ml (+) | 300 Patients | 40 Patients | 340 Patients |
| < 19 ng/ml (−) | 40 Patients | 20 Patients | 60 Patients |

TABLE 4.4 Self-reported CPD and Saliva Cotinine Exposure Levels

| CPD | N PATIENTS | MEAN S-COT | R | F | P |
|---|---|---|---|---|---|
| A. 1–10 | 100 | 141 ng/mL | 0.20 | 6.00 | 0.01 |
| B. 11–20 | 100 | 171 ng/mL | 0.25 | | |
| C. 21–30 | 100 | 180 ng/mL | 0.25 | | |
| D. Total | 300 | 163 ng/mL | 0.30 | | |

CPD = cigarettes per day; ng/mL = nanograms per milliliters

test, the independent criterion validity measure, is compared to patient self-reports. A cotinine value ≥ 20 ng/mL was defined in the literature to be the cutoff to document active smoking. Data in Table 4.4 indicated that the self-report plus the S-COT test were needed to determine, with a high degree of accuracy, the women's smoking status: PPV = 94%. The deception rate of this patient example (40/340) was 11.8%. Data in Table 4.3, based on the first 100 patients in each CPD group from the sample of 400, also confirmed a very weak or lack of association between the number of cigarettes smoked per day (CPD) by patients and the biochemical-cotinine values: $r = 0.10/0.05/0.15$. *Patient reports of CPD are very inaccurate.*

The mean cotinine value of these patients was not statistically different until you compared the cotinine values of CPD Group A (141 ng/mL) to those of CPD Group C (180 ng/mL). This methodology and type of pilot-test study needs to be conducted prior to the start of all evaluations to establish the validity of each core measure/variable, especially the dependent variables/rates. For an example using actual data, see Webb, Boyd, Messina, and Windsor, "The Discrepancy Between Self-Reported Smoking Status and Urine Cotinine Levels Among Women Enrolled in Prenatal Care at Four Publicly Funded Clinical Sites," *Journal of Public Health Management Practice* (2003).

## Measurement Validity: Patient Knowledge and Self-Care Skill Case Study 1

A measurement study was conducted at the Diabetes Hospital of the University of Alabama to assess the quality of patient education assessment methods and instruments for 100 Type 2 adult onset diabetic patients at admission. As noted in the discussion of content validity, a multidimensional instrument and measures were developed. Content validity was established by internal and external reviews by medical-nursing experts in diabetology.

The multitrait-multimethod approach was used to confirm the validity (Campell and Fiske, 1959) of different assessment measures and methods; for example, urine knowledge (UK) versus urine testing skill (UP), measured by different methods, for example, patient interview versus patient observation, were used. Associations between a characteristic, for example, urine testing knowledge, and a criterion, urine testing skill or routine testing behavior, for the same individual at one point in time, were documented. Data in Table 4.5 confirmed strong, direct relationships between past patient urine testing instruction (UI), urine testing knowledge (UK), ability to perform urine testing (UP), and self-reported, routine-urine testing behavior (UB). Within the concept area (trait) of urine testing assessment, all concurrent validity coefficients were much more strongly

TABLE 4.5 Validity Coefficient for Clinical Test Data of Diabetes Patients

| TRAIT | COGNITIVE INDEX | PERFORMANCE INDEX (PI) | URINE INSTRUCTION (UI) | URINE KNOWLEDGE (UK) | URINE TESTING PERFORMANCE (UP) | URINE TESTING BEHAVIOR (UB) |
|---|---|---|---|---|---|---|
| PI | 0.60 | | | | | |
| UI | 0.34 | 0.41 | | | | |
| UK | 0.80 | 0.64 | 0.42 | | | |
| UP | 0.56 | 0.82 | 0.39 | 0.65 | | |
| UB | 0.36 | 0.53 | 0.47 | 0.52 | 0.59 | |
| II | 0.34 | 0.32 | 0.66 | 0.37 | 0.29 | 0.31 |
| IK | 0.71 | 0.34 | 0.15* | 0.43 | 0.44 | 0.15* |
| IP | 0.31 | 0.67 | 0.32 | 0.26 | 0.45 | 0.23 |
| IB | 0.24 | 0.32 | 0.14* | 0.21 | 0.30 | 0.19* |
| DI | 0.42 | 0.20 | 0.45 | 0.38 | 0.14* | 0.24 |
| DK | 0.57 | 0.40 | 0.10* | 0.24 | 0.31 | 0.07* |
| DP | 0.46 | 0.50 | 0.09* | 0.27 | 0.27 | 0.13* |
| DB | 0.13* | 0.17* | 0.11* | 0.19* | 0.14* | 0.12* |

* Did not meet minimum item analysis criteria: r > = 0.20

IB: Insulin Testing Behavior; DI: Diabetes Instruction; DK: Diabetes Knowledge; DP: Diabetes Testing Performance; DB: Diabetes Testing Behavior inter-correlated within (r = 0.42, 0.39, 0.47, 0.65, 0.52, 0.59) urine mea-surement area (UI-UK-UP-UB) than for other content areas, for example, insulin testing instructions (II), insulin knowledge (IK), and insulin per-formance (IP). Data for the concept area (trait) in urine testing measure-ment, patient skill, and regular testing provided support for the concurrent validity of the instrument.

Statistically significant (> 0.01) moderately strong validity coefficients, blocked section, were found between the total diabetes knowledge and per-formance index scores, r = 0.60, and within subject areas, foot care instruc-tion and foot inspection behavior (r = 0.41), insulin instruction and insulin behavior (r = 0.50), and urine instruction and urine behavior (r = 0.34). Multiple positive associations were also documented (r ≥ 0.20) between overall self-care knowledge and performance for two core traits: UI-UK-UP-UB and II-IK-IS-IB. The results of these analyses provided good evidence of validity for selected diabetic patient self-management traits. Predictive validity, the strength of the validity coefficients significantly associated with reduced use of physician and/or hospital services for dia-betes care, was not assessed.

## Construct Validity: Factor Analysis

As knowledge of a variety of concepts, for example, depression and self-efficacy, increases, investigators learn more about how specific measures should relate to other measures. These relationships help to define the underlying construct, which cannot be directly measured. For example, people experiencing a high degree of stress should experience a variety of physiological responses, for example, rapid heartbeat and breathing, high blood pressure, and changed galvanic skin response, and are expected to be less efficient at cognitive tasks, such as memory and judgment. If an investigator believes that an existing stress measure is inadequate because it is highly related to some other variable not related to stress, she or he might develop and test the construct validity of a new instrument.

The investigator would expect to document two results. First, the new measure should correlate more highly with the physiological or cogni-tive changes (convergent validity) than the old measure. Second, the new stress measure should correlate less well with variables not related to stress (discriminant validity) than the old measure. If the new instrument demonstrates such convergent and discriminant validity, it is considered to have higher construct validity than the old measure. Good support for the construct validity of the diabetes assessment instrument presented in Table 4.5 was found. Significantly higher scores on the cognitive index, self-reported daily behavior, and the performance-skills indexes were noted for patients with higher levels of education, with more extensive exposure to diabetes education programs, and among patients who perceived little need for additional instruction. Construct validity also examines, by correlation analysis, hypothesized relationships between variables specified by a theory (see Figure 4.1).

## Case Study 2: Factor Analysis for Scale Development and Construct Validity Assessment

R. Windsor, S. Cleary, K. Ramiah, et al., "Development and Evaluation of the Smoking Cessation and Reduction In Pregnancy Treatment (SCRIPT) Adoption Scale (SAS) for Prenatal Care Programs and Providers," *Journal of Health Communication* (June 2013) (see publication for references).

### Introduction

When a new evidence-based patient education program is being considered for adoption by a public health-primary care agency, it is essential to determine provider perceptions of its acceptability for routine use. In 2007, the West Virginia Bureau of Public Health's Right From The Start (RFTS) program decided to adopt the AHRQ recommended Smoking Cessation and Reduction In Pregnancy Treatment (SCRIPT) Program for routine delivery by regular staff to pregnant smokers. RFTS, a state-wide Medicaid-supported program, is delivered by designated care coordinators (DCCs), registered nurses or social workers, a staff of 55 primary care agencies in West Virginia. They provide both home-based and clinic-based services to pregnant women. The authors developed the SCRIPT Adoption Scale (SAS) in the absence of a valid instrument to assess the attributes of a new treatment by DCCs.

The validity of the five constructs, Relative Advantage, Compatibility, Complexity, Observability, and Trialability, of Rogers's "Diffusion of Innovations Model in a Health Care Organization" to predict SCRIPT use by DCCs was evaluated. After reviewing the literature and developing 73 draft SAS questions, two expert panels, consisting of five external experts and five internal experts, reviewed the draft SAS to establish face and content validity. After two internal and two external panel reviews, the final draft SAS included 43 items.

## Methods

The SAS was administered twice by a mailed baseline assessment and a follow-up assessment survey < 30 days to 90% (85/90) of the RFTS-DCC population. Factor and psychometric analyses were conducted to confirm the validity and reliability of the 43-item scale. Confirmatory Factor Analysis (CFA), commonly used to assess convergent and divergent validity, was performed. Factor loadings of each item were tested against an a priori assumption about the domain area. A factor loading of > 0.40 confirmed that the item was part of the domain it represents. Internal consistency, test-retest stability, and item-to-total analyses were conducted.

## Results: Factor and Convergent Validity Analyses

As noted in Table 4.6, five factors were confirmed providing support for Rogers's Model. All 28 items had factor loadings > 0.40: range = 0.43 to 0.81. There was also a significant association (p = 0.01) between the DCC SAS score and DCC SCRIPTPII.

In addition to identifying a five-factor model, analyses of the relationship of all five factors provided additional evidence supporting the convergent validity of "Rogers's Diffusion of Innovation Theory." Data in Table 4.7 confirmed consistent and statistically significant (p > 0.01) relationships between the five-attribute SAS sub-scales.

## SAS Internal Consistency and Stability

The SAS internal consistency r was 0.93 and stability r was 0.76. All 28 item-to-total correlation coefficients were r > 0.30. As noted in Table 4.8, the final SAS scale consists of 28 items that had good validity, excellent overall reliability (alpha = 0.93), and borderline (0.67) to very good (0.88) sub-scale reliability. The sub-scale test-retest reliability was consistently below or at the cutoff for reliability: 0.60 to 0.73. The stability coefficient was adequate: 0.76. Although two of five subscales need to be improved by increasing stability, the SAS can be adapted by prenatal care programs to measure the attributes of adoption of new patient education methods.

Another excellent measurement study concerning how to establish the psychometric properties of a scale to measure adherence was conducted by Morisky et al., "Predictive Validity of a Medication Adherence Measure (MAS) in an Outpatient Setting," *Journal of Clinical Hypertension* (2008), 348–354. Analyses of an eight-item MAS from 1,367 low-income patients confirmed all factor loadings were > 0.40, the alpha r was 0.83, and all

TABLE 4.6 Factor Loading and T-values of the Five-Factor 28-item SAS Scale

| FACTOR ITEMS | FACTOR LOADING | T-VALUE |
|---|---|---|
| **Relative Advantage** | **9 Items** | |
| Q1 | 0.68 | 6.97 |
| Q2 | 0.72 | 7.40 |
| Q3 | 0.66 | 6.71 |
| Q7 | 0.71 | 7.32 |
| Q9 | 0.58 | 5.69 |
| Q11 | 0.48 | 4.49 |
| Q14 | 0.80 | 8.72 |
| Q23 | 0.72 | 7.42 |
| Q36 | 0.73 | 7.64 |
| **Compatibility** | **4 Items** | |
| Q5 | 0.67 | 6.75 |
| Q8 | 0.80 | 8.50 |
| Q15 | 0.76 | 8.00 |
| Q19 | 0.72 | 7.40 |
| **Complexity** | **7 Items** | |
| RQ22 | 0.81 | 8.80 |
| Q24 | 0.63 | 6.24 |
| RQ25 | 0.48 | 4.51 |
| RQ26 | 0.64 | 6.34 |
| Q29 | 0.77 | 8.16 |
| RQ34 | 0.70 | 7.16 |
| Q42 | 0.71 | 7.16 |
| **Observability** | **4 Items** | |
| Q33 | 0.43 | 4.06 |
| RQ38 | 0.61 | 5.91 |
| Q39 | 0.72 | 7.32 |
| RQ41 | 0.56 | 5.34 |
| **Trialability** | **4 Items** | |
| Q27 | 0.52 | 4.85 |
| RQ30 | 0.62 | 5.95 |
| RQ32 | 0.49 | 4.58 |
| RQ37 | 0.47 | 4.33 |

TABLE 4.7 SAS Sub-Scale Convergent Validity Correlational Analyses

| SUB-SCALE | ADVANTAGE | COMPATIBILITY | COMPLEXITY | OBSERVABILITY |
|---|---|---|---|---|
| Compatibility | 0.93 | | | |
| Complexity | 0.60 | 0.66 | | |
| Observability | 0.81 | 0.65 | 0.93 | |
| Trialability | 0.51 | 0.62 | 0.97 | 0.94 |

TABLE 4.8 Reliability Coefficients of the Final SAS Sub-Scales

| SCALE FACTORS: SUB-SCALES | CRONBACH ALPHA | TEST-RETEST RELIABILITY[*] |
|---|---|---|
| Relative Advantage: 9 Items | 0.88 | 0.74 (p < 0.0001) |
| Compatibility: 4 Items | 0.82 | 0.62 (p < 0.0001) |
| Complexity: 6 Items | 0.83 | 0.73 (p < 0.0001) |
| Observability: 4 Items | 0.67 | 0.60 (p < 0.0001) |
| Trialability: 5 Items | 0.71 | 0.67 (p < 0.0001) |
| Total Score: 28 Items | 0.93 | 0.76 (p < 0.0001) |

[*] Pearson Correlation

eight items had item-to-total correlations of > 0.30. The MAS predicted BP control.

## Reliability

*Reliability* is an empirical estimate of the extent to which an instrument produces the same result (measure or score), if applied two or more times. Using BP readings allows a clinician to decide with reasonable confidence whether the patient is troubled or not. Imagine taking a blood pressure (BP) reading twice on the same person. On the first administration, a BP reading was 140/100—hypertension. Worried, another BP reading is taken: 120/80—normal. If a BP reading produced measures with this much variability, the procedure or instrument used are not reliable. The patient's BP may be unstable, the instrument is not calibrated and needs to be recalibrated, or the patient assessor is poorly trained. Taking two or three BP readings should result in different measurement values, but they should be within +/- 5 mg/mL range.

Reliability may be better understood by considering the dimension of error. Think of most measures (M) as having a true score (T) component and an error (E) component: $M = T + E$. While we want a measure with a person's true score (T), all measures have some percentage of error. We assume that these errors are random. Random errors include any effects that introduce something other than a true measure. Suppose a patient takes the same blood or urine test on five consecutive days. The deviations of each of the test administrations (a) from the true response indicate random error. Thus, errors are randomly distributed (+ or -) around the true score.

The five measures may vary around the true response for many reasons, for example, the person got up late one day and was rushed, was too tired one day, or was anxious at work one day. Because of random error, the obtained scores vary around the true score. If a larger number of tests, two/day for 10 days, was performed on one person or group of 30 with a valid instrument and laboratory analyses, the mean of the measures would be very close to the true response.

The same test, however, will not be administered 20 times to document the distribution of scores around a true score. In administering a test once, the test result may be close to or far from the person's true score. We assume, with trained assessors and standardized methods, however, these errors are randomly distributed across all people tested. Because random error is assumed, the mean of the multiple administrations is used as a best estimate of the true score. There may not be a totally stable/true score for a person because a person's true score will vary from day to day. For example, how much fat/cholesterol is consumed on any day will vary. Errors decrease reliability, making it more difficult to detect a true score. Bias from error reduces statistical power, attenuates an effect size, and reduces or eliminates the probability of observing a significant impact. A reliable instrument will have less error and produce measurements close to true score.

## Methods to Assess Reliability

Reliability is an index of random measurement error. Reliability coefficients are highest with no error (r = + or - 1.0) and lowest with total error (r = 0.0). Does the instrument make distinctions between two or more behaviors with a reasonable level of confidence? Before using an instrument to collect baseline and follow-up program data, instrument reliability must be documented. For a few instruments, the reliability has been calculated with many different groups. For most instruments, however, it has not. There are multiple approaches to assessing instrument reliability. Two factors are important to consider: the type of instrument (observer or external source vs. self-report) and the times at which the instrument is applied (same time vs. different times). Table 4.9 shows the types of reliability.

## Inter-Rater Reliability

If two observers collect data at the same time, reliability can be estimated by having the two observers rate the same performance of a task, skill, or behavior: inter-observer or inter-rater reliability. This documents whether two people are seeing and interpreting the same responses or behaviors in the same way at the same time. Because both observers should measure the same actions, the perfect inter-observer reliability and instrument

TABLE 4.9 Types of Reliability

| | TIME MEASURE APPLIED | |
|---|---|---|
| TYPE OF MEASURE | SAME | DIFFERENT |
| Observed | Inter-observer | Intra-observer |
| Self-Reported | Internal Consistency | Test-Retest: Stability |

would produce an r = 1.0. The level of error variability decreases reliability downward from 1.0. Pearson correlation is the common technique for measuring reliability. Because most observation scales use nominal or ordinal rating categories, Cohen's kappa is an accepted statistical technique (Cohen, 1975). Kappa corrects the simple percentage agreement between two observers for chance agreement. Forms of Kappa have been developed to weight deviations from exact agreement and for multiple observers.

## Inter-Rater Reliability

### Methods

An observational study using nine insulin-controlled adult patients and three trained pairs (MPH students) of interviewers (A-B, A-C, B-C) was conducted twice on three consecutive days during a four-week period. It established the objectivity of rater assessments by three trained staff. The methods noted in Table 4.10 can be used to determine the degree of interview/observer agreement. A standardized instrument, discussed in the section on criterion validity, was used, and a series of questions were asked by rater pairs of the nine patients to determine (1) demographic, (2) educational, (3) instructional, (4) cognitive, and (5) self-care behavioral characteristics.

TABLE 4.10 Patient Assessment Methods to Establish Levels of Rater Agreement

| RATER PAIRS | PATIENTS | DAY | $O_1$ | | $O_2$ |
|---|---|---|---|---|---|
| A & B | 1, 2, 3 | 1 | 0 | x | 0 |
| B & C | 4, 5, 6 | 2 | 0 | x | 0 |
| C & A | 7, 8, 9 | 3 | 0 | x | 0 |

$O_1$ = observation; X = staff training; $O_2 = O_1 + 4$ weeks

All nine patients were also given a standard set of materials and were asked to show how they perform at-home insulin injection. After the baseline level of agreement in Week 1 for the patient-education assessment staff (Rater A-B-C) was established ($O_1$) for each category, using the standardized instrument presented in Table 4.5, a patient interview/observation training program was conducted in Week 2 and 3. The objective of this study was to reduce rater error in the patient assessment process noted in the first observational study (O1).

The rater-training sessions required approximately three hours. It consisted of systematic question-by-question discussions of the instrument and data of the nine patients among the three assessment staff, a group lecture-discussion of interview/observation techniques, and individual question-by-question discussions with the primary investigator (PI). After completion of the training, a second rater study of nine patients, replicating O1 methods, was performed one month after the first study: O2.

## Rater Reliability Results

Results of the first and second inter-rater studies are reported in Table 4.11 by data category.

Evidence from the first assessment study (O1) confirmed a high level of agreement for the first four categories examined: demographic, lifestyle, instructional/behavior, and cognitive index, but not for the patient performance-skill index. The mean percentage rater agreement was 90.9%. Data derived from the second observation ($O_2$), after staff training to eliminate error, showed a significant improvement in rater agreement using this instrument and method in each of the five data categories. The target percentage agreed upon before conducting the second assessment study was to increase the percentage agreement $\geq 99\%$ for each category. *The average level of agreement reached in the second study was 99%. A statistical analysis of the reliability of the performance indices produced an Inter-Rater Reliability Coefficient of $r = 0.93$ (Kappa statistic).*

Analysis of the percent increase from Study 1 to 2, using a $t$ test for independent samples, produced $t = 1.88$. This exceeded the 0.05 level of significance for a one-tailed $t$ test (1.64). A one-tailed test was used, because a positive (directional) impact of the staff training program (X) was hypothesized. This analysis confirmed a statistically significant, positive impact of the training program on assessment staff. Rater assessment error was almost eliminated. These data confirmed that the detailed discussions with all principal hospital staff involved in patient education,

TABLE 4.11 Percent of Rater Agreement and Change by
Category between O1 and O2

| CATEGORY | OBSERVATION (O) STUDY | | CHANGE (%) | GAIN (%) |
|---|---|---|---|---|
| | $O_1$ (%) | $O_2$ (%) | | |
| I. Demographic | 97.3 | 99.0 | + 1.7 | + 1.8 |
| II. Lifestyle | 89.7 | 99.0 | + 9.3 | + 10.4 |
| III. Instructional/Behavior Index | | | | |
| Foot/Skin Care | 93.3 | 100.0 | + 6.7 | + 7.2 |
| Urine Testing | 86.3 | 98.7 | + 12.2 | + 14.1 |
| Insulin | 89.0 | 99.3 | + 10.3 | + 11.6 |
| Reactions/Ketoacidosis | 94.7 | 98.7 | + 4.0 | + 4.2 |
| IV. Cognitive Index | | | | |
| Foot/Skin | 91.3 | 100 | + 8.7 | + 9.5 |
| Urine Testing | 96.0 | 96.7 | + 0.7 | + 0.0 |
| Insulin Injection | 98.0 | 100 | + 2.0 | + 2.0 |
| Reactions/Ketoacidosis | 96.0 | 100 | + 4.0 | + 4.2 |
| V. Performance Index | | | | |
| Urine Testing | 73.0 | 100 | + 27.0 | + 37.0 |
| Insulin Prep-Injection | 87.0 | 96.3 | + 9.3 | + 10.7 |
| VI. Total | 90.9% | 99.0% | + 8.1% | + 9.4%[*] |

O = observations; X = staff assessment training.
[*] 0.05, One-Tailed Test

including the patient assessors, prior to the first trial to standardize the instrument and procedures, were productive. This study confirmed that routine assessment of patients should be periodically monitored, using the quality control methods described, to ensure program data of high quality.

## Reproducibility-Consistency

Another dimension of inter-rater reliability is the consistency of measurement over two or more assessments. In this case, if more than two assessments have been performed, the Intra-class Correlation Coefficient is the appropriate analytical method. Measurement theory indicates total variance ($\sigma^2_x$) can be divided into true score variability ($\sigma^2_T$) (inter-individual variability) and the error portion of the scores ($\sigma^2_E$): ($\sigma^2_x$) = ($\sigma^2_T$) + ($\sigma^2_E$). Theoretically, reliability is the proportion of total variance accounted for by variance in the true scores. When multiple assessments are obtained per person, the error term can be further divided into variability due to raters and error. This is important to show that rater variability is based on the error term rather than the subject's term. Using mean squares within an ANOVA, the Intra-class Correlation Coefficient (ICC) is estimated.

The ICC is sensitive to differences in relative position and mean values over times of assessment (K). High ICC values indicate high levels of consistency across all assessments in relative position, with little or no differences in means. Multiple values may provide a more accurate estimate of quantity. For example, there is much day-to-day (intra-individual) variability in what people eat, how each metabolizes, and/or in how much physical activity a person experiences. One day's assessment is an unreliable estimate of consumption, because of intra-individual variance and error. A more valid and reliable estimate of what a person eats can be obtained by taking at least three- or preferably five-day assessments. More assessment days increases the reliability for a given level of accuracy, or increases the accuracy for a given level of reliability. Several methods can be used to assess reliability of self-report forms applied at the same time.

## Split-Half Reliability

If there are a large number of individual questions or items of an instrument, for example $\geq 30$ items that measure different dimensions of a core concept or construct, such as self-care knowledge or beliefs, you may decide to conduct a split-half reliability assessment. Randomly assign items in the instrument to two sets of scores and conduct a Pearson correlation for continuous variables or Cohen's kappa for discrete variables. This correlation should be high, $r \geq 0.80$, because both halves are supposed to be measuring the same variable's content. This type of reliability is typically used with knowledge tests or psychosocial scales and during scale development.

A statistical formula, **Spearman-Brown**, can be used to determine what effect lengthening a scale or test would have. If you had a "Self-Care Efficacy Scale" of 10 questions with a reliability of $r = 0.60$, but wanted the scale to have an $r \geq 0.80$, the following formula would be used: $N = P_D$ $(1-P_E)/P_D$ $(1-P_E)$ where $P_D$ = desired reliability, $P_E$ = existing reliability, and $N$ = the number of times the scale would be lengthened to obtain an $r = 0.80$... $N = 0.80(1-0.60)/0.60$ $(1-0.80) = 2.7$. You would need $>$ 27 items in the scale to achieve an $r = 0.80$, assuming at least an average inter-item correlation equal to or greater than items of the existing 10-item scale.

## Internal Consistency and Item Analysis

As discussed, the most commonly used method to assess reliability for continuous measures is internal consistency (r). This is often called Cronbach's alpha (1951), recognizing its originator (Lee Cronbach). The Kuder-Richardson (KR 20 or KR 21) is a form of internal consistency for dichotomous measures, knowledge, and skill, for which there is a correct and incorrect answer (Nunnally, 1978). With multi-item scales or tests, internal consistency analyses measure the extent of inter-item correlation among all items. Theoretically, multiple items in one test share true variation, or the extent to which they commonly measure an underlying construct. The higher the inter-item correlations, the more true variation is shared by the items.

Many textbooks indicate that the minimum internal consistency coefficient for a psycho-social scale, or knowledge-skill test, should be r > 0.70. This is too low, reflecting too much error and unexplained variance: $R^2 = 0.70 \times 0.70 = 49\%$. An evaluation to measure "HP-DP program impact" should produce an r > 0.80 for its psychosocial scales.

In conducting an "item analysis," items must have a minimum inter-item correlation, or item-to-total correlation coefficient, of r > 0.20: an $r \geq 0.30$ is preferred. The following is an example for calculating Cronbach alpha with a 10-item scale. Alpha increases as the inter-item correlation increases. A 10-item scale, with a mean inter-item correlation = 0.31, has an alpha = 0.82. If the mean inter-item correlation = 0.40, the same scale would have an alpha = 0.87. If the items are increased from 10 to 12, and $r \geq 0.40$ of each item, the alpha r = 0.89.

## Case Study 3: Internal Consistency and Item Analysis

An HP-DP evaluation may have as an objective to increase patient social support.

Data in Table 4.12 represent a psychometric analysis of an 18-item Social Support Scale (SSS), including internal consistency (Cronbach alpha) r = 0.90, item-to-total correlation coefficients, and test-retest scale stability r = 0.94. These data are based on assessments of 309 pregnant patients who smoked at the onset of care. Data in Table 4.13 are psychometric analysis of a 16-item Health Belief Scale (HBS), and internal consistency, Time 1: r = 0.83 and Time 2: r = 0.89,

TABLE 4.12  Social Support Scale For Pregnant Smokers

| ITEM-QUESTION | X | S.D. | VARIANCE | W/ITEM-TO-TOTAL |
|---|---|---|---|---|
| 1 | 6.2 | 3.5 | 12.3 | 0.74 |
| 2 | 7.4 | 3.0 | 9.0 | 0.69 |
| 3 | 5.6 | 3.5 | 12.3 | 0.49 |
| 4 | 5.7 | 3.8 | 14.4 | 0.57 |
| 5 | 5.0 | 3.6 | 13.0 | 0.59 |
| 6 | 4.1 | 3.6 | 13.0 | 0.59 |
| 7 | 7.6 | 2.8 | 7.8 | 0.62 |
| 8 | 6.9 | 3.0 | 9.0 | 0.58 |
| 9 | 6.8 | 3.2 | 10.2 | 0.55 |
| 10 | 6.6 | 3.2 | 10.2 | 0.72 |
| 11 | 4.6 | 3.5 | 12.3 | 0.79 |
| 12 | 6.5 | 5.2 | 27.0 | 0.46 |
| 13 | 4.4 | 3.6 | 13.0 | 0.24 |
| 14 | 3.7 | 3.5 | 12.3 | 0.67 |
| 15 | 4.4 | 3.5 | 12.3 | 0.79 |
| 16 | 8.7 | 2.1 | 4.4 | 0.59 |
| 17 | 7.9 | 2.6 | 6.8 | 0.61 |
| 18 | 6.9 | 3.2 | 10.2 | 0.75 |
| Score | 108.7 | 37.4 | 1398.8 | 0.90 |

Test-retest stability = r = 0.88.

with item-to-total correlation coefficients for both observations, and test-retest reliability: $r = 0.92$. When the poor items, $r = < 0.19$, were dropped at T1 and T2, reliability for T1 and $T2_2$ > from $0.78 > 0.83$ and $0.87 > 0.89$. The stability r increased by eliminating Items 2, 8, and 9: $r = 0.90 > 0.92$.

The item to total correlations, 2, 7, and 8, when dropped from the HBS scale, improve it.

## Factor and Psychometric Analyses of SSS and HBS of Pregnant Smokers

Factor analysis, not presented, of the Social Support Scale data in Table 4.11 documented that it had only one underlying factor. *All 16 SSS items had a factor loading > 0.50. All 21 HBS items had a factor loading > 0.50.* Factor analysis of the HBS data in Table 4.12 confirmed four independent factors: (1) susceptibility-harm to infant, (2) effects of smoking, (3) emotional concern about health of baby, and (4) general concern about health of pregnant women.

TABLE 4.13 Item-to-Total Correlation, Internal Consistency and Stability Coefficients at Baseline (O1) and Final Third Trimester Interviews (O2) for the Health Belief Scale (HBS) for 309 Pregnant Patients

| ITEM DESCRIPTION | ITEM-TO-TOTAL CORRELATIONS | |
|---|---|---|
| | $O_1$ | $O_2$ |
| MATERNAL HEALTH SUBSCALE | | |
| 1. Think about your health | 0.24 | 0.28 |
| 2. Follow doctor's advice | **− 0.01\*** | **0.08\*** |
| 3. Effects known about smoking and pregnancy | 0.51 | 0.63 |
| 4. Safe to smoke during pregnancy | 0.55 | 0.62 |
| 5. Smoking increases illness when pregnant | 0.35 | 0.46 |
| 6. Smoking can harm health when pregnant | 0.54 | 0.71 |
| FETAL HEALTH SUBSCALE | | |
| 7. Other women worry about fetal health | **0.09\*** | 0.21 |
| 8. You worry about fetal health | **0.17\*** | **0.12\*** |
| 9. Improve your health through actions | 0.24 | 0.24 |
| 10. Influence fetal health through actions | 0.33 | 0.40 |
| 11. Stopping smoking improves fetal health | 0.57 | 0.62 |
| 12. Fetus receives chemical from smoke | 0.46 | 0.58 |
| 13. Effects known about smoking and fetus | 0.59 | 0.71 |
| 14. Smoking increases illness for fetus | 0.47 | 0.62 |
| 15. Smoking can harm fetal health | 0.65 | 0.65 |
| Internal Consistency | 0.78 → 0.83 | 0.87 → 0.89 |
| $O_1$ = 1st Visit 1st Tri and $O_2$ = 3rd Trimester | Stability >>> | 0.90 → 0.92 |
| **\* Item dropped** | | |

## Item Analysis: Item Difficulty and Item Discrimination for Knowledge-Skills Tests

Tests relating to item difficulty and discrimination originated from the cognitive field, but are used widely. Item difficulty is defined as the percent of students (or respondents) correctly answering the item. The test reliability is higher when items of medium difficulty are predominant. But the optimal item difficulty varies from question to question depending on the number of choices. *Items with difficulties less than 30% or more than 90% definitely need to be reviewed and revised. Such items should either be revised or replaced. An exception might be at the beginning of a test where one or two easier items (90% or higher) may be desirable.*

## Test-Retest or Stability Reliability

Measuring reliability by using the same test at two different times with the same sample is test-retest reliability. Reliability scores from this method may be lower than the split-half method, because time has elapsed between the first and second assessment. The longer the interval between observations, the more likely it is that events will happen to some or all people in an evaluation to induce a real change in the measures of an instrument. *An r = 0.80 should be documented for a measure to have a minimum test-retest reliability.* If the coefficient is < 0.70, the measure has considerable variability, and should be improved, before use by an evaluation to document changes over time. Unstable scores from measures attenuates/ eliminates the opportunity for a program to demonstrate impact. Data in Table 4.11 and 4.12 confirmed high stability scores for Health Belief and Social Support scales of the patients assessed during their pregnancy.

## Relationships Between Validity and Reliability

Although developers and users of instruments must be concerned about both validity and reliability, validity is more important than reliability. If an instrument does not measure what it should be measuring, it is irrelevant that the measurement is reproducible. The procedures for evaluating an instrument used at two times are straightforward. Formulas exist to measure dimensions of reliability. Reliability sets an upper bound to validity. Thus, if $r^2_R$ is the reliability coefficient for a measure of a variable and $r^2_V$ is the reliability of a criterion variable, the correlation ($r_{RV}$) between the measure and the criterion has the following limit: $\frac{1}{2}r_{RV}\frac{1}{2} < (r^2_V)^{\frac{1}{2}} (r^2_V)^{\frac{1}{2}}$.

Empirically, the maximum correlation between two scales, used to measure the criterion or construct validity of one of them, is defined as the theoretically maximum correlation multiplied (reduced) by the square root of the product of the respective scale's reliability coefficients (test-retest or coefficient alpha). The maximum possible correlation between two scales with coefficient alphas of .60 and .80, even if the concepts they measure were perfectly correlated (1.00), would be only .69 (Carmines & Zeller, 1979). If a measure cannot be consistently reproduced from two assessments, it cannot accurately measure an underlying construct.

Reliability and validity tests should be conducted prior to an evaluation, to confirm that the instrument is measuring the desired variable(s) among a representative sample of participants at each evaluation site. Reliability and validity testing has to be repeated when used in a new setting. A valid and reliable instrument in one setting may not be reliable or valid in a different age group or a different ethnic group, for example. Pilot tests of instruments and data collection methods at all evaluation sites are critical before starting an evaluation of an HP-DP program.

## Systematic Sources of Error

Each source of error diminishes validity and reliability, attenuates potential effect, and reduces statistical power. Seven general sources of data error/bias and systematic variation have been identified. Possible sources of error should be anticipated and plans developed to avoid or minimize them. Measurement error will be produced from any and all of these sources:

- Chance variation
- Participant instructions
- The instrument
- The data collector
- The respondent
- The environment
- Data management errors.

## Common Biases to Valid and Reliable Measurement

All evaluations in which data are collected are subject to some forms of bias. Although controlling all sources of bias is impossible, minimizing error from *each* major source in an evaluation is critical. The literature has identified 12 common biases in human measurement:

1. *Subject effect*: People who are aware that they are being measured may respond in atypical ways.
2. *Role selection*: Awareness of being measured may influence people to play a special role.
3. *Measurement as a change agent*: Measurement affects a person's behavior.
4. *Response sets*: People respond to questionnaires and interviews in predictable ways that have little or nothing to do with the questions posed, for example, answering yes or no to most or all questions or giving a socially desirable response.

5. *Interviewer effects*: Interviewer characteristics, for example, age, gender, or dress, may affect the receptivity and answers of the respondent.

6. *Changes in the instrument:* When an instrument is used more than once, a learning effect is possible. Interviewers may become more proficient or tired of conducting an interview.

7. *Population restrictions:* The method of data collection may impose restrictions on the population to which the results can be generalized, for example, telephone interviews require phones.

8. *Population stability over time*: An instrument administered at different times may not be collecting the same data on different populations.

9. *Population stability over areas*: The same way of collecting data in two different geographic areas may assess different types of people.

10. *Content restriction*: Only a limited range of data can be reported by each method. Self-report questionnaires cannot be used to study cognitive mechanisms of short-term to long-term memory. Observational data cannot be used to study relationships among for values.

11. *Stability of content over time:* If a program restricts a study to naturally occurring behavior, the content of the studied phenomenon may vary over time.

12. *Stability of content over an area:* A program may not be uniform in content.

## Criteria for Selecting an Instrument and Data Collection Methods

There are many other issues to consider in the construction and implementation of an instrument. The procedures for each method should be explicitly written so they can be reviewed to assess appropriateness for a specific population. Each instrument is based on a specific method of collecting data, for example, interviewing, self-recording, observing, or obtaining data from medical records. How do you select an instrument and, by inference, a method for data collection? The primary concern in selecting an instrument and method is whether it has high validity and reliability from previous experience, especially for the population at risk and setting. Ask: What are the major purposes of the study? *Note*: Because an instrument has been documented to have excellent validity and reliability in published longitudinal or cross-sectional research in one or two cities does not mean that it automatically can detect changes over time in the independent or dependent variable(s) measured in an evaluation or for a new population.

You must consider the *precision* of the instrument and method. The *level of detail* of an instrument may not be sufficient to provide data about the variable needed. For example, if an evaluation needs to make fine distinctions in the level of nutrients consumed, a food-frequency questionnaire may not provide adequate detail to make a distinction. Alternatively, a measurement instrument/method, for example, a seven-day food diary, may require a level of detail beyond the capability of some respondents, such as children under 12, illiterate adults, or depressed patients.

When measuring behavior, we want to measure *routine behavior*: what people ordinarily do on a day-to-day basis. Just measuring behavior for three or four consecutive days (common in food or activity diaries) may miss differences in usual behavior on weekends, holidays, sick days, or season (validity issues). Research has shown very high level of day-to-day variability in behavior, which requires that multiple days be assessed to get an accurate estimate of that routine behavior (reproducibility issues). Examples of ethnic and regional appropriateness may also need to be considered. Food-frequency assessment technique includes documenting food common in a particular ethnic group or region of the country: greens in Southern China and greens in the Southern United States have a very different meaning. Assessments must be worded in a way understandable for a specific ethnic group or region.

As discussed under bias, the method of collecting data may be *reactive*; it may induce client behavior or other changes by collecting the data. The reactivity of an instrument will vary by population assessed and the situation in which the assessment occurs. The method should be selected to minimize reactivity for the population and settings to be studied. Instruments and methods may be appropriate or inappropriate for particular populations and settings. There are also issues of developmental appropriateness to be considered, that is, are the instruments and method appropriate to the cognitive and emotional abilities of respondents? What can be asked of normal adults may not be developmentally appropriate for children or the mentally impaired.

## Efficiency and Cost of Measurement

A common and significant issue when selecting an instrument is cost. The instrument and method may place undue burden on your budget and/or the participant or staff. Cost has several characteristics: (1) dollar cost, (2) time spent by the evaluation staff, (3) time spent by respondents, (4) training time, (5) ease of setting up instruments, (6) difficulty of getting individuals to participate, and (7) loss of accuracy due to increased workload. The key to selecting excellent measures is to choose a set sufficiently valid and reliable for your study's purposes, yet developed at an affordable cost to the project and burden to participants.

Another critical aspect of efficiency is collecting no more data than are necessary to achieve study purposes. There are numerous examples in the literature and from presentations at conferences that investigators have developed a 100+ question instrument requiring > 1 hour to complete. This assessment produces significant burden: costs in time, printing, collating, and data processing. Evaluation participants must also bear large burdens: time/costs, and possible frustration or disinterest in completing the questionnaire. Investigators typically collect far more data than they can reasonably analyze; the parties incur the costs of collection, but because of evaluation report deadlines, nothing is ever done with the data.

The most valid and reliable instruments and data collection methods always incur more financial resources, staff time, and costs to the investigator and time costs to the respondents. Sometimes an investigator must select a smaller set of the most valid and reliable instruments and methods for the amount of money and time available. *An evaluation should not be conducted if resources, funding, and time are not available for instruments and data collection methods that meet minimum global validity-reliability-representativeness criteria.*

## Purposes-Objectives of the Evaluation

A data collection method must clearly meet the purposes of an evaluation study, within your resource and time constraints. For a smoking cessation program, you might conduct an evaluation to assess impact (stopped smoking or not), the availability of resources in the environment (numbers of smokers willing to participate in a smoking-cessation program), the quality of the resources, the appropriateness of the structure (well-designed program), whether the processes are occurring as planned (conducted according to plans), and whether the processes are being related to outputs (attending more sessions increases quit rates). Each topic can be the focus for an evaluation in a specific program. The main purposes and type of question to be answered by the evaluation should determine the data-collection method. **Ask**: Why do we want answers to *this* question? Why are we collecting *these* data? How are we going to analyze the data?

## Quality Control in Data Collection

Because there are hundreds of books on this topic, in this section we briefly examine multiple, common methods of data collection, identify strengths and weaknesses (biases), consider issues in methods selection, and outline steps to develop an instrument and methods. There are many facets to collecting quality data. Quality control requires anticipating possible sources of problems, selecting the best methods for an evaluation, monitoring data collection quality, and minimizing problems before or as they occur.

## Sampling and Representativeness

Chapter 3 introduced methods to estimate needed sample size for each group to make the analyses and inferences, and discussed the salience of selection bias in accruing and retaining participants in an evaluation. A major assumption in performing an analysis to test a hypothesis or relationship is that a study is conducted to generalize to a defined population. While universally challenging, a primary objective of all evaluations is to recruit and to assess a representative sample of the target population. All samples of evaluation participants need to be assessed to determine how representative they are of the population at risk to which inferences of impact are to be made. Here, we briefly discuss one method to obtain a sample.

There are multiple types of random sampling techniques, such as simple random, clustering, or stratified. Randomness minimizes the likelihood that a systematic source of selection bias will occur among the sample, thereby influencing the degree of representativeness of a defined population at risk. It also minimizes confounding. If you could be sure that the entry of any person in your intervention program was a random event, then quota sampling might be appropriate. Selecting the next 50 participants in an HIV/AIDS disease management program at a hospital or from a community-based screening program (a quota sampling) may not be representative. Alternatively, the next 50 participants may all be obtained on Monday and Tuesday from 9 a.m. to 5 p.m. Patients who come to the hospital on Wednesday or Thursday, or from 5 p.m. to 10 p.m., may be different from those who use the clinic on other days of the week or at night.

Evaluators often collect data from record systems, for example, vital statistics for a defined geographic area or patient clinic records. A systematic sampling technique is often used to select cases from records. In systematic sampling, divide the population (e.g., 10,000 cases per year for a specific district) by the sample size needed (e.g., a 5% sample or 500 subjects). If every twentieth record is selected, 500 cases will be systematically obtained. Randomly select a number between 1 and 20—start with that case. Thus, if 17 were randomly selected, the study sample would consist of cases number 17, 37, 57. . . 9,097. A major strength of this sampling method is its ease of implementation. If the sequence of cases is random, such as by alphabetical order or by month or week of entry into a program, then systematic sampling is likely to produce an unbiased sample.

In developing sampling procedures, it is also critical to specify inclusionary characteristics (participants in the program to be evaluated) and exclusionary characteristics (characteristics of people used to keep them out of the sample and the evaluation). Inclusionary and exclusionary characteristics define the population to which data and results can be generalized. Consult any of a variety of texts on sampling and a biostatistician in developing your sampling procedures.

## Questionnaire Development

A questionnaire obtains information from a respondent through self-reported answers to a series of questions, usually using paper and pencil, administered by a computer, or by interview. Four general areas in questionnaire development are typically of concern to an evaluation:

- Instrument selection
- Instrument development
- Field testing
- Quality control.

### Instrument Selection

*Do not reinvent the wheel.* Meta-evaluation and meta-analysis of the global literature will confirm that many evaluations have developed and applied multiple types of instruments and measures for a wide variety of constructs, risk factors, diseases, and populations at risk. When an instrument has been shown to be valid and reliable and directly measures the variables of interest for a specific problem and target population of an evaluation, starting with that instrument as a draft makes good sense. Using developed instruments is also valuable for several reasons. First, you capitalize on the conceptual work of other experienced investigators in instrument design. Much time would have been spent by other evaluations reviewing the literature and considering alternative questions. Second, other investigators would have spent time revising, pilot testing, and evaluating the instrument to maximize validity and reliability. All evaluations go through multiple drafts of a questionnaire, typically at least five, to increase their quality.

Using an existing instrument should enhance some level of reliability and validity of measurement in a new application by a new evaluation. If you are using only parts of an instrument, there may be changes in the validity and reliability of the instrument. Third, using an existing instrument and the same question enables comparisons across evaluation studies. Developed instruments, however, should never be used without (1) thorough internal review by your evaluation team, (2) an external review by an expert panel, (3) a review and pilot test by staff at all sites who will use it and pre-test among participants from all sites who will be assessed, and (4) validity and reliability analysis, and psychometric and factor analyses of your sample.

## Instrument Development and Field Testing

In some cases, instruments have not been developed for a specific topic or subgroup, or existing instruments are not appropriate. Even when instruments are available, you almost always have to develop questions specific to your study. In general, almost all evaluations use close-ended questions. Respondents may not accurately understand an open-ended question, may not want to provide a full answer because it will take too much time, or may give a full and complete answer in his or her view. Developing close-ended questions, however, requires more time and attention to detail than open-ended questions. Review the literature to ensure that the response categories are mutually exclusive. Pilot test the questionnaire to ensure that the alternatives are understandable to the intended audience. When rating scales are used to obtain responses, the structure of the response scales can be important.

Open-ended questions can be useful in a questionnaire when you want to learn something about which little is known. In this case, a close-ended question is posed (usually in a yes-no format), followed by an open-ended question asking for an explanation. The questionnaire should be appealing to respondents. Keep the pages free of clutter and use empty space to make the form visually appealing. Asking several questions that are stimulating or pleasing early in the questionnaire increases the likelihood that respondents will maintain the motivation to complete the instrument. Developing and using clear and simple instruction increases the accuracy of questionnaire responses. Multi-item instruments should be constructed to avoid response sets that bias results. Windsor and colleagues have applied the following procedures in questionnaire-instrument development in multiple population health evaluation studies over a 40+ year period:

- Define your evaluation objectives and major types of data in specific measurable terms.
- Conduct a meta-evaluation and review of published instruments and the measurement literature to define the "measurement science" and "gold standard" for your evaluation and to select your measurement methods, instruments, and questions.
- Define the type, frequency, duration, and cost of data collection procedures.
- Draft and conduct an internal review of instruments/methods by evaluation staff and regular staff who will use the instrument; revise the instrument and methods.
- Conduct an external review of instruments and procedures by an expert panel; revise it.
- Train assessment staff at all evaluation sites.
- Pilot test the draft instrument and data collection procedures with ≥ 30 eligible participants and all staff at each evaluation site.
- Analyze the validity and reliability data, and qualitative data from pilot test and staff review.
- Revise the instrument and measurement protocol.
- Pilot test, again if necessary, the instrument with ≥ 30 participants at each site; revise it.
- Revise and finalize the instrument and implementation assessment and quality-control monitoring procedures for all staff and all evaluation sites.

## Quality Control

Selecting, developing, and field testing a questionnaire are necessary, but not sufficient, to collect valid and reliable data. Periodic quality control checks must be made of instruments. Conduct other data editing and cleaning procedures, after the data have been entered into the computer, for example, reviewing a 5% or 10% sample of the data-entry forms against hard copy of the data set. These checks detect data-entry errors, if a manual system is used. At a minimum, evaluators must conduct criterion validity studies, and conduct test-retest studies on all multi-item instruments, perform item analyses, and obtain an estimate of internal consistency and stability. Because there are many excellent textbooks on this topic and survey research courses, we present only a synopsis of several major methods.

## Self-Completion Questionnaires

A self-completion (or self-reporting) questionnaire is an instrument that the participants complete by reading almost all close-ended questions and answering all questions.

### Strengths

A self-completed questionnaire is a frequently used method of data collection for program evaluation because of convenience and efficiency. Almost all types of measures can be assessed by self-completed questionnaire, and 100% of evaluation participants can be exposed to the same instrument. Data can be collected from a large sample in a short period of time at a low cost/participant. Because no interviewer is involved, well-designed instrument controls for interviewer effects. The proportion of unusable data in a self-report questionnaire should be very low. All the questions are directed at the object of concern, and replicability is high. The questionnaire is particularly useful when the variables studied are amenable to self-observation. Specific answers can be elicited in simple, straightforward questions. Self-report questionnaires are most valid and reliable with short, simple, and straightforward questions. Numerous, excellent references on self-completion questionnaires exist.

### Weaknesses

A self-completion questionnaire is susceptible to biases. Respondents may fall into role selection when answering questions, because no one is present to observe, clarify, or challenge their role taking. Other problems include (1) the questionnaire may promote participant change, (2) changes may occur in the respondents' understanding of the questionnaire, and (3) limits may exist on the variables that a questionnaire is measuring. Although a self-completed questionnaire theoretically controls for possible interviewer effects, the person who distributes the questionnaire often answers questions about it. He or she may give subtle or overt cues about how it should be answered.

## Face-to-Face Interviewing

There may be no substitute for an interviewer-conducted personal survey. Literature on survey methods is too complicated to be easily summarized, so only a synopsis is presented.

### Strengths

Conducted face-to-face, the interview is preferable to a self-completion questionnaire.

- The content of the questionnaire may not be well defined;
- The questions are long, complex, or require subtle distinctions;
- The respondents have difficulty reading or writing;
- Personal effort may be needed to contact respondents; and
- Data on other variables, for example, blood pressure measurements, must be collected.

The primary strength of the face-to-face interview is the use of a well-trained interviewer to ask the respondent intensively and to detect, clarify, and follow up on confusing answers or questions. Interviewers can be trained to probe interviewees with a variety of questions, attempting to get below-surface responses, that is, flippant or simple answers that a respondent may provide. For example, if you are interested in why mothers decide to breast-feed or not, you could ask a simple question "Why did you decide to breast-feed or bottle-feed your baby?" and leave several lines for the unstructured response. Alternatively, you might use the power of having an interviewer ask the following series of questions:

- "What do you see as the benefits of breast-feeding (or bottle-feeding)?"
- "What do you see as the costs to you of bottle-feeding (or breast-feeding)?"

- "How important are the costs of bottle-feeding to you?"
- "Why did you select your method of infant feeding?"

Most respondents finding these questions on a self-response questionnaire answer them with the easiest responses. An interviewer can probe a little deeper, looking for things this mother might like about breast- or bottle-feeding. Interview questions are best formed when the investigator applies a theoretical model: questions are designed to assess key variables in a model. Probing respondents to collect the data of interest is appropriate for long and complex questions. The appropriateness of an interviewer for respondents who cannot read or write is obvious. Interviews provide the most flexible method for the use of descriptive cues. An interviewer can ask a variety of questions and make judgments about the state of the respondent. With careful attention to detail, an interview can almost always be replicated. This promotes reliability in data collection.

## Weaknesses

The face-to-face interview is susceptible to several biases. In an interpersonal situation, a percentage of respondents are likely to anticipate what the interviewer expects and respond accordingly (*role selection*). The probing of specific content areas is likely to focus the attention of the respondent on these issues (*social desirability*). This may change what respondents think about the issues and may confound future attempts at measuring this content area: (*measurement as change agent*). Interviewers become more proficient and ask more subtle questions. Later interviews may be different from earlier ones. The interview may not obtain as accurate information on highly sensitive issues, for example, regular sexual behavior or drug use. Realizing these biases, staff can take steps to counter or minimize these effects. The interpersonal interview, however, is an expensive method of data collection. Some combination of self-completed questionnaires and interviews may best achieve an investigator's objectives, within the available budget and time.

## Face-to-Face Interviews and Interviewer Training

A good face-to-face interview requires a well-designed interview schedule, a list of questions, and a well-trained interviewer. The guidelines presented in this chapter to develop questionnaires also apply to developing the interview. Training interviewers requires a substantial attention to detail. The qualities of a good training program are the following:

- Clear instructions to obtain and contact an eligible respondent;
- An understanding of the major objective of each part of the instrument;
- A guidebook or protocol on probing questions and on recording responses;
- Materials for clarifying responses;
- Detailed procedures for collecting other data;
- Experience in conducting the interview, especially probing;
- Common experiences in recording or coding self-report information;
- Sources of information to report or clarify problems; and
- Testing for validity and reliability.

Training should give participant interviewers enough knowledge of the subject area to enable them to ask intelligent questions. An answer to any question may be ambiguous, unless clear guidelines or categories of response exist for recording a response. For example, to the question "Why do you smoke after eating?" a new smoker might answer, "Well, I'm not too sure . . . well, it relaxes me right after a meal. I try to puff enough to feel good, but not keep that terrible smoke in my mouth." This is a complex response to a simple question. Some comments are positive, some negative. The basic response to the question is equivocal. Rules are needed to guide the interviewer about how to probe for classification and which parts of a response to record. An interviewer may need materials to show the respondent how to answer a question. Sometimes interviewers will collect data other than responses to questions. This might include blood pressure or saliva samples. Detailed guidelines, materials, and thorough training need to be provided.

Criteria need to be formulated for screening and rejecting potential interviewers who cannot collect data adequately. Interviewers need experience in conducting interviews on a pilot basis. The pilot interviews test the questionnaire and enable the interviewers to develop confidence in implementation. It clarifies issues that did not arise in review of materials and procedures. A sound procedure is to pre-test and record the interview and review the tape.

When evaluation staff is conducting a community survey, interviewers must be given a phone number to call when they need clarification on interview techniques, sample locations, or other problems. If physiological measures are collected, the interviewers' basic data-collection technique needs to be assessed at weekly intervals, and the machine used needs to be assessed to ensure calibration. Interview training time will vary and may take hours or days. Before being sent to the field, interviewers must have valid identification. The program staff, in some cases, should announce the interview schedule and locations to local authorities.

## Telephone Interviewing

Telephone interviewing is a good alternative to face-to-face interviewing. The information is cheaper to collect per interview, and greater control can be exerted by staff over the methods of data collection in a central automated center. It is also easier to conduct a large national sampling frame. Telephone survey research centers currently use computerized, random digit dialing centers for these interviews. There are three main types: traditional telephone interviews, computer assisted telephone dialing, and computer assisted telephone interviewing (CATI).

All comments made about face-to-face interviewing apply at some level to telephone interviewing, but telephone interviewing is susceptible to additional biases. A primary concern is population restrictions. Data reveal that > 95% of adults have home or cell phones. Further population-restriction problems arise when trying to reach people with unlisted phone numbers, those who have moved, and those who have changed phones for other reasons, since the last public listing of phone numbers. Investigators typically propose the random digit dialing method to overcome the latter two problems. The shortcoming of this approach is that it is not usable for contacting some known sampling of individuals, for example, all the former participants in a particular project, or contacting people in specific geographic areas, because the first local digits in the telephone number may not be specific to those areas.

There are greater restrictions on content on the telephone than in the face-to-face interview. A telephone interview should probably not last more than 30 minutes and is best conducted in ≤ 20 minutes. In contrast, face-to-face interviews could be ≤ 1 hour. Participant burden, data quality, and essential data needs, however, should be a concern of all evaluations. Some respondents may have gender preference while discussing sensitive issue. This may pose a challenge in anticipating who the respondent is going to be. Studies conducted on survey methods have not been clear if notifying by mail before increases or decreases of non-response. Receipt of advance notification may introduce bias to variables of interest.

## Direct Observations

Most evaluations need to conduct some type of direct observations. By definition, behavioral data are amenable to observation. Observational methods are most useful for collecting behavioral and skill data. Frequently the accuracy of self-reported behavior is biased. Ability, or skill, data often require a person to perform a task in a controlled circumstance to see whether the person can do it. For example, a diabetic patient is often asked to demonstrate that he or she can or does perform self-care management tasks (see Table 3.6). Direct observation includes a variety of methods. Observational data can be obtained directly by the observers, or by videotapes, audiotape recorders, and other mechanical means. In some methods, the observer attempts to be an objective recorder of phenomena; in others, the observer frequently interacts with the subjects and may, in fact, participate with the subjects in various key social events. Observational studies may be concerned simply with identifying the frequency of certain activities or, at a more complex level, with the relationships between events.

Direct observation is one of the most expensive methods to obtain data. One observer must be present for long periods of time. Extensive records must be maintained. Multiple coders may be needed to search the records and code the phenomena of concern, or expensive laptop computers must be used in the field to record observations. Using the self-report method, an investigator can use a questionnaire with multiple respondents, and < 1 hour obtain data from a respondent covering an hour, a day, a week, a year, or a lifetime of experiences. In contrast, a single observer in one hour can obtain data on one hour in the life of one person or group of people.

Observation can be cost-effective when used with small representative samples to validate data obtained using other methods. The assessment protocol must specify procedures for contracting, training, and/or interviewing people. The protocol should include definitions of items and examples of cases difficult to distinguish. It should clarify whether single or multiple checks or entries are disallowed, allowed, encouraged, or required. Procedures for recording field notes should be stated. The protocol should also specify periodic times for joint observations to obtain inter-rater reliability. Observer training is an essential method to promote the validity-reliability.

If not done by computer, people who code/enter information and data from the observation/instrument also may not agree on coding specifics, due to differences in interpretation or understanding of the coding task, temporary distractions, or errors in memory or perception. A protocol is needed for coding data from an observation instrument into meaningful variables. Many of the same issues covered in the observational protocol must be covered in the coding protocol. Coders need to be trained to perform each task, although the training may not have to be as long, because the task is more clearly defined and data are not lost once the coding is done. Coding of the same form by two coders must be built into daily tasks to obtain periodic estimates of inter-coder reliability. At least five key problems have been identified for observation methods:

1. Reliability estimates may not be made in the same coding and time units;
2. The days on which reliability in assessed may not be representative of other days;
3. Which observations are conducted; the instrument may decay due to the passage of time;
4. The observers may respond in some unknown way to being assessed; and
5. The people being observed may respond in some unknown way to being observed.

Methods for counteracting these problems have been developed.

The following components of training for a reliability monitoring system are recommended:

- Have all observers read and study the observation protocol.
- Have the observers complete programmed instruction materials on pre-coded interactions.
- Conduct daily, intensive training programs in pre-coded scripts enacted on videotape.
- Provide field training with an experienced observer, followed by reliability testing.
- Randomly assess inter-observer reliability in the field.

Observational techniques are very useful in assessing the extent to which self-report methods have provided valid data, and in assessing whether usual training provided to patients in clinics resulted in their having the skills necessary to perform the desired health maintaining behaviors.

## Health-Clinical-Physiological Measures

Clinical or physiological measures are used in almost all population health studies. In some cases, the physiological measure is the primary outcome measure, for example, blood pressure determinations as measures of effectiveness of programs to control high blood pressure. In other cases, physiological variables act as checks on the validity of self-reported measures, for example, urine or saliva cotinine levels to validate smoking cessation or significant reduction. In some studies, physiological variables reflect the subject's health status or disease risk, which may be affected by habitual behaviors. Examples included serum cholesterol or hemoglobin A1C (HA1C), which is affected by diet and exercise and is predictive of atherosclerosis or diabetes control, and a sub-maximal stress test, which measures physical fitness and is affected by aerobic activity.

The attraction of physiological measures is that they are not obtrusive in the many senses that directly observed behavioral measures are. It is not obvious to patients when collecting a blood sample for lab testing that they are being observed. The measures are reactive only to the extent that they encourage people to perform the desired behaviors when they are aware of the values. As discussed previously, despite the aura of the supposed objectivity of these "hard data" measures, they are subject to as many, but different, sources of error as the "soft data."

Physiological indicators vary daily, weekly, and by other cycles. Many published studies of blood pressure measurement, using continuous or frequent monitoring instruments, show marked variations between waking and sleeping hours, mornings and evenings, between conversation times and times alone. Blood pressure readings taken in an office or clinic may be 10 mm Hg higher than those taken in a home. Although physiological measures seem simple and straightforward to make, detailed protocols have been developed for obtaining them, including the following:

- Extended training procedures for even well-credentialed individuals;
- Specifications of the environmental conditions in which the measure is taken;
- Specification of the state of the subject, for example, an individual who has fasted for 12 hours before a blood sample for serum cholesterol analysis is taken;
- Procedures for handling the specimen if one was taken;

- Identification of the specific machine and how it should be run, periodically tested, and corrected; and
- Definer procedures for ongoing quality control of all elements of the data-collection process.

Blood pressures rise and fall in response to the person's emotional or arousal state. This systematic bias may occur in a study from simply taking a blood pressure measurement at different times in a day, different settings, and having it taken by a person of a different gender or age. Due to minute-to-minute variability, resting blood pressure readings should be taken over successive minutes to obtain estimates of blood pressure, and diastolic blood pressure readings obtained by auscultation may not reflect true diastolic pressures as assessed by intra-arterial sensors.

The primary difference between physiological measures and the behavioral and self-report measures is that the many sources of error in physiological measures are often known and more amenable to control, if highly structured quality control procedures are employed.

Human and other errors can occur at every stage in the taking of physiological measurements. Medication adherence provides an interesting example. Having enough medication flowing in a person's circulatory system to be effective in fighting a disease (a therapeutic plasma concentrate) requires (1) prescription of an adequate amount of medication for the size of the person's body or other personal characteristics (provider competence), (2) consumption of all the medication prescribed (patient adherence), and (3) action by the body to make the medication available in the bloodstream as expected (bio-availability). It is well documented that most physicians around the world have limited competency in pharmacotherapy to prescribe amounts that promote the therapeutic bioavailability for each patient. For many reasons, there is high variability from person to person in how the body absorbs, metabolizes, and stores the same medication. There are also serious problems in patient compliance.

Important sources of error often come to light from multicenter studies of inter-laboratory variability. The most common procedure for handling this source of error is for a central quality control center to prepare compounds with known, controlled levels of the chemical of interest, and to send samples of the compound to participating laboratories. Based on the values obtained at each laboratory in comparison with known values for each controlled compound, an adjustment value can be given to calibrate values obtained by laboratory machine and procedures. This calibration must be done periodically to control laboratory drift (similar to observer drift).

A variety of other errors can occur. The needle for taking a blood sample from a child may be too narrow, destroy red blood cells and contaminating the sample. The blood sample may be collected in an inappropriate test tube, leading to coagulation and destroying the sample for analysis. The centrifuge for separating red blood cells from serum may not work. These and a host of other errors should inform evaluation staff about physiological-clinical measurement.

## Abstraction of Existing Records: Medical and Clinical

Some investigators consider the medical record as a readily available and accessible source of rich data, at little cost. Imagine the millions of medical records across the country with millions of laboratory and physiological tests on a vast variety of health problems. A medical record abstraction is appropriate and valuable in certain scenarios. These occasions can be identified, after listing the biases in record abstraction.

### Strengths and Weaknesses

The critical issues in using an existing data set are availability, completeness, validity, reliability, and representativeness for a population, setting, and periods of time. Entries are made in one or more medical records each time a patient receives care from a healthcare provider. This produces an enormous quantity of data. If the healthcare provider or institution can be persuaded to share these records, the body of data may become available for evaluation purposes. Unless it is directly available from an existing information system, the primary cost is incurred by hiring staff to abstract and enter the desired data from all data available.

Another limitation is representativeness. Not every person receives medical care for a specific problem. Although some of the major barriers to care may have been overcome in many countries, multiple studies have indicated that the poor and minority groups in almost all countries are less likely to receive care for a health problem. This population restriction for results of studies made of only those receiving care may be more or less severe, depending on the topic. Because the evaluation team has little or no control over how much information gets recorded or over the quality of that recorded information, major problems can arise. Windsor, Gartseff, and Roseman, 1981 conducted a one-year retrospective medical record review of 996 diabetic in-patients in a tertiary care diabetes hospital at a major university medical center.

They documented the following: only 40% had a baseline admission behavioral-educational assessment—only 6% had at discharge from the hospital a patient behavioral-educational assessment for diabetes management.

The poor reliability of medical record information can be explained by examining the three major purposes of maintaining a medical record: patient management, legal, and science concerns. The way in which clinical facts are obtained in medical practice does not reflect the concern for validity and reliability given to data collected for scientific research. The stability of the content of medical records will vary over time and across diseases and medical conditions. For example, the International Classification of Diseases (ICD) is a set of codes for major categories of causes of death and disability. Hospitals use several ICD codes in the planning of health services. Moreover, the ICD codes are periodically updated to reflect the latest medial knowledge. Data collected before and after code changes are therefore not directly comparable because the diagnostic criteria for making a particular judgment may have changed.

## Steps in Abstracting Medical Records

A medical record abstraction can be useful when demographic data are simple, commonly recorded medical data are desired, and when attempts to control for reliability are made. Many studies have attempted to abstract relevant information on hypertensive patients in a family medicine clinic and have illustrated the steps required in conducting abstractions of medical records. Multiple drafts of a form are typically prepared. The first few drafts will be revised to reflect the purposes of the study more clearly, as these purposes became more clearly defined through staff decisions. Validity and reliability analyses will be conducted on the next two drafts by having sets of two abstracters jointly abstract 30 records. Reliability indices can be calculated on the 30 jointly abstracted records for each variable, and each pair of abstracters. All cases in which differing values are obtained need to be reviewed against the medical record. Rules can be generated to refine the search or the recording process. On the second set of reliability abstractions, rules for abstraction can be further refined. Variables for which a reliability of abstraction of $\geq 0.80$ or higher (kappa) is not achieved can be dropped. A final draft will then be produced for study.

## Summary

The issues related to selecting and developing data collection methods are complex. All methods are susceptible to threats to validity and reliability. Although many of these sources of error can be overcome, they are always overcome at an additional cost, time, staff, and processing. The responsibility of the evaluator is to select and develop the most valid and reliable methods and instruments appropriate to the questions to be answered, within the funding and other resources available. Many skills are involved at each stage in selecting and developing methods and instruments. The novice evaluator should not become intimidated or discouraged. Despite the collective skills and intelligence of teams of evaluators, anticipated and unanticipated problems occur in the best of evaluative studies.

No evaluation (or other) study has been perfect. Evaluators should, instead, have a realistic respect for the problems likely to be encountered, should build their skills to the maximum possible, and should involve biostatistical, computing, and information systems consultants who are knowledgeable in the specific type of evaluation contemplated. The best way to learn these skills is to participate in the selection and development of methods under the supervision of others skilled in these tasks.

# 5 | Process and Qualitative Evaluation

Linking Process and Impact Analyses should be an important
objective of Evaluation Research.

— *Thomas Cook and Charles Reichardt*

## Introduction

The need to document and know what program staff has provided to a
client, patient, student, or employee, and the acceptability of the program
and its assessment and intervention procedures, are the primary objectives
of process and qualitative evaluations. This chapter presents a discussion
of both types. Empirical evidence and insight from process and qualitative
evaluations, if well designed and successfully implemented, will provide
complementary results about staff performance and the acceptability of
participant assessment and intervention methods.

A process evaluation documents participant exposure to the core program procedures (Pn) to be routinely provided by regular staff. It describes
what actually happened as a new program was implemented. It applies
existing performance standards (Ps) for each core program procedure
(P1 + P2...) defined in the literature and/or derived by professional consensus through an internal and or external expert panel review. A process
evaluation also answers, in part, questions about why a program succeeded
or failed (efficacy or effectiveness) and documents which components
need to be revised and how. *While the HP-DP literature emphasizes the
need to conduct staff performance assessments and a process evaluation,
it continues to provide limited guidance about how to conduct a process
evaluation. This chapter begins to fill this deficiency.*

A process evaluation (1) defines the structure, process, and content of an HP-DP program to be delivered by designated staff; (2) documents the frequency of delivery of the first core procedure (P1) and all remaining procedures (P2 + P3 + P4...) for each provider, practice site, program, or a system of care; (3) conducts observational assessments of program sessions; and (4) monitors program-staff effort or activity. It provides routine empirical feedback, daily-weekly-monthly-quarterly-annually, of what is being implemented by staff at all program sites. Process evaluations provide data and documentation of the strength of the relationship between the intervention "process" and a significant increase (if observed) in a behavioral "impact" or health "outcome" rate.

In the planning phases, HP-DP specialists have the responsibility to define the salient structural and process components of a program. Staff should be able to describe what process data and information to collect, how they are going to be collected, who is going to collect them, and when they are going to be collected. Delineation of these steps should produce essential data and richer insight about what happened as a program is pilot tested and implemented.

Data and information from these methods also provide important insight about the sequence of events and interaction and linkage between participants, staff, and a program. They provide empirical data reflecting the qualitative aspects of program procedures and methods, including acceptance and participation rates by target groups for a specific setting. Data from these methods place the program manager in a more knowledgeable position to discuss how well the program and its parts are doing, what changes needed/were made, and how well the program worked. A process evaluation allows a manager to say with confidence that a significant 10% or 20% difference in impact and outcomes rates of an E and C group were attributable to the HP-DP and management program.

A detailed description of a Process Evaluation Model (PEM) and methods are presented in this chapter, as well as its application in multiple case studies. We identify normative criteria and procedures—professional standards and metrics—that a program should regularly consider during planning and implementation. Complementary process-quality control methods are also included:

- External program review,
- Program utilization and record review,
- Session or component observations,
- Program procedure pre-testing, and
- Readability testing and content analysis.

## Process Evaluation Methods and Quality

Several terms need to be defined in a discussion of process evaluation: quality, quality control, and performance (practice) standard or metrics. *Quality* can be defined as an assessment of the degree of appropriateness of a set of defined core procedures (P...), participant assessment, and intervention methods, delivered by a trained member of a program for a specific health problem, population, and practice setting. *Quality control* is the application of process evaluation methods to document the degree to which the program has been delivered with fidelity. A *performance standard or metric* ($P_s$) is the description of a minimum acceptable level of quality defined by experts in a specialty area of an individuals' level of professional practice in the delivery of program Procedures (P1 + P2 + P3...). A performance standard level may be absolute (100%) or variable (80% or 90%) for individual procedures. A quality assurance review of a program is a multidimensional process, including documentation of the level of professional preparation of program-service providers and the application of quality control methods to assess and to improve, if inadequate, critical procedural components of a professional practice. It identifies solutions to problems or barriers to program implementation by staff, acceptance of assessments methods, and level of client use of intervention methods.

Two concepts are frequently mentioned in discussions of program quality: efficacy and effectiveness rates. As noted in Chapter 1, **efficacy** is the capacity of a program, applied under optimal conditions by specialty trained staff, to significantly alter the normal history or rate of a behavioral risk factor for a specific health problem and population at risk. **Effectiveness** is the capacity of an efficacious program, applied under normal practice conditions by regular staff, to significantly alter the normal rate of a behavioral risk factor for a specific health problem and large, defined population at risk. Without documenting the fidelity of delivery-implementation by staff of HP-DP program procedures, significant changes in impact or outcome rates are unlikely to occur.

## Type III Error

A major concern in all programs is implementation success—the degree of program feasibility or failure. Basch, Sleipcovich, and Gold (1985) described the failure to implement a health education intervention as a "Type III Error." Steckler and colleagues (1998), in an insightful discussion of Type III Error, used the qualitative case-study approach to monitor data to complement an impact evaluation. They examined the implementation of a cancer control program at multiple industrial plants. Two types of process evaluation data were collected: each provided insight about the degree to which a Type III Error had occurred. The first type of data was from in-depth case studies from one intervention plan. The second type of data was based on records monitoring training activities and health educational events at all E and (C) industrial sites. Other process evaluation methods were used, including the following:

- Site visits,
- Participant observations,
- Interview with key decision makers, and
- Record reviews of reports and documents related to program planning and implementation.

Four additional types of process-monitoring data were also collected at all industrial study sites: running records, consultation logs, phone logs, and correspondence.

A general plan of how the project was intended to work was examined. This process evaluation example found that the cancer control programs were not used to any great extent by employees at the (C) group plant nor by employees at most of the E group plants. Significant change did not occur among intervention plant workers, because of inadequate implementation of the planned health education program. *The evaluation concluded that a Type III Error had occurred. The following conclusion, that the intervention content and structure were inappropriate for this type of industrial site and for these types of workers, should not be made about the program.* A more appropriate inference is that critical organizational barriers for this setting and time prevented the introduction of this type of program among and between management and workers.

Without process and qualitative data and insight, evaluators cannot know why an HP-DP program did or did not produce a behavioral impact. With such empirically based insight, however, an evaluation is in a stronger position to attribute observed significant change (if any) to an intervention. In cases where implementation is not successful, process and qualitative evaluations may explain what happened and why.

## Provider Technical Competence and Education

The need to examine program procedures and skill and training levels of staff that plan and deliver health-related programs is well established. A judgment based on existing performance standards is required to evaluate the structure, content, and quality of the planning and delivery process. As noted in Chapter 1, there is a long-standing, historical concern in the United States and globally about the need to improve the quality of professional preparation and practice in health promotion and education. The connections between structure-process-impact-outcome continue to be an issue in examinations of the quality of health services and HP-DP programs.

Provider skill to deliver a program can be assessed through internal and external peer review methods. This requires examining the professional education and experience of staff and current performance levels in the implementation of an existing program. If an individual has the responsibility to plan, manage, and evaluate a HP-DP program, the type of graduate academic credentials, competencies, and the credentialing process for an MPH or Certified Health Education Specialist (CHES) are well defined. *Although codification of the competencies for health education–promotion practice, like all professions, continues to evolve, widely disseminated documents confirm that competencies to evaluate an HP-DP program have been established for > 30 years.*

Although the evidence base continues to mature, the HP-DP literature and behavioral and social science–related disciplines offer a body of knowledge about human behavior in sickness or health for most major diseases and behavioral risk factors for almost all large populations at risk. A competent practitioner should be knowledgeable about how to access and use the most up-to-date literature and methods applicable to each program. Accordingly, program directors of any HP-DP program need to know what has been done, what can be done, and how it should be done for a specific problem: a meta-evaluation. Commonly cited reasons for program failure include the following:

- Lack of academic coursework or field experience in applying HP-DP program planning-evaluation skills;
- Lack of knowledge by program staff of what level of impact is possible or probable;
- Ignorance or incomplete knowledge of published literature;

- Insufficient theoretical grounding about behavior change; and
- Weak-insufficient technical skill in planning, measurement, and evaluation.

Knowledge, skill, and experience in performing meta-evaluation and meta-analysis are essential competencies of a HP-DP specialist. These types of deficiencies often exist, in part, because of the diverse backgrounds of mid-level to senior staff engaged in directing the planning and provision of HP-DP programs without adequate graduate academic training. In addition, employers usually do not hold common views about what are appropriate academic and professional credentials in the recruitment and appointment of HP-DP program personnel.

Planners, directors, and coordinators should be able to provide evidence that programs under their direction reflect high standards of practice and, within the context of available resources, reflect the knowledge base. The level and type of academic training that should produce a person with these competencies is the master's degree (MPH, MSPH, or MS) in health education, or health promotion. Staff responsible for planning, managing, and evaluating HP-DP directors or managers of HP-DP programs should provide documentation of appropriate baccalaureate and master's degree training and skills to meet performance standards identified in Table 5.1

## Cultural Competency

Understanding the unique characteristics of communities, groups, and individuals is an established principle of HP-DP planning and evaluation. The evaluator's technical skills need to be complemented by an appreciation for the range of characteristics of different social groups. Many excellent examples of how to systematically plan and evaluate a health promotion program for diverse populations are presented in multiple governmental and nongovernmental publications.

## Quality Control Methods

Practitioners need to be able to conduct assessments of specific HP-DP program components in a systematic and technically acceptable fashion. Project staff can use a number of techniques to gain insight into how well each part of a program is being implemented, how well it is being accepted

TABLE 5.1 Practice Standards for Health Education Specialists

| PERFORMANCE STANDARD | CATEGORY |
|---|---|
| 1. Interpret data on the distribution of a selected health problem/ risk factor for a defined geographical area, setting, and population, using available and/or derived sources of data | POPULATION ASSESSMENT |
| 2. Describe, from available or collected evidence and expert opinion, the behavioral and non-behavioral risk factors associated with a specific health priority | PRIORITY SETTING |
| 3. Describe, from the related literature, the meta-evolution/ meta-analysis, the current knowledge about interventions for the specified risk factor or health problem and defined population at risk and the degree to which a behavior or risk factor(s) is amenable to change | DEFINING OBJECTIVES |
| 4. Describe, from the scientific evidence in the literature and from an educational – behavioral assessment, the contributing factors found to be causally associated with the health behavior/risk factor(s) defining the population, including: <br> a. Target group: predisposing factors—attitudes, beliefs, values, etc. <br> b. Setting: enabling factors\availability, accessibility, services cost. <br> c. Program/provider: reinforcing factors – staff attitudes, beliefs, etc. | CONTRIBUTING FACTORS |
| 5. Synthesize and translate the information and data from Steps 1–4 into a program plan | INTERVENTION PLANNING |
| 6. Design, implement, manage, and evaluate appropriate communication, community organization, and organizational development-training and education-behavioral methods to produce change in the contributing factors and the behaviors identified in sites 3–5, in partnerships with other health professionals, organizational personnel, and consumers | EVALUATION PLANS |
| 7. Prepare reports of a publishable quality based on appropriate analytical methods | EVALUATION REPORTS |
| 8. Conduct professional activities in an ethical manner | ETHICS |

by a target group, and what adjustments in methods and procedures might be made. One quality control technique is not necessarily superior to another. Each is useful in planning and implementing. Each serves a specific purpose and provides unique information about the structure, content, and process of an ongoing program. All require resources, staff, and time. Selecting the most appropriate and feasible methods for a specific program is important. A combination of quality control methods are recommended to review program components during planning or implementation: (1) expert panel review, (2) program utilization and record review,

(3) program/session observation, (4) community and participant surveys, (5) component-instrument pre-testing, (6) readability testing, and (7) content analysis.

## Internal and External Program Reviews (EPR): Evaluability Assessments

The importance of an internal and external review of an evaluation plan during the early stages of preparation, especially in the first year of the introduction of a "new" program, cannot be overstressed. An External Program Review (EPR) is an efficient way to assess the overall quality of a program. It assumes that a written program plan exists: structure, objectives, methods, activities, procedures, and tasks are described in detail. A complete plan delineates the target group, staff, time, place, budget, and resources. An EPR will determine if staff has followed a systematic process to plan a program and are following implementation plans.

An EPR examines all major components, activities, materials, and procedures during planning and program implementation. It compares written documents, and documentation data with a set of performance standards, using professional ratings. The total program and individual procedures are reviewed, for example, the implementation plan, evaluation design, data-collection procedures, mass-media components, and content of the intervention. The "Evaluability Assessment Form" in Table 1.4 in Chapter 1 is a useful referent for drafting a review plan.

An EPR is particularly useful during planning and during the early stages of implementation. Practically speaking, it is important to have a small review panel. Two experts from the local area or state university can be asked to examine a program. A review by two experienced consultants, once in the first six months and again each year for a project, should provide sufficient, independent insight into program progress. Although EPR panel members need experience with the health problem and the target population the program is serving, they need not be national leaders in HP-DP.

Common standards used by staff and expert panels for an Evaluability Assessment by an internal or external expert panel are listed in Chapter 1's "Evaluability Assessment Form" (Table 1.4). The panel provides comments on the degree of adequacy and suggests program revisions. This information gives program staff an overall qualitative judgment of the structure and process of the ongoing program. The review should be a collaborative activity between staff and external reviewers, providing practical suggestions as part of a formative assessment for program improvement.

## Program Utilization and Record Review

HP-DP programs often collect too much or too little information on participants. The information collected is often not used. Despite the difficulty that may be encountered, a record-keeping system is an essential component of program implementation. All program-monitoring and data-collection systems should be compatible with ongoing data systems. Program utilization and record reviews encompass four topics:

1. Monitoring program participation or session exposure,
2. Improving record completeness,
3. Documenting program or session exposure, and
4. Monitoring the use of information services.

### Monitoring Program Participation

Inherent to setting up a monitoring system is the need to define who the program is attempting to serve and an estimated number of eligible participants for the target area or location. All target populations need to be enumerated in the development of a plan. This allows you to answer the following questions: How many of those eligible were served? Where are they located and how many sites? Were the people who participated members of the target group for whom the program was designed? For some programs, standard record forms are often mandated. Programs always need minimum demographic and psycho-social characteristics and data concerning participants. Although this responsibility may seem to present major difficulties, if staff agree about the most important type of information needed on each participant and pay particular attention to efficiency in information collection, they should be able to gather complete documentation on service use.

From the standpoint of assessing educational needs, preparing a counseling plan, or evaluating program effectiveness, data abstracted from the forms for this period were of no value. Serious questions about the quality, validity, and reliability of the data collected were apparent. Although this reference is dated, it continues to be an excellent illustration of just how poor a "record system" can be. *Current record reviews that yield incomplete or missing data or data of such poor quality are common in public health settings. The completeness and validity of all data sets for all assessment years must be confirmed, not assumed.*

HP-DP programs will improve their recording systems by developing a monitoring mechanism to meet staff and evaluation needs. It should be compatible with data processing for quick periodic assessment, for example, monthly or per session. A record-keeping system is the only mechanism by which program evaluators can confirm how many of which demographic groups of clients were served. It is an essential program evaluation element.

Table 5.2 illustrates the amount of information lost by a poor instrument and record-keeping system. A retrospective 12-month review of medical

TABLE 5.2 Rank Order of Completed Items in Patient Records

| ITEM | DECILE OF FORMS: ITEM COMPLETED |
|---|---|
| Diabetes Instructor + Age | 90%–100% |
| Put on _____ calorie: ADA diet | 80%–89% |
| Diabetes mellitus diagnosed _____ year | |
| Demonstrated drawing up and injection of insulin | 70%–79% |
| Has been taught to use _____ urine test | |
| Personal hygiene/foot care items taught; educated in diabetic control | |
| After learning to use a urine test, knows how and when to test urine for sugar | 60%–69% |
| Knows how/when to test for acetone + use dextrosix | |
| Understands causes and symptoms of reactions, acidosis | |
| Understands need to call doctor if acidosis develops | |
| Attitude on admission | 50%–59% |
| Understands insulin adjustment for reactions, etc. | |
| Attitude on discharge | 40%–49% |
| Can test urine for sugar accurately | |
| Knows how to use booklet to follow diet | |
| Patient or member of family has been taught to use glucagon | |
| Pre-test score: Admission | 30%–39% |
| Class attendance—insulin injection | |
| Personal hygiene and foot care, acidosis, diabetes | 20%–29% |
| Urine checks + Diet restrictions, and diet | |
| Patient's physical or learning handicaps | 10%–19% |
| Post-test score: Discharge | 0%–10% |
| Incapable of drawing up own insulin or testing urine | |

records at a 40-bed hospital was conducted by Windsor, Gartseff, and Roseman, Diabetes Care, 1981 to determine the completeness and quality of patient education assessment data for diabetic patient admits. Although it was hospital policy to assess each patient on admission, only 394 of 996 patients (39%) had a baseline assessment form. The 394 baseline forms were reviewed to determine the quality of the assessments. A major problem identified, beyond not performing the assessment, was 50%–80% data incompleteness for most categories.

## Documenting Program-Session-Component Exposure

Another dimension to examine is records confirming participant exposure to program sessions. Baseline and follow-up assessments of participants or a representative sample should be conducted. Without exception, an HP-DP program must document who received how much of what from whom, where, how, and when. The Form in Table 5.3 was used to confirm patient exposure to a closed-circuit patient educational television program on the

TABLE 5.3 Observation Form for Closed-Circuit Television Patient Education Programming

Rm, Patient No _____

| Monday | Tuesday | Wednesday | Thursday | Friday | Saturday | Sunday |
|--------|---------|-----------|----------|--------|----------|--------|
| A.M. | | | | | | |
| P.M. | | | | | | |

Rm, Patient No _____

| Monday | Tuesday | Wednesday | Thursday | Friday | Saturday | Sunday |
|--------|---------|-----------|----------|--------|----------|--------|
| A.M. | | | | | | |
| P.M. | | | | | | |

Rm, Patient No _____

| Monday | Tuesday | Wednesday | Thursday | Friday | Saturday | Sunday |
|--------|---------|-----------|----------|--------|----------|--------|
| A.M. | | | | | | |
| P.M. | | | | | | |

Rm, Patient No _____

| Monday | Tuesday | Wednesday | Thursday | Friday | Saturday | Sunday |
|--------|---------|-----------|----------|--------|----------|--------|
| A.M. | | | | | | |
| P.M. | | | | | | |

TABLE 5.4 Patient Exposure to Closed-Circuit Television Programming

| DAY | PROGRAM | PATIENTS EXPOSED | POTENTIAL PATIENTS | PERCENT EXPOSED |
|---|---|---|---|---|
| Monday | 1 | 10 | 29 | 34% |
| | 2 | 3 | 31 | 10% |
| Tuesday | 3 | 5 | 31 | 16% |
| | 4 | 3 | 29 | 10% |
| | 5 | 6 | 27 | 22% |
| Wednesday | 6 | 6 | 28 | 21% |
| | 7 | 6 | 30 | 20% |
| Thursday | 8 | 4 | 30 | 13% |
| | 9 | 7 | 31 | 23% |
| Friday | 10 | 4 | 30 | 13% |
| | 11 | 10 | 31 | 32% |
| Saturday | 12 | 6 | 31 | 19% |
| Sunday | 13 | 8 | 31 | 26% |
| | 14 | 7 | 30 | 23% |
| Total | 14 | 85 | 419 | 20% |

treatment, management, and control for diabetic in-patients for a 40-bed hospital. Patients' rooms were observed for seven days to determine if they were viewing the TV programs presented daily at 10:00 a.m. and 2:00 p.m.

Using this method, staff confirmed the percent of patients exposed to each program, and the proportion of programs to which each patient was exposed during the one-week observation period. As Table 5.4 indicates, on average, only 20% of approximately 30 eligible patients/day watched the closed-circuit programs. This documented a very low level of patient exposure to this channel of communication-counseling. The data in Table 5.4 confirmed a need to examine why so few patients used all patient education programs, and to review program content and structure.

## Focus Group Interviews

A focus group interview is a group session method used to explore insights of target audiences about a specific topic. Social marketing researchers and advertisers use this method to derive the perceptions, beliefs, language, and interests of an audience to whom a product or service would be marketed. The focus group interview usually involves eight to ten people. Using a detailed discussion outline, a moderator keeps the group session within the appropriate time limits but gives considerable latitude to participants to respond spontaneously to a set of general or specific questions. The moderator has the opportunity to probe and gain in-depth insight from the interviews. These sessions are often video- or audiotaped.

Particularly used in the concept development stage of the communications development process, focus group interviews help health communications/media planners identify key concepts that may trigger awareness and interests in participation. This method is often used to complement population-based, representative-sample surveys on specific topics. Qualitative information is issued, in combination with the survey data, to make judgments about the perceptions, beliefs, and behaviors of the target population and subgroups within it.

## Component Pre-testing

Pre-testing is a quality control method used to document perceptions of target audiences. All programs should have core assessment and intervention elements pre-tested prior to routine application. Good pre-testing is a continuing issue in the field, because it requires technical skill from the staff, resources, and time, which is often not available. The three most common program elements that should be pre-tested are instruments, media, and materials, both written and visual. The following sections discuss the purposes and methods of pre-testing these elements. Detailed procedures for developing instruments are presented in Chapter 3.

### Instrument Development and Pre-testing

In conducting a process evaluation, the quality of the evaluation instrument (questionnaire) must be determined. A well-documented deficiency in the literature is the failure of many program planners to establish the reliability and validity of their instrument. Examine all instruments to determine their relevance to the specified program objectives. In the development and pre-testing of an instrument, program planners must demonstrate concern for the consumer, especially burden. The instrument should be a manageable length: shorter is better. Collect only essential information from participants.

Pre-test instruments for such characteristics as time of administration, ease of comprehension, readability, sensitivity, reactivity of questions, organization of questions, and standardization of administration and scoring. First, select a sample of individuals who are representative of the population for whom the instrument is prepared. Then test the instrument under conditions comparable to those in which it will be applied in the program setting.

As a preliminary step (before a pilot test), in order to eliminate glaring problems of omission or commission, four or five people from the target group can be asked to review and complete the instrument. The target group should identify ambiguous questions, lack of clarity, or insensitivity in word choice. Usually 30 to 50 people participate in a pilot test to ensure the distribution of responses across characteristics. Pilot test at all sites and with all staff using the forms and methods. If the pilot test is self-administered, provide a set of written instructions on how to complete the form. Respondents should be able to provide reactions/suggestions for changes.

Instrument pre-testing is a critical first step to ensure data quality and competencies. Rely heavily on instruments used by comparable programs. No planner should develop a new instrument unless absolutely necessary. If, for example, a program is attempting to change the participants' personal health practices or beliefs, the staff should adapt forms identified in the literature or available from national agencies for surveying health risk factors, practices, knowledge, and beliefs. Examples of types of pre-testing questions are presented in Table 5.5.

TABLE 5.5 Pre-Testing Message Characteristics

| CHARACTERISTIC | QUESTIONS |
| --- | --- |
| Attraction: | Is the presentation interesting enough to attract and hold the attention of the target group? Do consumers like it? Which aspects of the presentation do people like most? What gained the greatest share of their attention? |
| Comprehension: | How clear is the message? How well is it understood? |
| Acceptability: | Does the message contain anything that is offensive or distasteful by local standards? Does it reflect community norms and beliefs? Does it contain irritating or abusive language? |
| Personal Involvement: | Is the program perceived to be directed to persons in the target audience? In other words, do the consumers feel that the program is for them personally, or do they perceive it as being for someone else? |
| Persuasion: | Does the message convince the target audience to try the desired behavior? How favorably predisposed are individuals to try a certain product, use a specific service, originate a new personal health behavior? |

## Media and Messages

Pre-testing systematically gathers target audience reaction to written, visual, or audio messages and media. In assessing the quality of media, program staff should document their having followed procedures that meet professional standards and that follow well-established steps to create media. Program planners who do not pre-test media lose the opportunity to gain valuable insights into the quality of those methods of communication. A thorough review of formative evaluation methods for media is provided in "Making Health Communication Programs Work" (US Department of Health and Human Services, 2005).

Pre-testing media is designed to improve communications before diffusion and to document which alternatives will be most efficient and effective. The concept of pre-testing is simple; it involves measuring the reactions of a group of people to the object of interest, such as a film, booklet, or TV announcement. Pre-testing should be done not only with members of the target audience but with staff. Obviously, the sophistication and budget that can be applied to conducting a pre-test seem infinite. The resources expended by the advertising industry each year confirm this fact.

In developing health information programs and revising existing messages and media, pre-testing is an essential method to assess ease of comprehension, personal relevance, audience acceptance, recall, and other strengths and weaknesses of draft messages before production. A pre-test should establish a target audience baseline and should determine if there are large cognitive, affective, perception, or behavioral differences within the target audience. Planners should design pre-tests of media to provide information on the following components of effectiveness.

No absolute formula can be used to design a pre-test or field trial. All ongoing programs need to have their media examined carefully before using them with an audience. Simple or highly technical and costly methods and procedures are available. The acceptability and memorability of selected media and products may often be improved, however, without a major allocation of time or resources. A pre-test should be tailored to objectives and should consider time, cost, resources, and the availability of a target audience. Planners may have to decide which media will be formally pre-tested and which will undergo only internal review. This decision must be tempered by the risk of creating active opposition responses. The following are suggested steps for developing media:

- State briefly the program topic;
- List the primary and secondary program audiences;

- Select the medium;
- State why the program is important;
- Specify expected objectives for consumer and provider;
- Specify what the viewer should know, do, or believe from media exposure;
- Prepare a 10- to 30-minute instructional program;
- Provide information on why this is an important information source;
- Prepare script content based on characteristics of the audience;
- Plan visual materials and develop a storyboard;
- Describe the evaluation procedures to assess cognitive, belief, skill, and impact;
- Conduct and evaluate the program; and
- Revise the product.

### Written Materials

Written materials are almost always used in health promotion and education programs. The major concern is whether people can read and understand the material. Written materials should serve as aids to information transfer and should clarify and reinforce the principal messages specified in the program objectives. Using written materials as principal behavior-change elements of your program is, however, archaic. Many professionally developed and field-tested written materials are available for most health problems and risk factors. To assess program materials, use a three-step process: (1) assessment of reading level, (2) content analysis, and (3) review by content and health education specialists. The following are recommended steps for preparing written materials:

- Use one-and two-syllable words if appropriate;
- Write short, simple sentences with only one idea per sentence;
- State the main idea at the beginning of each paragraph;
- Break up parts of the narrative with subheadings and captions;
- Use the active voice;
- Highlight important ideas and terms in boldface or italic type;
- Leave plenty of "white space" on the printed page;
- Add the phonetic pronunciation of key technical terms;
- Define difficult words; and
- Summarize important points in short paragraphs.

The program staff must first gather materials and review them thoroughly to determine which might serve the program objectives best. Some can be modified for the target audience. Design written materials for efficient, low-cost distribution. They must be capable of capturing the interest of the audience and should be presented in an imaginative yet simple fashion. It is important that terms, word choice, and other characteristics be chosen to promote reading. Ask several major questions to assess the quality of materials: (1) What are the objectives? (2) Why use this medium to communicate this information? (3) For whom are the materials intended? (4) Under what circumstances will people read it? (5) What languages or ethnic perspectives need to be considered? Use pre-testing to gather words, phrases, and vernacular from target audiences, so an appropriate language can be used, and to determine effective methods for communicating.

"Making Health Communication Programs Work" (USDHHS, NCI, 2005) provides information on the content and methods used to assess printed materials. If a program uses written materials extensively, as aids to the reinforcement of its educational and counseling efforts, staff may want to assess whether participants are accessing and using the information. A random sample of program participants at each program site can be asked a set of basic questions to determine their behavioral responses to written materials:

- Do you remember a brochure that came with your prescription?
- Did you read it before you started taking your drugs?
- (If no): Did you get a chance to read it later?
- After you read it, did you ever go back and read it again?
- Did you keep the brochure, throw it away, or give it to a friend?
- Did anyone else read the leaflet from your prescription?

Although many questions can be asked, and these may be tailored to variations in format, length, content, and style, the basic process is designed to determine what document worked best. An HP-DP program can conduct a qualitative assessment of participants, asking each to rate different pamphlets on the basis of thoroughness and clarity of explanation, degree of stimulation, simplicity or complexity, level of reassurance, and factuality. Many ongoing programs that use written information could use the questions, documentation, and formative evaluation design applied to determine how effective written components of a program are in communicating information to program participants.

### Visual Materials-Radio-Television

In pre-testing visual aids (e.g., posters), a principal aim is to assess their ability to attract. In general, they should be attention getters, conveying one single idea. The extent to which they are comprehensible, educationally and ethnically acceptable, and promote audience involvement should be assessed. If a major fiscal expenditure is being made, multiple samples from the target audience at different locations may be needed. To pre-test a poster, however, a small number of people may be sufficient (5 to 10). Although many questions can be asked, the 10 presented here are often used by an interviewer or in a self-administered questionnaire to determine an individual's response to a visual aid:

1. What is the most important message presented?
2. Is this visual aid asking you to do something?
3. Is there anything offensive to you or other people who live in your community?
4. What do you like about it?
5. What do you dislike about it?
6. In comparison to others you have seen before, how would you rate it?
7. Is the information new to you?
8. Are you likely to do what the visual aid asks?
9. Do you think the average person would understand it?
10. How would you improve it?

These questions and others that staff may consider appropriate should be asked as the visual aid is shown to the individual. Responses will provide insight into the attractiveness, comprehensibility, and acceptability. The pre-testing of radio and television announcements follows the general principles outlined for other categories of media. One difference, however, is the need to produce and pilot test an announcement. Cost is a major factor to consider. A radio announcement can be easily taped on a recorder and a poster designed to rough form, but producing a TV announcement or program, even in preliminary form, can be expensive.

### Health Message-Testing Service

Some large programs for a specific health problem, for example, smoking cessation, breast self-examination, physical fitness, may have the budget and resources to use a commercial health message-testing service. This service provides a standardized system to assess audience response to mass media messages about health to gauge the communication effectiveness of these messages. The system informs program planners of the audience's message recall, comprehension, and sense of the personal relevance and believability of the message, as well as identifying strong and weak communication points. In testing a message, the major concern is its appropriateness for its intended subgroup. A testing service examines the attention-getting ability of the message and audience recall of the main idea. Overall, a health message-testing service can provide invaluable insights to refine draft message announcements, alternative messages, and planning future HP-DP campaigns. But it is very expensive.

### Media Program Evaluation and Computer Analysis

Current technology provides the most sophisticated evaluation and research of media productions through the application of microcomputer technology. Electronic analyses can be made of the effects of any media presentation, documenting an audience's reaction second by second. This technology can document the effects of minute changes in presentation on audience attitudes, skill, and knowledge. Program staff has the opportunity to manipulate covertly what the audience sees and to analyze responses instantaneously. It allows a program to collect instant feedback data on an infinite number of visual, graphic, and verbal configurations. It is a powerful technique to conduct formative media evaluations during the pre-production stage. Before investing in production costs that could run in the millions, agencies need to perform careful preliminary assessments.

### Readability Testing

Readability is another important aspect of pre-testing written materials. Readability tests are available and easy to apply. Readability tests determine the reading grade level required of the average person to understand the written materials. Readability estimates provide evidence of only the structural difficulties of a written document: vocabulary and sentence structure. They indicate how well the information will be understood but do not guarantee comprehension. Many readability formulas exist (Dale and Chall, 1948; Flesch, 1948: Fry, 1968; Klare, 1974–1975), but the Simple Measure of Gobbledygook (SMOG) grading formula for testing the readability of educational material is one of the most commonly applied. Generally considered an excellent method of assessing the grade level a person must have reached to understand the text, it requires 100% comprehension of the material read. To calculate the SMOG reading-grade level, program staff should use the entire written work being evaluated using these steps:

- Count 10 consecutive sentences at the start, in the middle, and the end of the text.
- From this sample, circle all words with > 3 syllables, including repetitions of the same word.
- Total the number of words circled.
- Estimate the square root of the total number of polysyllabic words counted.
- Find the nearest perfect square and calculate the square root.
- Add a constant of 3 to the square root to calculate grade (reading-grade level) that a person must have completed to fully understand the text being evaluated.

Sentence and word length and difficulty affect the readability score. The SMOG formula ensures 90% comprehension; that is, a person with a tenth-grade reading level will comprehend 90% of the material rated at that level. This procedure can be applied to all texts prepared by a program for public consumption. "Making Health Communication Programs Work" (USDHHS, 2005) presents useful discussions of readability in general and in health-related literature.

Another readability method increasingly being used by health education specialists is the Flesch-Kincaid Readability tests. This method has a long history, dating to 1948, when Flesch published the Reading Ease test. The formula for the test produces a score ranging from 0 to 120. A higher score indicates material easier to read, while a lower number indicates material more difficult to read. For example, reading ease scores of 90–100 indicate the material can be read and understood by the average 11-year-old. Reading ease scores of 0–30 mean the passage is understood by university graduates. In 1975 Kincaid, working under a US Navy contract, developed the Reading Grade level. It translates the Flesch Reading Ease to actual grade levels in US schools. These formulae were combined and are now known as the Flesch-Kincaid Readability tests. They are widely applied by writers of self-help booklets, brochures, and pamphlets. The Flesch-Kincaid formulae can be accessed on a number of computer software programs and no longer require hand calculation of reading levels.

# A Process Evaluation Model: Documenting Fidelity and Quality of HP-DP Program Delivery

In a structural assessment of a program, an evaluator examines the resources, personnel, facilities, and equipment to deliver services and asks: Are they adequate? In a process evaluation, the ultimate questions are: What program procedures were delivered by each member and all members of a program staff to all eligible clients? Are the core procedures based on normative criteria or professional practice standards (criteria developed by a consensus of experienced peers in health education and health promotion with established professional credentials)? A process assessment, using normative performance criteria, is a direct examination of program quality.

The following section describes a model that can be used to plan and assess implementation of HP-DP program intervention and assessment procedures.

Process evaluation data provide essential data and insight about what types of client assessment and intervention procedures can (and cannot) be routinely delivered for specific settings, behaviors, types of providers, and participants. Process evaluation methods should be used as a routine quality control mechanism to assess staff provision of core program procedures. They also have a very practical function. They provide empirical evidence and information about salient structure and operational procedures within and across HP-DP programs in different sites.

Process evaluation data documenting the level of client exposure to each health education method are also critical to making a conclusion about efficacy-effectiveness, internal and external validity, and costs and cost-effectiveness of an HP-DP intervention. For example, in a meta-evaluation of 31 evaluation studies of cessation methods for pregnant smokers, serious process evaluation deficiencies were reported (Windsor, Boyd, and Orleans, 1998). Although space limitations in a publication often restrict a study from providing a complete description of its intervention methods, most of the evaluation studies lacked an adequate description and/or documentation of the delivery of experimental and control group intervention methods. Only 12 of the 31 evaluation studies reviewed adequately described the specific characteristics of core program methods, such as number, type, frequency, and duration of client counseling contacts.

The following section provides explicit practice guidelines and examples of how to systematically evaluate program implementation using (1) a framework to describe client assessment and intervention procedures; (2) a description of the program (site) flow analysis method; (3) a description of a process evaluation model (PEM); and (4) examples of applications of the PEM, using data from two different patient education projects.

## Definition of HP-DP Intervention and Measurement Procedures

One of the first planning tasks that all programs must perform is to describe what assessment and intervention procedures (Pn) clients with specific characteristics are supposed to receive as part of routine care and as part of an evaluation. E–C–(C) group intervention procedures need to be described, specifying the following: (1) what, (2) who, (3) when, (4) how much, and (5) where. Descriptions of these process variables are essential to standardize methods, develop staff training programs, recommend specific modifications of methods during pilot testing and at the end of an evaluation study, and replicate methods by future intervention programs and evaluation studies. Because "normal" health education methods and staff behavior will typically change from the presence of an evaluation, documentation of salient clinical procedures at each client contact is essential before and during an evaluation study.

Information in Table 5.6 describes the core HP-DP procedures, the staff providing the procedures, methods and materials, and time. Cost can be estimated for each procedure. This description helps project staff to define client procedures, personnel methods, and materials, and to estimate time for each client contact. As noted in Table 5.6, this method defines what methods were supposed to be provided by whom at each visit/contact. It is also an excellent

TABLE 5.6 Specification of Intervention Procedures

| PROCESS VARIABLE | PROGRAM TASK |
| --- | --- |
| What: | Describe the structure-procedures-content of the health education program used, including, e.g., audiovisuals, written materials, and telephone counseling methods. |
| Who: | Name each member of the staff by degree/title who provides each procedure. |
| When: | Specify the time (estimated or observed) to deliver each health education procedure at each contact. |
| How much: | Specify the frequency, duration, and periodicity of procedures for each patient contact by the type of method and type of provider. |
| Setting: | Specify where and how the procedures are delivered, e.g., group, one-to-one format, video, text messages, or interactive computer. |

method to document labor and non-labor costs for an intervention. Separate forms should be used to describe procedures for the experimental group and control group in an evaluation study. Each intervention program needs to provide descriptions of their core clinical practice procedures.

## Program or Practice Flow Analysis (PFA)

After describing the core intervention and assessment procedures to be provided to clients at each site (*what*), program staff must define *how, when*, and *who* would deliver the new methods (*how much*). Program (Practice-Site-Client) Flow Analysis (PFA) is an excellent method to be applied when a program is considering the introduction of new client assessment or counseling methods into program services, for example, improving blood pressure. PFA documents exposure to specific services and staff at each contact from start to end of contact. It examines the average client time by type of contact, time for specific services, and proportion of time in contact and not in contact with each provider. It also helps site program managers and staff to document who can deliver what kinds of services to whom. It can be used to estimate cost for each participant and provider. A sample of five to ten clients for each provider for a one-week period at each site where the new methods are being considered for adoption is needed to document the type of services received and specific time (in minutes) that a participant spends with each provider.

### Organizational Development and PFA

The introduction of any new set of procedures into a patient care, worksite, or school system requires policy, management, and practice support. PFA involves a collaborative process between program staff and managers who deliver and plan services. A PFA study should start with a careful examination of current program, policy, structure, process, and content to determine what will be delivered, where, and by whom. Without participation of staff from each practice setting/site, it is very unlikely that a site flow analysis will be conducted and/or that its results will be useful or used by staff to plan the integration of the new methods into that setting. A PFA helps to identify normal patterns to gain insight about possible adjustments to that pattern to maximize the opportunity for routine delivery of new procedures. Evaluation staff should review program procedures with managers and regular staff to determine how best to integrate new methods into a practice and site.

## Case Study 1: Process Evaluation Model, Smoke Free Families Program

R. Windsor, H. Whiteside, Jr., L. Solomon, et al. "A Process Evaluation Model for Patient Education Programs for Pregnant Smokers," *Tobacco Control* (2000) 9, Supplement III (see publication for references).

The following case study presents an example of the application of the PEM by the Smoke Free Families (SFF) Program of the National Program Office (NPO) funded by the Robert Wood Johnson Foundation (RWJF). The primary questions in a process assessment evaluation of a patient education program for pregnant smokers are the following: (1) What procedures should a trained professional routinely provide to a pregnant smoker at her first visit and at follow-up visits? (2) What is excellent clinical practice standard for counseling for this risk factor and patient population? (3) Were the new procedures based on normative criteria (evidence based) developed by a consensus of experts? (4) Did staff participate in the development of the implementation plan? and (5) Did staff perform/provide the procedures to patients as planned at each OB or prenatal care visit?

Identification of the number of patients screened and recruited each week who smoked—Procedure 1 (P1)—was the first task for all projects. Baseline data on patients who were screened and recruited, as well as refusals, documented the daily, weekly, monthly, and annual census for each project by site. Among each eligible cohort of 100 patients who smoke (A), a number of patients accept the program at each site (B). These criteria produce information to compute an exposure rate for each procedure (B/A = C). As noted in Table 5.7, each SFF study had planned at the first visit a smoking status and psychosocial assessment of patients—Procedures 2 (P2) and 3 (P3). Patients in this example were scheduled to receive each of the next seven procedures at future visits. This example indicates that intervention-patients will receive Procedures 7, 8, 9, and 10.

Under the National Program Office Process Evaluation Guidelines (1994–2004), each of the RWJF- SFF grantees had to define and to implement a set of new patient education and counseling procedures. As noted in Table 5.7, one of the first steps in the preparation of a process evaluation plan was to require each RWJF program to define its essential new patient assessment and intervention methods for each visit, and by patient-staff contact. A practice Performance Standard (D), based on Guidelines and

TABLE 5.7 Patient Education Procedures for Pregnant Smokers

| PROCEDURE | STAFF | METHODS + MATERIALS | TIME | COST |
|---|---|---|---|---|
| 1st Visit Obstetric ☐ Pediatric ☐ | | | | |
| I. Patient Assessment Procedures | | | 5 min | ? |
|   a. Smoking status | RN or SW | Screening Form (self-report) | | |
|   b. Collection of fluid | RN or SW | Vials, Cotton Rolls, Saliva | | |
|   c. Psycho-social assessment | RN or SW | Baseline Form | | |
| II. Patient Education Procedures | | | | |
|   a. Component 1 | RN or SW | *A Pregnant Woman's Guide to Quit Smoking* | | |
|   b. Component 2 | RN or SW | Brief Patient Counseling + Patient Education Prescription | 1–2 min | ? |
| 2nd Visit | RN or SW | Self-Report | 1 min | ? |
| III. Patient Assessment Procedures 2 | | | | |
| | RN or SW | Chart Reminder Form | 1 min | ? |
| 3rd Visit | RN or SW | Self-Report | 1 min | ? |
| IV. Patient Assessment Procedures 3 | | | | |
| | RN or SW | Staff Reinforcement-Chart | | |
| 4th Visit | RN or SW | Self-Report and Vials Cotton Rolls, Saliva | 1 min | ? |
| V. Patient Assessment Procedures 4 | | | | |

an expert panel review, defined the expected level of provider performance and levels of patient exposure to each procedure (P).

The National Program Office (NPO) used 100% as an absolute practice standard (D) for each procedure. An Implementation Index (E) for each procedure is derived by dividing the exposure rate (C) by the practice-performance standard (D). In this example, where the practice-performance standard (D) is 100%, the Implementation Index (E) and exposure rate (C) are equal. A composite of all Implementation Indexes (☐E) provides a summary index of the successful delivery of a patient assessment and education program: a Program Implementation Index (PII). *A PII > 0.90 is an excellent level of implementation for a multi-component program.*

## PEM Application

Illustrative data for the 10 clinical practice procedures for the E group patients are presented in Table 5.8. These data indicated that the project needs to increase patient exposure to Procedures 6-7-8-9-10. Each SFF grantee had the responsibility to apply the PEM to patients at all sites to produce implementation data for its procedures. A staff training plan can be prepared to improve a specific exposure rate (C) or implementation index (E), when problems are documented: for example, when an exposure rate or Implementation Index falls < 90%.

## Patient Assessment and Counseling Procedures (P...)

An example of an unsuccessful implementation is presented in Table 5.9.

Data and the PII in Table 5.9 are excerpted from the publication. Although >100 was the target sample size for an E and C group, this process evaluation included only 42 E group patients.

After patients had undergone a telephone screening for inclusion in this study, each was asked to set a quit date within the next two weeks and mailed treatment materials. Women in the E group (usual care plus video) received the calendar, tip guide, and the six-video

TABLE 5.8 Process Evaluation Example

| PATIENT CLINICAL | ELIGIBLE PATIENTS | EXPOSED PATIENTS | EXPOSURE RATE (B/A) | PERFORMANCE STANDARD | IMPLEMENTATION INDEX (C/D) |
|---|---|---|---|---|---|
| Procedures (P) | (A) | (B) | (C) | (D) | (E) |
| 1. Smokers Recruited ($S_1$) | 100 | 90 | 90% | 100% | 0.90 |
| 2. Baseline Form ($O_{1A}$) | 100 | 100 | 100% | 100% | 1.00 |
| 3. Baseline Cotinine ($O_{1B}$) | 100 | 100 | 100% | 100% | 1.00 |
| 4. E group ($X_1$) | 100 | 100 | 100% | 100% | 1.00 |
| 5. E group ($X_2$) | 100 | 95 | 95% | 100% | 0.95 |
| 6. E group ($X_3$) | 100 | 95 | 95% | 100% | 0.95 |
| 7. Follow up $O_{2A}$ | 100 | 80 | 80% | 100% | 0.80 |
| 8. Follow up $O_{2B}$ | 100 | 80 | 80% | 100% | 0.80 |
| 9. Follow up $O_{3A}$ | 100 | 70 | 70% | 100% | 0.70 |
| 10. Follow up $O_{3B}$ | 100 | 70 | 70% | 100% | 0.70 |

Program Implementation Index =
$\Sigma e/P_n = 0.90 + 1.00 + 1.00 + 1.00 + 0.95 + 0.95 + 0.80 + 0.80 + 0.70 + 0.70/10 = 0.95$
X = intervention group-component; O = patient observation-smoking status; P = procedure.

TABLE 5.9 Case Study: Experimental Group Process Evaluation

| PATIENT CLINICAL PROCEDURES (P) | ELIGIBLE PATIENTS (A) | EXPOSED PATIENTS (B) | EXPOSURE RATE (B/A) (C) | PERFORMANCE STANDARD (D) | IMPLEMENTATION INDEX (C/D) (E) |
|---|---|---|---|---|---|
| 1. Base: Psychosocial (PS) | 42 | 42 | 100% | 100% | 1.00 |
| 2. Saliva Collection | 42 | 26 | 62% | 100% | 0.62 |
| 3. Patient Education | 42 | 42 | 100% | 100% | 1.00 |
| 4. Video 1 | 42 | 31 | 74% | 100% | 0.74 |
| 5. Video 2 | 42 | 26 | 62% | 100% | 0.62 |
| 6. Video 3 | 42 | 22 | 52% | 100% | 0.52 |
| 7. Video 4 | 42 | 13 | 31% | 100% | 0.31 |
| 8. Video 5 | 42 | 6 | 14% | 100% | 0.14 |
| 9. Video 6 | 42 | 8 | 19% | 100% | 0.19 |
| 10. Follow-up 1: PS | 42 | 31 | 74% | 100% | 0.74 |
| 11. Follow-up 2: PS * | 42 | 27 | 64% | 100% | 0.64 |
| 12. Postpartum PS follow-up | 42 | 21 | 50% | 100% | 0.50 |

PII = 1.00 + 0.62 + 1.00 + 0.74 + 0.62 + 0.52 + 0.31 + 0.14 + 0.19 + 0.74 + 0.64 + 0.50/12 = 0.56

program. All follow-ups were conducted by telephone. Major patient assessments were conducted two to three days after a quit date, four to five weeks after the quit date, and one month postpartum. Abstinence, negative affect, coping stress, and self-efficacy were obtained by phone interviews only. No counseling was provided during any of the phone follow-up visits.

As noted in Table 5.9, the most significant difficulties encountered in this study were patient recruitment and retention. While there may be some appeal for using videos as a minimal intervention, the lack of personal contact may have contributed to very poor compliance. As noted, very low patient adherence was an issue in this study. Multiple factors, including poor commitment, high nicotine dependence, and affective disturbance, may have contributed significantly to the overall poor adherence to the patient education procedures and low cessation rates. The limited value of planning a future patient education program using six videos is self-evident.

## Discussion

As documented in the case study, the primary value of the PEM is that it can and does provide data for weekly and/or monthly progress reviews for each site and individual providers. It can be used to identify specific implementation problems by site and specific staff. In case study 1, for example, six videos for patients were created. The process data confirmed almost no use of the videos beyond video 3 or video 4. These data, combined with patient feedback, require a reduction of the number of videos. The routine application of the PEM documented the degree to which the clinical staff of the example had implemented all procedures as planned. The PEM provided empirical data about the feasibility of routine delivery and replicability of procedures at comparable settings. It is also the primary method used to prepare a cost analysis of new and existing health education programs. Future studies should apply the PEM in planning an evaluation.

## Case Study 2: A Peer-Delivered Health Promotion Program

J. Williams, G. Belle, C. Houston, et al. "Process Evaluation Methods of a Peer-Delivered Health Promotion Program for African American Women." *Health Promotion Practice* (2001) (see publication for references).

### Introduction

This case study, based on the Eat Well, Live Well Nutrition Program, is an excellent example of translating public health science into practice. The results of the impact evaluation were presented in *Research in Social Work Practice* (2000). It represents a partnership between university faculty and a social service agency with extensive history in providing services to African American (AA) communities in a large Midwestern city. The objective of the program was to reduce cardiovascular disease (CVD)-related risks primarily through diet and weight control. This community-based peer-delivered nutrition program was designed to promote dietary change among low-income AA women by "activation."

The program director recognized that a major weakness in community-based programs was the lack of attention to evaluating program delivery with fidelity: **Process Evaluation**. She acknowledged that often much effort is placed on evaluating impact and not process. As noted, "The critical product from process evaluation is a clear, descriptive picture of program quality." African-American (AA) women who agreed to participate in the Nutrition Program were randomly assigned to either an E group (n = 154) or C group (n = 148). The program was delivered by peer educators in three-month intervals to 80 individuals to each group. The program was administered in 12 group sessions; peer educators led 6 sessions (4–6 participants) and 6 individual sessions.

## Peer Training

African American women in the community were trained as peer educators to deliver a program designed to reduce high-fat dietary patterns among obese women at risk for developing non-insulin dependent diabetes. They were recruited to serve as educators, based on leadership and communication skills, and their ability to make their own dietary changes. The training program, four-hour sessions delivered three days/week for 16 weeks, was designed to improve the knowledge, dietary changes, basic nutrition, and teaching methods of peer educators. They received 48 hours of nutrition-specific training, 48 hours of communication and group-facilitation training and problem-solving skills training, and 24 hours of administrative training. Peer educators were provided one-hour weekly supervision meetings during the implementation phase.

## Process Evaluation

A detailed checklist and rating procedures were developed. The checklist was used as a guide by the peer educators in conducting each of the 12 sessions. A total of 144 sessions over four cohorts, 36 sessions per cohort, were delivered. For each cohort, 12 of the 36 sessions were randomly selected; 33% of the 144 sessions were audiotaped. Sessions typically lasted 45–90 minutes. Two outside raters independently rated the "comprehensiveness" of the content delivered. Kappa ($k$) statistics were used to assess the % of content delivered. A registered dietitian conducted a third review to assess the "accuracy" of the nutrition content delivered.

## Results

The Eat Well, Live Well process evaluation had two objectives: (1) to document the comprehensiveness of content delivered; and (2) to assess the accuracy of the nutrition information delivered. Data in Tables 5.10, 5.11 and 5.12 are a synthesis of the data from the original article.

TABLE 5.10 Comprehensiveness of Program Items Delivered per Session

| SESSION | COMPREHENSIVENESS (%) | PERFORMANCE S (%) | IMPLEMENTATION INDEX |
|---|---|---|---|
| 1 | 88.0 | 95% | 0.93 |
| 2 | 81.1 | 95% | 0.85 |
| 3 | 93.0 | 95% | 0.98 |
| 4 | 90.5 | 95% | 0.95 |
| 5 | 96.8 | 95% | 1.02 |
| 6 | 90.3 | 95% | 0.95 |
| 7 | 97.1 | 95% | 1.02 |
| 8 | 95.6 | 95% | 1.00 |
| 9 | 93.1 | 95% | 0.98 |
| 10 | 87.4 | 95% | 0.92 |
| 11 | 94.3 | 95% | 0.99 |
| 12 | 95.2 | 95% | 1.00 |
| Overall | 91.4 | 95% | 0.96 |

PII = 0.93 + 0.85 + 0.98 + 0.95 + 1.02 + 0.95 + 1.02 + 1.00 + 0.98 + 0.92 + 0.99 + 1.00/12 = 0.97 = PII

TABLE 5.11 Accuracy of Program Items Delivered per Session

| SESSION | ACCURACY (%) | PERFORMANCE STANDARD (%) | IMPLEMENTATION INDEX |
|---|---|---|---|
| 1 | 81.0 | 95% | 0.85 |
| 2 | 88.0 | 95% | 0.93 |
| 3 | 74.9 | 95% | 0.79 |
| 4 | 93.1 | 95% | 0.98 |
| 5 | 96.7 | 95% | 1.02 |
| 6 | 84.8 | 95% | 0.89 |
| 7 | 93.8 | 95% | 1.04 |
| 8 | 87.2 | 95% | 0.99 |
| 9 | 81.5 | 95% | 0.92 |
| 10 | 87.4 | 95% | 0.92 |
| 11 | 97.3 | 95% | 1.02 |
| 12 | 96.8 | 95% | 1.02 |
| Overall | 88.5 | 95% | 0.93 |

PII = 0.85 + 0.93 + 0.79 + 0.98 + 1.02 + 0.89 + 1.04 + 0.99 + 0.92 + 0.92 + 1.02 + 1.02/12 = 0.95 = PII

This process evaluation provided an excellent example of how to gain very explicit insight into the implementation of a community-based program. Although others may be available, it is among the most comprehensive process evaluations available in the health promotion–health education literature. As noted, "Studying the implementation of a program can also

TABLE 5.12 Items Delivered by Peer Educator; Comprehensiveness and Accuracy

| PEER EDUCATOR | COMP. (%) | PERFORMANCE STANDARD | IMPLEMENTATION INDEX + | PERFORMANCE STANDARD | ACCURACY (%) | IMPLEMENTATION INDEX+ |
|---|---|---|---|---|---|---|
| A | 95.4 | 95% | 1.00 | 95% | 92.9 | 0.98 |
| B | 88.4 | 95% | 0.93 | 95% | 83.4 | 0.88 |
| C | 89.4 | 95% | 0.94 | 95% | 85.1 | 0.89 |

+ Based on a 95% Peer Educator Performance Standard

help planners learn how to modify programs and policies to improve their effectiveness." This article reaffirmed that from an evaluation perspective, a process evaluation is necessary to ensure that a Type III error does not occur, "we did not make conclusions about the program's effectiveness until we evaluated the extent to which the program was delivered." The authors perceived that a process evaluation was an integral part of an overall evaluation plan.

## Case Study 3: The Partners for Life Program

N. Boyd, R. Windsor, "Formative Evaluation in Maternal and Child Health Practice: The Partners for Life Nutrition Education Program for Pregnant Women," *Maternal & Child Health Journal* (2002) (see publication for references).

### Introduction

Public health interventions often fail to have an impact for many reasons, including failure to deliver program components, failure to pilot test E group methods, and/or failure to monitor the delivery of core procedures. These problems may be avoided, if a pilot test is conducted. The following discussion provides data and insight about a program that was not implemented with fidelity.

### Background

The Mississippi Department of Health identified patients' lack of knowledge, skill, and poor overall nutritional status at conception and during pregnancy as primary contributing factors to high rates of low birth-weight and infant mortality. The Freedom From Hunger Foundation of California (FFHF) joined with the Mississippi Cooperative Extension Service and Department of Health to establish the Partners for Life Program (PFLP) to address nutrition problems in the Delta region. Over 95% of pregnant women in the Delta region received MCH services at the county health department. These women were eligible for the Special Supplemental Program for Women, Infants, and Children (WIC) services. WIC policy recommends that clients receive at least two 15-minute educational sessions for every six months of participation. A meta-evaluation confirmed that the behavioral impact of nutrition education had not been documented (Boyd and Windsor, 1989).

The PFLP decided that because of the successful evaluations of the Expanded Food and Nutrition Education Program (EFNEP), which involve a more personalized instruction, changes could be made in EFNEP to meet local health department project needs. The primary aim of the PFLP project was to build a partnership between the WIC and EFNEP program staff. The PFLP project was established to plan and evaluate the impact of nutrition education on the dietary-related behaviors associated with infant and maternal health.

## Study Location

Leflore County, a county representative of a six-county Delta region, was selected as the pilot site for a two-year Formative Evaluation by the FFHF. The Formative Evaluation was designed to assess intervention strengths and weaknesses to revise the program prior to implementation it in a multi-county, Phase 2 Efficacy Evaluation. Its objectives were the following:

- To develop a new EFNEP curriculum tailored to pregnancy;
- To recruit and train peer EFNEP educators;
- To develop and validate patient assessment instruments;
- To pilot test the new curriculum under normal conditions to determine impact;
- To convene focus groups to determine the usefulness-acceptability of the new curriculum;
- To conduct a review of intervention forms-procedures to determine data completeness.

## Methods

### Program Development

An advisory committee of physicians, nurses, nutritionists, health educators, and other health professionals with MCH expertise was established to provide guidance about content validity, structure, and program process. It defined eight essential content areas. The EFNEP content was altered to meet the specific nutritional needs of pregnant women and was designed to be delivered in eight consecutive weekly sessions of 60 minutes. The delivery format was discussion and demonstration in the clients' homes, creating an interactive education/teaching style. A draft of the PFLP was revised, based on the comments of two external nutrition education evaluators.

## Peer Educator Recruitment and Training

The PFLP staff recruited five local female peer educators with qualifications that included being African American, being a mother, and being a high school graduate. They received an intensive three-month training program from the PFLP staff. The five peer educators completed their training by delivering the new intervention to a sample of 25 WIC-eligible pregnant women in the homes of the clients by the same peer educator. The PFLP director was present to critique peer educator presentations. Strengths and weaknesses of delivery were discussed after each presentation.

## Instrumentation and Measurement

The lesson objectives and content were used to develop a 28-item nutrition in pregnancy patient knowledge test. Two experts in nutrition education and instrument development reviewed the test for content validity. This instrument was administered to a sample of 63 pregnant women in Leflore County who met the eligibility criteria. The test Internal Consistency analysis was: $r = 0.71$ (Kuder-Richardson 21) and all items retained had an item to total correlation of $r > 0.20$. A 24-hour dietary recall instrument was administered to a pilot sample of 63 patients to assess dietary behavior. A random sub-sample of ten 24-hour recalls was independently rated by two nutritionists to determine inter-rater reliability: Kappa (K). Inter-rater reliabilities were marginal to excellent: meat: $K = 0.50$; fruits and vegetables: $K = 0.60$; milk and dairy products: $K = 0.65$; and breads and cereals: $K = 0.90$. The data confirmed that the ratings varied considerably.

## Formative Evaluation Design and Sample Size Estimation

A randomized design assessed the impact of the nutrition education program. All women receiving maternity care at the Leflore County Health Department were eligible to participate. The C group received the standard WIC education and the E group received the standard WIC education *plus* the new PFLP nutrition education program. Two behavioral outcomes were assessed: nutrition knowledge and 24-hour dietary recall score. With an alpha = 0.10 and power = 0.80, > 120 subjects/group were needed to evaluate E versus C group impact differences.

## Measurement and Analysis Methods

All women completed the following: a baseline questionnaire with demo-graphic information, a nutrition knowledge test, and a 24-hour dietary recall. C group women received *only* educational sessions required by the WIC program. At the completion of the eighth nutrition education lesson for E group women, all were scheduled for the post-test assessment. An Analysis of Covariance, with the pre-test scores as covariates, assessed group post-test differences

Focus group discussions with patients were convened to provide infor-mation about clients' use, acceptance, satisfaction, and recommendations for change in the new curriculum

## Process Evaluation

The Process Evaluation Model developed by Windsor et al. (2000) moni-tored implementation of the 12 core procedures. As shown in Table 5.13,

TABLE 5.13 Process Evaluation: Leflore County Nutrition Education Program

| PROCEDURES (P) | (A) ELIGIBLE | (B) EXPOSED | (C) RATE-B/A | (D) STANDARD | (E) INDEX-C/D |
|---|---|---|---|---|---|
| 1) Pre-test: 01-K | 240 | 236 | 98 | 100% | 0.98 |
| 2) Pre-test: 01-24Hr | 240 | 238 | 99 | 100% | 0.99 |
| 3) Lesson 1 | R 120 | 85 | 71 | 100% | 0.75 |
| 4) Lesson 2 | 120 | 81 | 68 | 100% | 0.71 |
| 5) Lesson 3 | 120 | 76 | 63 | 100% | 0.67 |
| 6) Lesson 4 | 120 | 69 | 57 | 100% | 0.61 |
| 7) Lesson 5 | 120 | 59 | 49 | 100% | 0.52 |
| 8) Lesson 6 | 120 | 59 | 49 | 100% | 0.52 |
| 9) Lesson 7 | 120 | 50 | 42 | 100% | 0.44 |
| 10) Lesson 8 | 120 | 46 | 38 | 100% | 0.40 |
| 11) Post-test: 02-K | 240 | 115 | 48 | 100% | 0.53 |
| 12) Post-test: 02-24Hr | 240 | 101 | 42 | 100% | 0.47 |

Program Implementation Index (PII) =
$$\frac{0.98 + 0.99 + 0.75 + 0.71 + 0.67 + 0.61 + 0.52 + 0.52 + 0.44 + 0.40 + 0.53 + 0.47}{12} = 0.63$$
(A) Eligible Patients . . . (B) = Exposed . . . (C) = Exposure Rate—B/A
(D) = Performance Standard . . . (E) = Index—C/D

the clients exposed to each procedure were divided by the clients eligible to participate to compute an Exposure Rate (B). The Implementation Index for each procedure was calculated by dividing the Exposure Rate (B) by the Performance Standard (C) established prior to program implementation. A Performance Standard of 100% was set for Assessment Procedures 1 and 2. A Performance Standard of 95% exposure was set for Procedures 3 to 10. A standard of 90% was applied for Assessment Procedures 11 and 12.

## Results

### Process Evaluation

As shown in Column A, 240 patients were randomly assigned to the E (120) or C (120) group. For assessment Procedures 1–2 and 11–12, all 240 patients were eligible. Only the 120 women assigned to the E group were eligible for exposure to Procedures 3–10. A decrease in exposure was documented between Procedures 2 and 3: PII = 0.75 and PII = 0.71 for all intervention–eight sessions: Procedure 3 (PII = 0.75) to a low for Procedure 10 (PII = 0.40). Compared with the final intervention delivery procedures, the PII increased slightly for Procedures 11 and 12 to PII = 0.53 and PII = 0.47. The PII was 0.63: a much lower rate than the recommended PII > 0.90.

## Discussion

Many public health programs are implemented without a formative evaluation. The formative evaluation of the PFLP demonstrated limited behavioral impact, and identified large problems with the intervention delivery, participant attrition, and measurement. The Program Implementation Index (PII = 0.63) confirmed it was substantially below the recommended: PII = 0.90.

A record review of program delivery by the peer educators revealed that the average time taken to deliver the sessions was 134.6 days, or approximately 19 weeks. This dramatically exceeded the time planned, 8–10 weeks, by the program developers. Unfortunately, the PFLP peer educators altered the delivery policy and plan. They decided to spread out the eight lessons to maintain client contact during the prenatal period. The failure to complete program delivery during the planned time frame prevented additional E group nutritional behavior changes from occurring.

Focus groups indicated that the increased length of time between lessons caused a loss of interest and made their time commitment too great. And, over 20% of the women moved during pregnancy.

A retrospective record review revealed that only 15 E group clients completed five lessons or more, but could not be located for the post-test. In addition, 55 C group clients could not be located for the post-test assessment. Lack of follow-up measurement introduced a significant methodological bias to the evaluation. The number of sessions also contributed to attrition. Focus group discussions with participants revealed that many felt the time commitment was too much. A reduction in the number of E group sessions from eight to six should make it more attractive to clients.

## Conclusion

This Formative Evaluation of a component of a prenatal care program in a public health clinic demonstrated that despite thorough planning, implementation problems occurred. Only when all major implementation problems have been addressed will the intervention be sufficiently strong to have the potential to produce the desired behavioral effect and to then be evaluated.

## Case Study 4: A Diabetes Disease Management Program

Nursing Disease Management Program Adults with Diabetes, G. Berg and S. Wadha, "Health Services Outcomes for a Diabetes Disease Management Program for the Elderly," *Disease Management* (2007), 226–234 (see publication for references).

### Introduction

The incidence and prevalence rates of adult onset Type 2 diabetes has significantly increased in the United States and is expected to continue for the foreseeable future. The US Task Force on Community Preventive Services has recommended the dissemination of "Diabetes Disease Management (DM) Programs" as an important solution. This case study presents an example of a successful DM program, Medicare+ Choice Health Plan, for elderly patients with diabetes. This case study focused only on the "process of care" measures and results for the target group.

## Background

Members of the health plan in Indiana, Kentucky, and Ohio, who met eligibility criteria (N = 610) were recruited by registered nurses. This cohort (E group) was stratified by risk, and agreed to receive a tailored self-management intervention (X. . .). It included formal RN counseling sessions by telephone, 24-hour access to $RN_x$, printed action plans, medication reminders, and a variety of other appropriate methods. Patient MDs/RNs communicated regularly about DM for each patient. A health plan Case Manager was available to assist all DM program participants. The DM program was based on the American Diabetes Association counseling guidelines.

A Comparison (C) group cohort of 610 patients was established by systematically reviewing the records of health plan members in the same state and year who did not participate in the DM program. Using an extensive database on all members, (C) group patients were matched with E group patients on baseline "Propensity Scores." This included risk stratification, and multiple demographic and clinical variables. The primary difference between the E and (C) group patients was that the (C) group represented the cohort who could not be reached by phone.

## Evaluation Design

This evaluation applied a quasi-experimental design: a non-randomized comparison (C) group design. Once E group patients were enrolled, each was assessed at baseline, 6, 12, 18, and 24 months. Following creation of the E group, the (C) group was established electronically. All E and C group patients continued to receive care from their regular, within-system providers.

## Process Evaluation Results

Data in Table 5.14 (excerpted from Table 1 from the report) confirm E and (C) group comparability. Data in Table 5.15 (excerpted from Table 2 in the report) are presented for the E and (C) group using the Process Evaluation Model (PEM). These data documented the impact of the DM program on changes in the "processes of care." It is important to note that 477 (78.2%) actually received the DM program of the original E group cohort of 610.

TABLE 5.14  E and (C) group Baseline Comparability

| VARIABLE | E GROUP | (C) GROUP | P VALUE |
|---|---|---|---|
| Male | 38.0% | 38.5% | 0.86 |
| Age | 73.9% | 73.8% | 0.45 |
| COPD | 14.3% | 13.3% | 0.61 |
| Diabetic Retinopathy | 12.5% | 11.3% | 0.54 |
| Medical Admissions | 605 | 612 | 0.66 |
| Diuretics | 37.3% | 39.8% | 0.38 |
| Antihypertensives | 47.7% | 49.8% | 0.46 |
| HbA1c | 77.0% | 73.6% | 0.16 |
| | **N = 610** | **N = 610** | |

TABLE 5.15  A Process of Care Evaluation of the Diabetes
DM Program

| PROCEDURES | E GROUP | (C) GROUP | P VALUE | % CHANGE |
|---|---|---|---|---|
| ACE inhibitors | 34.3% | 27.7% | 0.013 | + 23.7% |
| HbA1c | 71.3% | 63.0% | 0.002 | + 13.3% |
| Lipid Panel | 62.0% | 55.4% | 0.020 | + 11.8% |
| Eye Exam | 52.8% | 47.9% | 0.086 | + 10.3% |
| Maculopathy | 41.3% | 32.8% | 0.002 | + 26.0% |
| Flu Immunication (Im) | 16.9% | 12.5% | 0.029 | + 35.5% |

The E group received an average of 3.5 patient education and monitoring calls per patient, and 1.4 MD alert calls per patient. Although improvement was not documented for two measures, the average process measure improvement for six of the process of care procedures was 18%. These data provided good evidence that the DM program was acceptable to a high percentage of elderly patient with diabetes and was deliverable by phone. The DM program appeared to have reduced the use of acute care services.

## Summary

This project represents a very good example of methods to conduct process, impact, and outcome evaluations of a disease management program. Although a quasi-experimental design was applied, the propensity scoring and matching methods are good examples of how to address the issue of selection biases.

## Case Study 5: Friendships and Dating Program

K. Ward, R. Windsor, and J. Atkinson, "A Process Evaluation of the Friendships and Dating Program for Adults with Developmental Disabilities: Measuring the Fidelity of Program Delivery," *Research and Practice for Persons with Disabilities* (2012) (see publication for references).

### Introduction

Adults with intellectual and developmental disabilities are frequently abused in dating and partnered relationships. Research has repeatedly shown that interpersonal violence negatively impacts the abilities of persons with developmental disabilities to work, live independently, and maintain their health. Very few studies, however, have rigorously evaluated interventions to prevent partner violence. Our review confirmed the lack of process evaluation models, and weak evaluation designs, poor validity and reliability of measurement, small sample size, and lack of statistical power. Empirical evidence documenting the feasibility and fidelity of successful implementation of programs for persons with intellectual disabilities that prevent interpersonal violence have not been reported. Confirmation of the acceptability by participants and fidelity of implementation is needed to establish the feasibility and replicability of a program.

### Friendships and Dating Program (FDP)

The Friendships and Dating Program (FDP), developed to prevent violence in dating and partnered relationships and to teach social skills needed to develop healthy, meaningful relationships, was designed at the University of Alaska Anchorage (UAA) Center for Human Development (CHD). Development of the FDP included three pilot tests to determine whether the intervention session topics and activities were acceptable, appropriate, and beneficial to participants. The FDP could be delivered by community-based direct service personnel: 25 facilitators and 65 participants were involved in the pilot tests. The FDP requires a modest level and intensity of training: 14 hours. The program consists of 20 sessions delivered twice each week over a 10-week period in a small coed group format of 6–8 participants. Each session is approximately 1.5 hours, for a total of 30 hours over the 20 sessions. Odd-numbered sessions are delivered in a classroom setting, and even-numbered sessions are practiced in situ in the community. The FDP uses a multi-modal approach.

## Importance of Process Evaluation

Due to the large deficit in the literature regarding the documentation of acceptability and routine delivery of programs for people with developmental disabilities, it is critical to conduct a process evaluation, in addition to an impact evaluation. Process evaluation data provide essential information and insight about what types of participant assessment and intervention methods can (and cannot) be routinely delivered for specific settings, behaviors, types of providers, and program participants. Process evaluation data provide information about the degree to which a program was implemented at each program site.

While the literature has consistently indicated a need for evaluations of abuse-prevention programs for adults with intellectual disabilities and has stressed the importance of providing empirical evidence to confirm program exposure, no specific methodological guidance has been presented about how to conduct a "process evaluation." A "Process Evaluation Model (PEM)" applied by Public Health Programs, developed and applied by Windsor, are presented as an excellent planning model to address the methodological deficiency noted in the disability literature.

## Methods

### Training Facilitators for Program Delivery

In 2009–2010 CHD worked with five community agencies serving people with intellectual and developmental disabilities throughout Alaska to document the fidelity of delivery of the FDP. Communities included a combination of both urban and rural communities from different regions of the state. Eleven direct service personnel from community-based service agencies serving people with intellectual and developmental disabilities across Alaska were recruited and trained by CHD as facilitators to deliver the FDP. Facilitators attended a two-day, 14-hour, face-to-face training. Technical assistance was provided through conference calls twice a month and as needed.

The *Friendships and Dating Manual* organizes materials for facilitators to easily conduct sessions. The *Manual* presents the key content and related activities in a logical, sequential order. Each session in the manual is outlined in detail and contains objectives, activities, and handouts for that session. Facilitators receive a CD with all session materials and additional resources, such as DVDs, slides, posters, and games. A *Facilitator's*

*Training Guide* includes supplemental materials to assist facilitators in the preparation of delivering the FDP.

### Participants

Facilitators were responsible for recruiting participants. Participants were required (1) to be over 18 years of age; (2) to have experienced an intellectual or related developmental disability; and (3) to not have a history of inappropriate sexual behaviors. The five sites recruited 31 adults with intellectual and related developmental disabilities. Group sizes ranged from three to eight. All groups were mixed-gender, resulting in 14 female and 17 male participants. All of the participants met the eligibility criteria, and informed consent was obtained from the participants (and their guardians when appropriate).

### Outcome Measures

Two measures were used to assess outcomes: the Social Networks Measure (SNM) and the Interpersonal Violence Interview (IVI). Facilitators collected data at baseline, after the completion of FDP (post-test), and 10 weeks following the end of the program (10-week post-test) to check for maintenance. Each data collection point examined the previous 10-week timeframe.

#### Social Networks Measure

The Social Networks Measure (SNM) was developed to examine possible changes in the size and composition of the social networks of participants.

#### Interpersonal Violence Interview

The Interpersonal Violence Interview (IVI) was developed by project researchers, since a review of the literature found no evidence-based measure. A modified Delphi Technique was used to develop a 30-item questionnaire to measure the incidence of interpersonal violence among adults with intellectual and related developmental disabilities.

### Process Evaluation Model

The Process Evaluation Model (PEM) and methods used in this study are based on those developed for a Robert Wood Johnson Foundation (RWJF) National Program Office (NPO). The primary objective of a process evaluation was to document specific levels of exposure to the core procedures ($P_n$) of the FDP delivered by community agency facilitators. Data for this process evaluation metric document the degree of fidelity of program delivery for each site and all sites. It is an excellent method to routinely monitor and give feedback to program leadership and staff on a weekly, monthly, quarterly, and annual basis. It can also be used to compare rates at any location, or for any geographical area for a city-wide, system-wide, or state-wide HP-DP program for any target population and problem.

Exposure rates to the FDP were documented weekly to monitor the implementation of procedures by site. Facilitators provided detailed information about the number of participants exposed to each procedure and the amount of content delivered at each session through online surveys. The PII documented the exposure level of 23 FDP procedures: baseline measures, sessions 1–20, post-test measures, and 10-week post-test. In this case, PII = (P1-Index + P2-Index ... + P23-Index)/23. These data also document the performance levels of facilitators implementing the FDP. Individual implementation indices of > .90 and an overall PII ≥ .90 provide empirical data that a high level of implementation success was achieved.

Data were aggregated to produce an overall PII. Assuming that measurement is excellent and selection biases are controlled, if a PII > 0.90 is documented for a program, and if a statistically significant difference in outcome measures is documented, the PEM provides strong evidence that the intervention is one of the most plausible explanations for observed effects.

## Results

### Social Networks and Interpersonal Violence Outcome Results

The average social network size of 6.48 at baseline was significantly increased by a mean of 2.34 ($p = .002$) at the end of the intervention with no significant subsequent change at the 10-week follow-up ($p = .470$). Results of a repeated measures ANOVA and post hoc analyses showed the number of instances of interpersonal violence significantly decreased during and after the FDP, $F(1.21, 19.42) = 7.84, p = .008$. A description of the outcome results is presented in the article.

### Process Evaluation Results

Facilitator feedback documented the number of individuals exposed to the core measures and intervention program procedures. The PEM was used to monitor the delivery of the 20 FDP sessions and the administration of the pre-test–post-test outcome measures. The PEM examined a total of 23 FDP Procedures. As shown in Table 5.16, in Column A, 31 individuals participated in the FDP. An Exposure Rate (C) was calculated by dividing the number of participants exposed to each procedure (B) by the number eligible of participants (A). The Implementation Index (E) for each procedure was calculated by dividing the Exposure Rate (C) by the Performance Standard (D) established prior to program implementation. A Performance Standard (D) of 100% was set for Procedure 1, baseline outcome measures (P1).

Given the reality of program delivery and follow-up in community settings where attrition is typically observed, a Performance Standard of 95% exposure was set for Procedures 2 to 23 (P2... P23). The overall PII was 0.98 (greater than the recommended rate PII > 0.90). The PII provided specific evidence that direct service personnel can be trained to use the FDP and can deliver it to a group of adults with developmental disabilities. Participants continued to engage at high rates in the program over a 10-week period. While most programs delivered over an extended period of time tend to see participation rates decrease, this was not observed by the FDP.

## Discussion

This evaluation confirmed that an abuse-prevention program for adults with developmental disabilities can be successfully delivered to them by facilitators at community service agencies with minimal training. The FDP Implementation Index (PII = 0.98) documented that the intervention was delivered with a very high degree of fidelity to our planning model; participants of the program attended all 20 sessions. A Comprehensiveness Program Implementation Index (PII = 0.96), not presented in this case study, confirmed that facilitators were able to deliver the FDP content as intended, as it is significantly greater than the recommended PII > 0.90. The comprehensiveness results show that the facilitators followed the *FDP Manual* to deliver the program with fidelity.

The process and outcome evaluation results from the FDP Formative Evaluation were encouraging. While some variation in Implementation Indexes existed, the results from the FDP PEM were similar across the five sites. Clients engaged in the FDP at high rates at all locations, and all of the facilitators were able to deliver FDP content. These results help to document the acceptability of the program by the participants and how well facilitators delivered the content. They represent empirical building

TABLE 5.16 Process Evaluation of the Friendships and Dating Program: All Sites

| PROCEDURE | PARTICIPANTS | | EXPOSURE RATE—B/A | PERFORMANCE STANDARD | IMPLEMENTATION INDEX—C/D |
|---|---|---|---|---|---|
| | ELIGIBLE | EXPOSED | | | |
| (P) | (A) | (B) | (C) | (D) | (E) |
| 1. Baseline (O1) | 31 | 31 | 100 | 100% | 1.00 |
| 2. Session 1 (X1) | 30 | 30 | 100 | 95% | 1.05 |
| 3. Session 2 (X2) | 30 | 29 | 97 | 95% | 1.02 |
| 4. Session 3 (X3) | 29 | 29 | 100 | 95% | 1.05 |
| 5. Session 4 (X4) | 28 | 27 | 96 | 95% | 1.01 |
| 6. Session 5 (X5) | 28 | 28 | 100 | 95% | 1.05 |
| 7. Session 6 (X6) | 28 | 27 | 96 | 95% | 1.01 |
| 8. Session 7 (X7) | 28 | 25 | 89 | 95% | .94 |
| 9. Session 8 (X8) | 28 | 25 | 89 | 95% | .94 |
| 10. Session 9 (X9) | 28 | 27 | 96 | 95% | 1.01 |
| 11. Session 10 (X10) | 28 | 25 | 89 | 95% | .94 |
| 12. Session 11 (X11) | 28 | 28 | 100 | 95% | 1.05 |
| 13. Session 12 (X12) | 28 | 27 | 96 | 95% | 1.01 |
| 14. Session 13 (X13) | 28 | 27 | 96 | 95% | 1.01 |
| 15. Session 14 (X14) | 28 | 28 | 100 | 95% | 1.05 |
| 16. Session 15 (X15) | 28 | 27 | 96 | 95% | 1.01 |
| 17. Session 16 (X16) | 28 | 27 | 96 | 95% | 1.01 |
| 18. Session 17 (X17) | 28 | 23 | 82 | 95% | .86 |
| 19. Session 18 (X18) | 28 | 26 | 92 | 95% | .97 |
| 20. Session 19 (X19) | 28 | 22 | 79 | 95% | .83 |
| 21. Session 20 (X20) | 28 | 24 | 86 | 95% | .91 |
| 22. Post-Test (O2) | 28 | 26 | 92 | 95% | .97 |
| 23. 10-Wk Post-Test (O3) | 28 | 25 | 89 | 95% | .94 |

Program Implementation Index (PII)= $(\Sigma E)/P_n$ = 22.62/23 = 0.98

blocks for future research to conduct an efficacy evaluation with a much larger number of sites and participants using an experimental design. The results and insight from a well-planned efficacy evaluation that builds on the literature would provide the type and quality of evidence needed to begin to define the feasibility, impact, and cost of tailored programs such as the FDP for people with developmental disabilities. This study illustrated how process evaluations can be applied to programs for people with developmental disabilities.

## Small Group Class Exercise

V. Sanchez, L. Stone, M. Moffett, et al., "Process Evaluation of a Promotora de Salud Intervention for Improving Hypertension Outcomes for Latinos in a Rural-Mexico Border Region," *Health Promotion Practice* (May 2014).

This community-based public health program, "Corazon por la Vida" for 115 adults in three communities, is an excellent example of how to assess program delivery and quality, client adherence, exposure, and participant qualitative assessments. Using the Process Evaluation Model (PEM) presented in this chapter and data in Table 1 of the Sanchez et al. article, prepare a Summary Table for the nine-session program. Use a Performance Standard = 100% for P1 (Baseline Assessment) and for each of the nine Sessions, P2 to P10. Use a Performance Standard = 90% for P11 (Follow-Up Assessment). Include in the Summary Table the Program Implementation Index (PII = ?).

## Qualitative Evaluation Methods

The next section of this chapter briefly discusses a range of useful qualitative methods to assist program staff in assessing the acceptability of HP-DP program by key stakeholders. Qualitative evaluation methods do not seek to collect or compare categorical data sets, including measures of quantity, but to answer questions about the contextual dimensions of a program or intervention that defy structured categorization. This situation exists in the early phases of a project, when researchers are developing appropriate metrics for an evaluation, and throughout the collection of structured evaluative data to explore and explain structured, categorical findings.

Many disciplines have contributed to the development and refinement of the qualitative strategies described in this text. This section summarizes specific qualitative techniques for designing and conducting qualitative data collection in evaluation.

## Collecting Qualitative Data for Evaluations

Quantitative research should be designed to collect data that can be generalized to a larger population. For this reason, the study sample must be as representative as possible of the cases in that population. Qualitative research designs prioritize depth as well as breadth, and thus a qualitative study sample must consist of study participants who can provide a range of meaningful insights into the study variables of interest. Although such samples can be identified randomly, most are selected according to conceptual rather than numerical considerations.

The nature of your evaluation questions, and resources available to conduct the study, determine which qualitative sampling strategy is most appropriate for you. The random sampling strategy employed in quantitative research could be employed if the majority of the study population from which the sample is to be derived possesses the depth of information required to satisfy study objectives. For example, a descriptive qualitative process evaluation of a national disease prevention program could include a randomly selected subsample of program directors with knowledge of the processes by which their respective programs were implemented. Unlike in quantitative research, the size of the subsample is driven by the data collected; qualitative researchers continue randomly selecting study participants until they are no longer collecting new information-insights. The random sampling strategy will be time-consuming and expensive.

A purposive sampling strategy is often employed to maximize the range of a study with a limited set of participants. This strategy defines a generalized sample that includes as many different kinds of experiences as possible within the larger study population. The range of purposive sampling attributes should be based on previous studies and likely variables of relevance to study objectives. For example, a formative evaluation intended to develop metrics for a structured evaluation of a community-based intervention could include participants representing leadership, staff, and community perspectives across demographic or geographic dimensions of relevance to a program. While not a random sample, purposive designs can be roughly generalized to a larger population. Another strategy commonly employed in qualitative research is convenience sampling. This strategy is appropriate in those evaluative designs that preclude the use of a completely random survey or the identification of the entire range of experiences within a larger study population. The commonly employed "snowball" sample is one example of a convenience sampling strategy whereby the researchers build their study sample iteratively, progressively identifying additional study participants who can offer insights relevant to the overall study population. For example, a qualitative evaluation component nested within a structured program evaluation might identify study participants for interviews in meetings of program staff or community members. Although convenience sampling is not as representative as the first two methods, it provides a relatively inexpensive and intuitive strategy to identify unexpected or emergent themes that would otherwise go undiscovered in an evaluation.

## Analyzing Qualitative Data for Evaluations

Qualitative research often results in complex, large, and richly detailed data sets. These data must be coded, or reduced to major themes or categories of relevance to the evaluation objectives. Rather than describe the process in detail, this section highlights methods to code raw qualitative data into evaluative findings, to document the analytic process so that others may evaluate the credibility of your findings, and to assess such studies by other researchers.

All qualitative data analysis should involve the development and maintenance of a structured coding protocol, which can sometimes be referred to as a codebook. The coding protocol should include a *label*, or name for each conceptual category of data; a *definition*, or list or characteristics or issues that constitute that category; a *description* of how that category occurs in the data; and finally, some *examples* of these categories from the data set. These conceptual categories are often developed iteratively, and organized hierarchically, such that initial coding would arrive at general summary category of data and then over time specific sub-categories would emerge. For example, a process evaluation might begin with a descriptive code "administrative concerns" and over time various sub-codes of administrative concerns, such as "budgeting," "management," and "working environment," would emerge from the data. Secondary codes need not be simply descriptive, but can include inferential codes referring to patterns that emerge in the data over time. These codes, and the relationships between them, should be carefully recorded and summarized along with your findings.

When working as part of a team of coders, a researcher should carefully track *intercoder reliability*, or the consistency with which team members apply the coding protocol. To do this, at least two team members need to independently code segments of the data set, such as an interview, and then their work should be compared. Cases of inter-coder conflict require careful deliberation and discussion among the team and prospective refinements to the codebook to maintain reliability.

Many types of software programs can assist the researcher with the coding and management of qualitative data. They can facilitate the development and application of coding protocols across large data sets, and provide measures of inter-coder reliability. Regardless of the technology, the researcher is responsible for the interpretive development and refinement of the coding scheme, and the final development and presentation of the findings. The human dimension can be either the greatest strength or the greatest weakness of qualitative data analysis.

## Structured Observations

Social and behavioral scientists have developed a variety of nonreactive research methods with applicability in evaluation research. Anthropological methods include the collection of structured or systematic observations of social dynamics in community settings. Observational data are less vulnerable to many biases that confound the collection of interview or survey data, but must be conducted in a systematic or structured fashion to avoid bias. This section provides a brief description of how structured observations can be collected and employed in an evaluation.

The systematic collection of observational data is founded on the application of a structured observational research guide. These guides assist in the collection of objective facts rather than subjective perceptions by specifying categories of observational data with specific definitions and the inclusion of examples. One fairly common conceptual framework employed in anthropology separates observations into three analytic domains: actors, actions, and settings. The first set of observations describes the study participants present and those with whom they interact, the second describes behaviors of research interest and the consequences of these behaviors, and the third set describes the physical spaces of the interaction, technology employed, and other contextual details.

The objectives of your evaluation will determine the categories of observational data to be collected, along with the level of detail required in each category. Regardless of the categories employed, recording observational data systematically should be akin to coding than to narrative descriptions. In other words, the structured observation guide should be as specific as possible regarding the types and nature of observations sought. Depending on the nature of the study objectives, these categories can be recorded as nominal or quantitative variables.

## Case Study 6: Observational Data in Evaluative Research

M. Eisenberg, C. Ringwalt, D. Driscoll, et al., "Learning from Truth (sm): Youth Participation in Field Marketing Techniques to Counter Tobacco Advertising," *Journal of Health Communication* (2004), 223–231 (See publication for references).

In 2000, the American Legacy Foundation (Legacy) launched truth [sm], a national tobacco control social marketing campaign targeting youth aged 12–17. This study evaluated one aspect of that campaign, the *truth [sm] tour*, in which convoys of young people traveled to and staged street-level events in communities across the nation. The objectives of these events were to educate young people about tobacco industry practices and to promote the *truth [sm]* social marketing campaign. The evaluative strategy employed systematic observations of the field marketing activities by the tour riders as youth ethnographers; the structured observation guides collected data on the number and demographic profile of young people participating in the event, the manner of their participation, and content of discussions with the riders, and provided space for a sketch of the event layout, the locations of social encounters, and other contextual information that riders considered important for the evaluation. The systematic observations were integrated and analyzed by experienced anthropologists in a process evaluation of the field marketing campaign, and the results employed to refine and improve the effectiveness of the tour riders approach. Finally, the structured observations allowed for an outcome evaluation of key nominal and numerical metrics between tours and within the same tour over time, and informed the development of subsequent field marketing efforts.

### In-depth Interviews

Program evaluators often need to interview participants in a program, both those within the organization and in communities served, to determine their attitudes about the program or knowledge about it objectives. Although the purposes of such interviews vary, they include attempts to determine whether a program has

- Reached a target audience,
- Increased the target audience's awareness of the program,
- Increased the level of community interest,
- Increased the number who use the program or service, and
- Provided a satisfactory service.

In-depth interviews incorporate structured questions to elicit key information about a proposed or ongoing program, along with contextual probes, or follow-up questions that may or may not be used, depending on the response to the key question. This method allows for an interview process sufficiently flexible to better understand expected responses and to collect information on emergent or unexpected responses. Such detail can be invaluable in identifying program barriers, acceptability, and initial participant satisfaction. Using this method, program planners should be able to document community and organizational input and support.

## Individual Interviews

Individual in-depth interviews have the advantage of allowing for extensive probes of structured responses, and eliciting confidential information that might be problematic in a group format. An important difference between in-depth interviews and structured individual surveys is the use of open-ended questions. When conducted properly, interviews should provide study participants with the opportunity to determine the most appropriate response to a question, and allow for the collection and exploration of unexpected or emergent findings. These interviews can be readily biased by over-zealous interviewers employing close-ended questions, or probes.

Individual interviews can be conducted in community settings, such as heavily trafficked locales, including shopping centers, movie theaters, hospitals, or other pedestrian high-traffic areas in a metropolitan city or rural county. One common form of individual interviews are intercept interviews, in which people who possess the characteristics of the target audience for the health promotion program, for example, women of a certain racial, ethnic, or age group, are recruited on the spot for short, two- to five-minute interviews. Formal in-depth interviews require more time than intercept interviews, but can also be scheduled to take place in community settings where participants are comfortable and are thus more likely to provide contextual details important to a program evaluation. In both strategies, key questions may concern the person's familiarity with a health problem, knowledge of the availability of the program and its purpose, or interest in a special program. Probing questions might consist of queries into the source of knowledge or the basis for perceptions about or interest in a program.

## Opinion Leader Survey

Generally, data from this survey are generated from person-to-person interviews. Using a nominal group process is also effective. Written questions should be prepared to elicit key information from leaders about their impressions of a proposed or ongoing program. An opinion leader survey usually solicits a range of information. Results reflect the degree of consensus about the program from knowledgeable community people. This method plays an important role in assessing political support for a program. It may be invaluable to an innovative program in identifying barriers, acceptability, and initial participant satisfaction. This method will help program planner document community-organizational input to and support for a program.

## Community Forum Survey

In the community forum approach, several locations are selected for public meetings with a specific target audience. Community forums are inexpensive and are usually easy to arrange, and typically take one to two hours. The meetings may be open or by invitation. The method can be used to educate current participants and to gather their impressions of the acceptance, diffusion, and levels of participation in the program. A list of key questions must be prepared to elicit audience input. The forum method is most efficient when the meetings are small or the audience is divided into smaller groups of 20–25. A staff member or trained layperson should facilitate and maintain records to ensure participation. The forum encourages a range of community expressions about a problem. Its major disadvantages are (1) one group or individual may control the discussions or use the forum exclusively for expression of a grievance or opposition to the program, and (2) attendance may be limited and information covered may be biased.

## Central Location Survey

The central location survey is another technique commonly employed to gather information quickly and efficiently from a large number of people: 100 to 200 in a community. Two to ten sites, visited by a large number of people who possess the characteristics of the target audience for the health promotion program, for example, a shopping center, movie theater, beach, or other pedestrian high-traffic areas in a metropolitan city or rural county, are typically selected. Interviewers identify a specific group, for example, women of a certain racial, ethnic, or age group, and conduct short two- to five-minute interviews of the people on the spot. Questions may concern the person's familiarity with a health problem, knowledge of the availability of the program and its purpose, or interest in a special program.

## Case Study 7: Individual Interviews

D. Driscoll, C. Rupert, L. Golin, et al, "Promoting Prostate-Specific Antigen Informed Decision-Making: Evaluating Two Community-Level Interventions." *American Journal of Preventive Medicine* (2008), 87–94 (see publication for references).

This study evaluated two community-level interventions to promote informed decisions about whether to be screened for prostate cancer with the prostate-specific antigen (PSA) test. Both interventions promoted informed PSA decision-making. One intervention (PSA-Only) consisted of educational information about prostate cancer and PSA test. The other (Men's Health) included additional information about recognizing and preventing heart attack, stroke, and colon cancer. Data collected from in-depth individual interviews were collected from participants 6–12 months post-intervention to assess pre-/post- changes in PSA knowledge, intentions, and behaviors. An interview guide consisting of structured key questions and contextual probes was employed in interviews conducted in community settings, such as churches, hospitals, and community centers. The results were integrated with structured observations and survey results to assess the utility of both interventions in promoting informed PSA decision-making. The community-level interventions successfully engaged community participants in discussions, educated individuals, encouraged deliberation of information, and facilitated PSA test discussions with physicians.

## Group Interviews

There are several methods for collecting in-depth interview data in group settings. This section will describe two methods differentiated by the venue and objectives of the data collection process. The first method is a town hall-style group interview that can be employed to collect information quickly and efficiently from a large number of people in a community context. These can be a relatively inexpensive and usually easy to arrange, and typically take one to two hours. The meetings may be open or by invitation. This method can be used to educate the current participants and to gather their impressions of the acceptance, diffusion, and levels of participation in the program. A list of key questions must be prepared to elicit audience input.

The method is most efficient when the town hall meetings are divided into smaller groups of 20–25 for break-out discussions and reconvene into a larger group for final conclusions. A staff member or trained layperson should facilitate and maintain records to ensure participation. A forum encourages a wide range of community expressions about the problem. Its major disadvantages are (1) one group or individual may control the discussions or use it exclusively for expression of a grievance or opposition to the program, and (2) attendance may be limited and information covered may be very biased.

## Case Study 8: Town Hall-Style Interviews

D. Driscoll, M. Lynch, M. Burke, et al., "A Formative Assessment of Knowledge and Beliefs Regarding Pandemic Influenza Mitigation Among Culturally Distinct Audience Segments," Report to the Centers for Disease Control (2009).

This study evaluated the utility of various non-pharmaceutical mitigation measures, such as school closings, to reduce the rate of infection during an influenza pandemic. The study objectives were to assess knowledge and beliefs about pandemic influenza and the mitigation measures across audience segments. First individual and then group interview data were collected with residents of culturally distinct communities across the United States. The town hall interview featured a formal presentation that included mock news broadcasts describing each mitigation measure, and a summary of results from individual interviews conducted with residents of the community about these pandemic mitigation measures. Participants were organized into breakout groups to discuss their responses to the mitigation measures and the individual interview findings. At the conclusion of the town hall meeting, community members were invited to describe their thoughts and concerns about pandemic influenza, and a researcher answered all questions and distributed educational materials. The study revealed important population-level differences in the likely utility of non-pharmaceutical mitigation measures by culturally distinct audience segments.

A second style of group interview is the focus group. Unlike a town hall, focus group interviews involve smaller numbers of participants and are focused on a specific topic. Social marketing researchers and advertisers use this method to assess the perceptions, beliefs, language, and interests of an audience to whom a product or service would be marketed. The focus group interview usually involves 8–10 people. Using a detailed discussion outline, a moderator keeps the group session within the appropriate time limits, but gives considerable latitude to participants to respond spontaneously to a set of general or specific questions. The moderator has the opportunity to probe and gain in-depth insights. These sessions are often video- or audiotaped.

Focus group interviews help health communications/media planners identify key concepts that may trigger awareness and interests in participation. This method is often used to complement population-based, representative-sample surveys on specific topics. Qualitative information is elicited in combination with the survey data to make judgments about perceptions, beliefs, and behaviors of a population or subgroups.

## Case Study 9: Focus Groups

D. Driscoll, S. Rojas-Smith, K. Sotnikov, et al., "An Instrument for Assessing Public Health System Performance: Validity in Rural Settings," *National Rural Health Association* (2006), 254–259 (see publication for reference).

This study evaluated the Local Public Health System Assessment Instrument (Local Instrument) of the National Public Health Performance Standards Program. The objective was to compare the Local Instrument of those public health systems. Focus group and individual interview data were collected with department staff in each public health system, and community partners and constituents.

Archival data were also collected and integrated with the interview data. The focus group data revealed that, despite differences in Local Instrument scores, the representative public health systems in each state provided roughly the same levels of public health service. Sites varied considerably in the percentage of survey items rated highly or less relevant. Conclusions: The National Public Health Performance Standards Program Local Instrument can provide a useful structure and process for assessing public health system performance at the local level.

## Mixed Methods Research

Program evaluators may find it helpful to integrate qualitative data collected by one of the strategies described in this section with quantitative data from structured surveys or archival reviews described elsewhere in this text. These procedures can be particularly employed when evaluative researchers have collected qualitative data from a randomly selected or purposive sample representative of the population from which the quantitative data were collected. The complexities associated with the development and application of mixed methods designs precludes a detailed description of such designs in this section, and interested researchers should review one or more of the references cited here.

*Mixed methods research* employs procedures for collecting and analyzing both quantitative and qualitative data in the context of a single study. The prospective mixed methods researcher will find a variety of classificatory metrics by which mixed methods research designs can be described. There is as of yet no discrete list of mixed methods design options, and so researchers should plan to develop a design that answers their own research questions within the constraints and boundaries of the study context. Some researchers suggest that the term *mixed model* be used to differentiate research designs integrating qualitative and quantitative data from those that merely employ both types of data. These include transformative designs that change one form of data into another (most often qualitative to quantitative data) so that the data collected by mixed methods designs can be merged. (The term *quantitizing* has been coined to describe the process of transforming coded qualitative data into quantitative data and *qualitizing* to describe the process of converting quantitative data to qualitative data.)

## Case Study 10: Mixed Methods

D. Driscoll, Appiah-Yeboah, P. Salib, and D. Rupert, "Merging Qualitative and Quantitative Data in Mixed Methods Research: How To and Why

Not," *Ecological and Environmental Anthropology* (2007), 19–28 (see publication for references).

This study employed transformative mixed methods evaluative designs to evaluate the utility of vaccine-safety reviews conducted by the Institutes of Medicine for promoting effective vaccination practices among health-care providers. The two designs fall on somewhat different ends of the mixed methods design spectrum related to when the data were collected. The first was a concurrent mixed methods design employed to validate one form of data with the other. We employed a Web-based instrument to collect both structured and unstructured data to collect and compare perceptions of vaccine safety among an extensive and varied set of non-governmental advocacy groups. Each topic-specific set of structured questions in the survey instrument was followed by at least one open-ended and unlimited comment field, which was explicitly linked to the question set immediately preceding it.

In most cases, an open-ended question asked: "What additional information would you like to provide to explain these responses?" This strategy has several advantages for mixed-methods applications. First, they can be fairly intuitive for participants. In the study described, the Web-based format was easy to understand and open-ended response fields were unlimited. Many respondents took advantage of the resource to post extensive comments. Also, these fields were overtly linked to the preceding structured responses, facilitating linkage both by the participant during data collection and by the research team in relating the structured and unstructured responses. However, concurrent data collection designs precluded follow-up on interesting or confusing responses. In our study we relied entirely on respondents to augment survey answers by following up on issues. Many respondents provided follow-up; some did not.

The other mixed methods design employed in this evaluation was a fairly complex sequential one in which one quantitative data set were employed to shape the collection and integration of a subsequent qualitative data set. This design was employed to collect perceptions and attitudes regarding the utility of vaccine-safety guidelines from staff of several federal agencies with vaccine safety missions. The study participants had various roles and disciplinary backgrounds and were associated with a host of federal agencies. Further, the prospective participants had very limited time available to respond to the study. For these reasons we chose to employ a flexible and iterative data collection strategy consisting of two data collection phases. In the first phase, we collected survey data; in the second phase, in-depth interview data.

The survey questions were entirely close-ended, and the response categories were developed in consultation with representatives of the various federal agencies. The subsequent in-depth interview instruments consisted of individualized questions intended to explore particularly interesting or ambiguous survey responses, as well as standard questions exploring general perspectives on the purpose and future utility of vaccine safety guidelines. This two-phased approach allowed study participants to respond to the survey on their own time and reduced the time required for in-depth discussions of emergent themes.

It provided members of the research team with the opportunity to review and analyze the survey results and to tailor the subsequent in-depth interview instrument to follow up on confusing or significant responses. This iterative analytic approach also simplified subsequent attempts to integrate the coded qualitative data collected in in-depth interviews with survey data. A primary disadvantage of this strategy is the time required to design and conduct separate tailored instruments for each key informant. A second complicating factor is the lack of overt linkages between the structured and unstructured responses compared to the concurrent design.

This study demonstrated some techniques for and outcomes from mixed methods evaluation research designs. The opportunity to provide additional qualitative information augmenting structured responses can provide key insights into unexpected relationships between local resource use patterns and community factors. Program evaluators interested in applying such designs should be responsive to their particular study objectives and parameters.

# 6 | Basic Cost Analysis and Economic Evaluation

> Cost analysis studies should be made to determine the long term
> effectiveness of health education programs in reducing personal health
> care costs for persons with specific types of health problems.
> —*President's Committee on Health Education, 1971*

## Introduction

Because of the complexity of the topic and the large literature base, it is beyond the scope of this chapter to present a comprehensive review and examples of all types of cost and economic evaluation methods and case studies. Complete discussions are available in multiple health economics texts, and health services research literature. *This chapter presents a synthesis of basic principles and methods, and provides examples of the application of common cost and economic evaluations of Health Promotion–Disease Prevention and Management (HP-DP) programs.* It builds on the evaluation methods and case material presented in Chapters 1 through 5. The primary purposes of Chapter 6 are to assist the HP-DP professional (1) to become a more knowledgeable and informed consumer of cost and economic evaluation methods and oral and written reports, and (2) to be a more confident participant in discussions of cost-effectiveness analysis (CEA) and cost-benefit analysis (CBA), and planning of HP-DP programs. Although the chapter is designed for the MPH/MSPH/MS students in training, master's trained HP-DP specialists, or staff working in public-population health programs, students in a DrPH/PhD/DSc program will also find its content and methods useful.

A decade after the President's Committee on Health Education Report, Warner and Luce in "Cost-Benefit and Cost-Effectiveness Analysis in Health Care" (1982) indicated, "The potential significance and nature of CEA-CBA contributions to healthcare resource allocation have yet to be established." While there have been a multitude of CEA and CBA studies since these publications, many contemporary sources in Health Promotion–Disease Prevention (HP-DP) reflect ambivalence about progress in this area. In approaching a discussion of economic evaluation of an HP-DP program, it is important to emphasize that cost is only one dimension of decision-making about a programs' value. While cost will usually (but not always) be an issue in the development of a new program and health policy or a significant revision of an existing program, quality, effectiveness, and equity should be the primary criteria when an agency is deciding what interventions should be routinely delivered. Unfortunately, political issues play a dominate role, often regardless of the cost, in the decision to create and introduce new HP-DP, public health, or new healthcare policies or services programs (e.g., ObamaCare?).

At least two basic questions need to be asked and answered in planning and defining an HP-DP program and its costs. What do specialists in a field define as the most appropriate, minimum "best practice or evidenced-based" intervention that trained, regular staff, or HP-DP specialist staff should provide to eligible individuals who should receive it? If an impact evaluation and meta-evaluation confirm that a new multi-component intervention is significantly more effective than an existing program, what will the HP-DP program cost an agency, system, or organization to introduce, to improve, or to significantly expand an existing program? This chapter describes methods to help answer these questions and other pertinent issues.

## Development of Cost and Economic Evaluations of HP-DP Programs

Cost effectiveness analyses began to be discussed in a wide variety of fields, including HP-DP in the United States, Canada, and Europe in the 1960s. As noted, *Report of the President's Committee on Health Education* (USDHEW, 1971) recommended that "Cost analys is studies should be made to determine the long term effectiveness of health education programs . . . " This report represented the first national (US) consensus statement from the government about the need and utility of economic evaluations of HP-DP programs. Very few economic evaluations, however, were conducted and published in the health promotion literature in the 1970s (Thompson and Fortress, 1980; Rogers et al., 1981; Warner and Luce, 1982).

Few reports in the 1980s in journals such as the *American Journal of Public Health, American Journal of Health Promotion, Health Education and Behavior, Health Education Research*, and related journals presented economic analyses of HP-DP interventions (Barry and Defriese, 1990). The Report from the Brookings Institution, *Evaluating Preventive Care*, by Russell (1987), was one of the first to review the efficacy, cost, and cost-effectiveness of health promotion programs to improve the health of older people in six areas: (1) drug therapy for hypertension control, (2) smoking, (3) exercise, (4) dietary calcium uses, (5) obesity counseling, and (6) alcohol use. "Guidelines for Cost Effectiveness Evaluations" were also presented by Russell. A frequently cited, comprehensive synthesis of the economic evaluation literature was presented by Tengs, Adams, Pliskin, et al. (1995), "Five Hundred Life Saving Interventions and Their Cost Effectiveness." This sentinel report evaluated 587 interventions for a wide variety of problems, and provided a reference base for discussions about HP-DP program costs and cost-effectiveness.

While a large number of cost and economic analyses and evaluations of individual HP-DP programs and systematic reviews of the literature have been published since 2000, an array of issues continue to be barriers to wide-scale, routine use of CEA and CBA. "A Strategic Plan for Integrating Cost-effectiveness Analyses Into the US Healthcare System," prepared for the Panel on Integrating Cost-Effectiveness Consideration into Health Policy Decisions, Neumann, Palmer, Daniels, et al., *American Journal of Managed Care* (2008), presented a country-level perspective about economic evaluation in primary care and public health. This report provided the HP-DP field, especially disease management programs as a core component of primary care, with a basic discussion of enduring issues and barriers facing future CEA applications. The Panel identified six barriers to the integration of CEA into healthcare systems (and HP-DP) planning and evaluation: (1) lack of cultural acceptance, (2) inadequate evidence base, (3) lack of infrastructure, (4) weak/conflicting incentives, (5) regulatory/legal issues, and (6) ethical concerns.

A synthesis of five systematic reviews by Weatherly, Drummond, Claxton, et al., "Methods for Assessing the Cost-Effectiveness of Public Health Interventions" in *Health Policy* (2009), indicated that the empirical literature was also disappointing for the United Kingdom and other high-income countries. *The report noted: very few of the 154 studies reviewed demonstrated methodological rigor.* Suhrcke, Nugent, Stuckler, and Rocco, in "Chronic Disease: An Economic Perspective," oxa. org, (2006), and Lewin, Lavis, Oxman, et al, "Supporting the Delivery of Cost-Effective Interventions in Primary Health-Care Systems in Low-Income and Middle Income Countries: An Overview of Systematic Reviews" in *Lancet* (2008) presented comprehensive reports on economic evaluations in low- and middle-income countries. *All reviews emphasized how much more we need to learn about what interventions, at what cost, can reduce the severity of chronic and acute diseases.*

Each report, as well as many other sources, reflected the global attention to the evaluation of interventions to improve health and prevent diseases, and confirmed the enduring challenges to conducting sound economic analyses. These sources in the literature present the global-population health student or HP-DP specialist with a synthesis of the state of the science and practice for CEA. They also provide insight about the usefulness of CEA in improving the efficiency of primary care, and HP-DP programs, policy and professional practice. Many reviews noted that relatively few rigorous economic evaluation studies were available for low-, middle-, and high-income countries. While the current literature informs the HP-DP specialist about how to conduct cost-economic analyses and evaluations as a component of professional practice, multiple sources indicate considerable inconsistency in the application of well-established CEA-CBA methods.

## Is HP-DP Cost-Effective?

Documentation of the level of program implementation, associated costs, degree of behavioral impact or health outcome, and analyses of intervention cost, effectiveness, cost-effectiveness, and cost-benefit are recognized as important, if not essential, sources of evidence, information, and insight for decision-making. As the cited reports have noted, a discussion of this topic must be approached with care. Far too often, a valid effectiveness evaluation and/or CEA are not performed, or inaccurate statements are made about the cost-effectiveness and potential savings that could be produced by the HP-DP interventions. *Candidates for senior political offices and elected national and state officials in high-income countries, especially in the United States, are routinely prone to declare that investments in health promotion and disease prevention or healthcare services will automatically save many lives, improve health, reduce healthcare utilization rates, and significantly reduce associated costs.* These types of statements about the potential individual and societal economic benefits/savings from HP-DP programs (or a new healthcare system) are misleading exaggerations of weak, invalid, or nonexistent evidence by elected officials. They need to be critically evaluated and rebutted.

Two editorials, by Cohen, Neumann, and Weinstein (*NEJM*, 2008) and Woolf (*JAMA*, 2009), present thoughtful commentaries in response to the tendency by some individuals to state that federal agencies or nongovernmental organizations (NGOs) are missing an opportunity to save millions of dollars by not investing in more HP-DP programs. *These two reports (and many others) noted that although many HP-DP interventions may save money, many will not. And it is possible for an intervention to be cost-effective and not save money (cost-benefit).* All reviews on this topic stress the need to consider interventions, evaluations, and cost-economic analyses contextually. The existing healthcare system, program, and infrastructure, level of organizational development, staff competency/training, and capacity and resources to deliver an HP-DP program will always vary. A HP-DP intervention impact-effect size, and direct and indirect program costs, will also vary dramatically for each health problem, country, region, target population, and practice-program delivery setting. Extrapolation and generalization of impact and economic evaluations from a similar population, even in the same state, should be approached with cautious skepticism.

While there are a large number of options as initial referents to learn more about cost analyses and economic evaluation methods, two choices are available for US programs: (1) "Framing an Economic Evaluation: A Self-Study Guide," and (2) "Applying Cost Analysis to Public Health Programs: A Self-Study Course" (CDC, 2008) by the Health Economics Research Group of the US Centers for Disease Control: epopeb@cdc.gov. Among the many references for additional insight about the application of economic evaluation methods in low- or middle-income countries, the following is an excellent guide: *Disease Control Priorities in Developing Countries* by Jamison, Breman, Measham, et al., (Oxford University Press, 2nd ed., 2006), especially Chapter 2: "Intervention Cost-Effectiveness" by Laxminarayan, Chow, and Shahid-Salles. It provides information on the cost-effectiveness estimates of 319 interventions.

An informative and readable publication for a public audience is "Millions Saved: Proven Successes in Global Health (2008)" by Levine et al., of the Center for Global Development, Washington, D.C. These publications identify an insightful list of effective and cost-effective methods to substantially improve the health of millions of people throughout the world, especially women, infants, and children. While much work is still needed, examples of the effectiveness and cost-effectiveness of HP-DP programs in high-income countries such as the United States and low-income countries throughout the world are presented in these and other publications.

Almost all reports indicate a clear need for sound cost analyses and economic evaluations. As noted, the cost and economic evaluation literature cited emphasize the need to carefully consider contextual factors when examining the program effectiveness, cost, and cost-effectiveness. The internal and external validity of the results from even the most rigorous, prospective randomized clinical trial (RCT) or group randomized community trial (GRCT) and economic evaluation for a problem, and/or economic evaluations from a meta-evaluation, need to be carefully considered before making any conclusion about effectiveness and efficiency: the cost per unit of effect, or return on investment (ROI). Program and scientific leadership needs to be more critical and assertive in translating evidence to political and organizational leadership. Leaders need to be much more thoughtful about making statements about the generalization of the results of any HP-DP impact and/or cost evaluation to a *new* target population, and *new* program delivery setting.

## Purposes of Cost Analysis and Economic Evaluation

The general purposes of cost analyses and economic evaluations are to serve as tools to provide data and empirical insight about cost per participant and program efficiency. Thus, a valid economic evaluation (in theory) should yield valid results to help program leadership make better or fairer decisions about resource allocation to the broadest range of people. Cost and economic evaluations apply a set of standard methods to define, measure, value, and compare the costs and negative or positive consequences (impact) produced by alternative HP-DP interventions.

The CDC identified five areas where an economic evaluation would be useful to program and policy leadership: (1) planning-cost projections, (2) efficiency estimation, (3) priority assessment and decision-making, (4) public accountability, and (5) equity. A valid economic evaluation should provide timely documentation of expended resources to answer questions about HP-DP program implementation in each area. Multiple methodological issues, however, identified in Chapters 1 through 5 of this volume, must be addressed first to confirm the "effectiveness" of an HP-DP program. Data confirming measurement validity, successful program implementation, and internal validity of results need to be available before conducting an economic evaluation of an intervention.

## Types of Economic Evaluation

There are three primary types of economic evaluations that HP-DP programs will typically conduct: (1) cost-effective analysis (CEA); (2) cost-utility analysis (CUA); and (3) cost-benefit analysis (CBA). Cost of illness or cost-minimization evaluations would not be a method typically used by an HP-DP program. The following are brief descriptions of CEA, CUA, and CBA.

### Cost-Effectiveness Analysis (CEA)

CEA is an evaluation method designed to assess program alternatives according to effectiveness and costs in the production of behavioral impact or health outcome rates, measured in salient units of effect. The objective of an HP-DP program evaluation is to determine which intervention produced a significant change (+ or -) in a behavioral impact or health outcome rate from a baseline rate: for example, increased self-care/disease management skill, increased medication adherence, decreased or increased utilization of health services, and/or decreased workdays lost. Typically, a program evaluates the impact of a combination of different health education, behavioral treatment, or health communication interventions designed to change client behavior of an experimental (E) group or a control (minimal intervention; C) group.

In performing a CEA, E and C groups are compared, using common measurement or metrics, to confirm the level of impact. Behavioral impact or health outcome rates (**Output**) are compared in the context of personnel and non-personnel resources-costs expended (**Input**) to accomplish the observed degree of change in effectiveness rates. This "process evaluation" (see Chapter 5) should answer the following question: How much did it cost to produce each percent of change for a specific unit of effect, for example, percent of behavior change, or percent of high blood pressure or diabetes controlled, over what time period, at what types of practice setting? This computation enables the evaluator and leadership to identify, with sensitivity analysis, which intervention is more likely to provide the optimal/threshold effectiveness levels in relation to HP-DP program costs.

A cost analysis should be based on a complete process evaluation, described in Chapter 5, for an ongoing or new HP-DP program. It provides current data and valuable information to HP-DP practice, program, and policy leadership about what level of impact may be possible at what cost per unit of effect for current and future annual planning and budgeting. A CEA is especially useful as a micro-level decision-making tool for a program for a well-defined population in a city, county, or for a defined public health or primary care system and population. Valid cost-effectiveness information should be used in combination with a meta-evaluation, and judgment by HP-DP program leadership to make resource allocation decisions.

## Cost-Utility Analysis (CUA)

This is a form of CEA that measures outcomes in quality-adjusted life years (QUALYs) or disability-adjusted life year (DALYs) gained. A summary measure is the cost-utility ratio, expressed as the dollar value per QUALY/DALY. *A methodological issue with CUA is that "quality" is a subjective concept, and its measurement is complex.* As discussed in Chapter 4 (Measurement and Analysis in Evaluation), the validity-reliability-representativeness of any construct such as "quality adjusted life years" needs to be documented for each CUA for each problem and population. The very wide variations in the assumptions, and the potential for inaccuracies about effectiveness and cost used to derive DALYs and QUALYs, are enduring issues.

The concept of "utility" in a CUA refers to the process of deriving from the literature and/or a representative sample of a reference population perceptions of the value of several alternative activities relative to the potential impact and cost of each. Each respondent is asked to rate alternative interventions and cost on a "1(low) to 10 (high)" scale. Converting and interpreting the qualitative, subjective responses and ordinal ratings into a "quality of life score" for different problems and populations, however, is problematic. Converting the product of this process into a numerical score and "intangible costs (dollars)" represents to many social scientists, health services researchers, and economists an imperfect methodology. The problems of the validity of measurement and cost analysis of "utility" are beyond the scope of this chapter.

*Because there are a variety of major assumptions and complex pro-cedures in the production of a QUALY or DALY, and CUA does not pro-duce documentation of actual economic benefits or savings to an HP-DP program, a CUA example is not presented in this chapter.* This chapter focuses primarily on Health Promotion Practice at the micro or program level. Thus, only CEA and CBA studies are presented that produce data about impact and efficiency in the near or intermediate term, for example, 12–36 months, for a specific evaluation. A synopsis and primary differ-ences in the definition of CEA and CBA are presented in Table 6.1.

## Cost-Benefit Analysis (CBA)

This is a method in which two or more intervention alternatives are com-pared according to monetary costs (*input*) and monetary benefits-savings attributable to the significant changes in an impact or outcome rate (*output*) produced by alternative HP-DP interventions. A *CBA measures both pro-gram costs and program consequences-benefits in actual monetary terms.* A CBA determines which intervention has the lowest cost-to-benefit ratio (CBR) and produces a return on investment (ROI). Because CBA com-pares alternatives in monetary terms, the evaluator documents whether a method has economic benefits ($$$) exceeding costs.

One issue raised about a CBA is that, for some problems, it may be difficult, philosophically and methodologically, to place a dollar value on *all* program consequences. The documentation of cost and economic ben-efits for a very large majority of impact or outcome rates produced by an HP-DP evaluation, however, are readily measured and translated into a CBR and ROI. In the last decade, multiple meta-evaluations and economic analyses of interventions for specific problems and target groups have been

TABLE 6.1 Measurement of Costs and Consequences in Economic Evaluations

| TYPE | MEASUREMENT OF COST | IDENTIFICATION OF CONSEQUENCES | MEASUREMENT OF CONSEQUENCES-EFFECTS |
|---|---|---|---|
| Cost-Effectiveness Analysis | Dollars | Single effect of interest common to both to different degrees | Natural units, >>> blood pressure, <<< NCD rates |
| Cost-Benefit Analysis | Dollars | Single or multiple effects, not neces-sarily common to both alternatives; common effects may be by degrees by the alternatives | Dollars |

published. Multiple CBAs have documented the cost and potential and actual savings from reducing workdays lost, reducing the use of health-care services by high-risk patients or employees, significant reductions of risk among target groups, and significant increases in disease management and adherence rates, especially for chronic diseases such as diabetes, high blood pressure, and asthma. Although most of the technical issues in conducting a CEA and CBA are readily understandable by graduate-trained staff, it is prudent to seek graduate-level expertise in health economics to plan and conduct cost-economic analyses of a program (see Table 6.2). The following is a brief description of each step.

## STEP 1: Define the Economic Evaluation Question-Population-Problem

The first step in a cost and economic evaluation is to state the question to be answered. For example, What is the behavioral impact and cost-effectiveness of a standard, brief parent information intervention (X1) versus a tailored, multi-component parent counseling-communication intervention (X1 + X2 + X3) to reduce injuries among infants and children (age 1–5 years) in the home? Or, What is the cost-effectiveness of two different asthma management interventions, standard (X1) versus enhanced methods (X1 + X2 + X3), for either adults with asthma in primary care practices or children with asthma in elementary schools? Having stated the economic evaluation question, the extent of the problem among the population needs to be well defined for the target group.

TABLE 6.2 Cost Analysis (CA) and Economic Evaluation Methods

| | |
|---|---|
| There are a series of **STEPS** to conduct an economic evaluation of an HP-DP program: | |
| **STEP 1** | Define the cost analysis question for a population-problem-setting |
| **STEP 2** | Define the usual care and "best practice" intervention methods for comparison |
| **STEP 3** | Define the cost perspective: Agency–Societal–Client |
| **STEP 4** | Define from a process evaluation program-intervention costs (input) |
| **STEP 5** | Define from a meta-evaluation the estimated levels of behavioral impact or health outcome rates from an HP-DP intervention for specific problems, and/or confirm the behavioral impact or health outcome rates attributable to an intervention from a prospective HP-DP program evaluation (output) |
| **STEP 6** | Perform a CEA and/or CBA |
| **STEP 7** | Perform a sensitivity analysis, varying plausible cost and impact assumptions. |

Incidence and prevalence rate and trends, and estimated total number of eligible people among the target population, need to be defined in epidemiological, behavioral, and clinical terms. This defines, in theory, how much of what percent of a health status rate is caused by a modifiable risk factor(s). Significant reduction and/or elimination of a risk factor(s), in theory, reduces or eliminates the population attributable risk (PAR). *If the incidence rate or level of risk is significantly reduced or eliminated, it is likely that the immediate or intermediate associated excess costs and positive or negative consequences/benefits (economic and health) can be documented.*

For example, if infant and child injuries in the home are the target population and setting, what are the injury rates and trends, associated types of morbidity, and incidence rates of use of child health services attributable to the problem? Changes in an incidence rate, if significantly improved, probably represent an opportunity to confirm associated economic benefits or savings. An ROI may be documentable. In this chapter, the primary risk factors associated with adverse health outcomes are assumed to be behavioral, and amenable to significant changes.

## STEP 2: Define the Program-Intervention Methods-Setting

In Chapter 2 and Chapter 5 of this volume, considerable emphasis was placed on the need to define all major HP-DP procedures (P. . .). Routine empirical documentation of the extent to which core program assessment and intervention procedures (P1 + P2 + P3. . .) were delivered to the target population by staff with fidelity (as planned) were identified as essential tasks. When conducting an economic analysis, in order to define all costs, the analysis must delineate the type, number, frequency of contact, and duration of exposures from program staff to major HP-DP program assessment and intervention procedures (P. . .). The type(s) of routine procedures, the population, practice setting, and type of staff used to deliver how much of what, where, when, and how need to be thoroughly described.

The evaluation team also needs to describe the program delivery setting and typical HP-DP intervention methods (X1) currently provided. It needs to define the structure and procedures of the proposed, new "best practice" intervention to be introduced (X1 + X2 + X3. . .) and evaluated. A program needs to state the following: *who* will deliver the various components of the new intervention and *when, how,* and *where,* (e.g., health clinics, schools, home visits, worksites, or community health centers). The available staffing, infrastructure, and capacity to deliver the existing or new HP-DP program practice setting needs to be described. This level of detail regarding the intensity, frequency, and duration of contact is essential to plan a cost analysis as a core component of an evaluation.

It is presumed from a meta-evaluation of the literature and/or from a prospective, experimental evaluation study that the "efficacy or effectiveness" of a new HP-DP program has been confirmed for a specific problem and target population. The intervention methods have demonstrated at least a moderate probability of significantly modifying a behavioral impact rate above a base impact rate. There will be at least two intervention alternatives in an HP-DP program cost-effectiveness evaluations. One alternative will be the usual intervention group (C group) and at least one special intervention group (E group). In the decision to develop and evaluate an HP-DP program, interventions should be selected and tailored so that they are a reasonably good fit for a problem, program setting, and population at risk: feasible, sustainable, and affordable/efficient.

## STEP 3: Define the Cost Perspective

There are several perspectives that can be used in cost analysis.

### Societal Perspective

All costs for healthcare, hospitalization, and related services would be included in this perspective. In addition, client or patient costs would be defined, such as out-of-pocket payments. In the societal perspective, other indirect costs may be included, for example, gains or losses in employment that are directly associated with the morbidity-mortality of the target audience.

### Client Perspective

All costs borne by the client within a target group, such as out-of-pocket payment for drugs, medications, transportation costs, child-care expenses, and loss of work due to the condition or participation in the HP-DP program would be included. It is more difficult to measure client costs, such as pain or anxiety, which may also be included, with a monetary value placed on these. Client copayment costs would be included in this category.

### Agency Perspective

An economic analysis of an HP-DP program using an "agency perspective" would only include direct and indirect costs associated with the expenditure of resources to create, manage, and provide the program. This perspective asks the following: How much will it cost the agency funding the HP-DP program to routinely deliver it to the people and locations for which it was designed? The principal foci of this perspective are the direct costs associated with services consumed for a specific health problem, and the potential healthcare expenses avoided (or increased) as a result of an intervention. Other costs, such as patient loss of productivity, travel, out of pocket costs, and so on, would generally not be part of an agency perspective. Health maintenance organizations (HMOs), managed care organizations, and federal-state-local governments may pay for and/or reimburse related costs for an HP-DP intervention for specific problems among a target group. In most economic evaluations of HP-DP programs primarily designed to counsel participants to modify individual risk factors, or to change their self-care or health services utilization behaviors, an agency perspective will be typically taken.

## STEP 4: Define Program Costs (Input) and Cost Analysis Methods

In the specification of costs, all budgetary resources expended to implement the HP-DP program are documented. As defined in Chapter 5, a successfully implemented process evaluation will provide this information and data. Staff needs to prepare a cost inventory of all resources required to provide the program, define the units of measurement for each resource category, and assign a monetary value to each resource unit. This step requires documentation of the costs associated with program delivery: staff time/group or individual contact, number of contacts, and total amount of resources expended and cost per client. The following is a synopsis of the main cost/budget categories. Costs are segmented into two categories: direct and indirect.

### Direct Costs

These are expenditures for staff training and staff time to deliver the intervention, and non-personnel costs, such as tests, and program materials.

### Indirect Costs

These are expenditures for facilities rent, maintenance, security, and so on. Whether to use indirect costs is an individual program judgment and depends on the extent to which the organization requires these costs to be used.

## Personnel Costs

The major cost associated with the delivery of most HP-DP programs is personnel time, typically 70%–90% of a budget. If mass media and/or specific materials are used, the proportion of a budget for staff may be lower. A detailed description of the HP-DP program specifies how much individual staff time is expended to provide the different assessment and intervention components. As noted in Chapter 5, a program-provider flow analysis (PFA) of what is being delivered on a typical day to 10–30 clients (varies by census) at each site, and > 5 clients per provider for a typical workday, should provide this information.

A basic example of the costs of a program is as follows. In an employee wellness program, a graduate-trained exercise physiologist might use 20 hours to deliver twice a week a one-hour aerobics class for each group of 10 employees over a period of 10 weeks. The instructor may have to spend an additional 20 hours in preparation: 60 minutes/session. If you assume a $50,000 per year salary for this person, with a 20% fringe benefit rate (0.20 x $50,000 = $10,000), the total salary costs would be $60,000 per year. The rate for the staff would be about $30/hour ($60,000; 2,080 hours). Thus, the total staff costs to deliver this type of program to 10 employees would be about $1,200 ($30 x 40 hours): $120/employee. It is assumed that equipment cost is minimal, and not a direct cost.

Additional costs to the company could be considered, depending on whether the program was delivered on company time or employee time. It would be zero, if on employee time, or based on the average hourly wage of the 20 employees, if conducted on company time. If the average wage (salary + fringe) was $50/hr, the company direct cost for lost employee time would be $10,000: 10 X 20 X $50/hr. In this example, employees do not participate during company time.

Although probably small, costs for staff to communicate to employees about the program and/or to schedule the facilities would also be incurred and counted. Another dimension of a cost analysis may be participant copayment. If each employee had to pay $50 to enroll, the income would be $500, and total net cost of the program to the employer would be $700, or $70/employee.

## Equipment and Material Costs

In marketing and delivering a program, materials (e.g., books, hand-outs, leaflets, and posters) may be used. In addition, special equipment may be needed (e.g., for an exercise class). Some HP-DP programs would incur cost for drugs, lab tests, and transportation. Equipment costs used for multiple programs and purposes can be estimated with the amount of dollars equivalent to that proportion of the time the equipment is used by the program.

## Facilities Costs

Facilities costs reflect the monetary value of the use of the space in which a program is provided. A company could define the cost of space used (rent/sq. ft.) for employees HP-DP classes, because it could be used for profit-making activity. The current rate of the cost/square foot for classroom or meeting space would be available. The cost/square foot times the hours of use divided by the total number of possible hours of use would produce an accurate accounting of facilities costs. In situations in which facilities are rented, a lease contract should specify facilities costs. A budget worksheet (see Chapters 2 and 4) can be constructed to estimate the total personnel or non-personnel input costs allocated to deliver an employee health promotion program.

## Adjusting Costs: Inflation and Discounting

### Inflation

Inflation in an economic evaluation of the impact of an HP-DP intervention is typically adjusted to by using the Consumer Price Index (CPI) rates for healthcare costs from the US Bureau of Labor Statistics (BLS). It is used to adjust and compare cost over a defined period of time. Monthly and annual rates are available for the last 30 years, and are current to the latest month. An example, using the BLS-CPI data, is presented in the CBA in Case Study 3 on smoking and pregnancy in this chapter.

### Discounting

A discussion of costs should also include consideration of the value of monetary resources for purposes other than allocation to the HP-DP program, that is, an opportunity cost. Simply put, if a managed care organization or public health agency budgets (invests) $100,000 annually in a specific intervention program, it is not available for other programs or income-producing opportunities. It is also important to recognize that all program costs and expenditures are not incurred at the present time. Costs are incurred over a period of years, and the benefits (real or estimated savings) typically occur over a longer period of time. The issue is estimating the costs and benefits of a program throughout its effective lifetime. The term used to consider the value of current and future dollars in an economic analysis is *discounting*.

Future dollar costs and benefits are reduced, or "discounted," to reflect the assumption that dollars spent or saved in the future are not worth as much as dollars spent or saved today. The basic premise of discounting is that an organization has the option to use money for different purposes or to invest, for example, $100,000, in different units of an activity. If $100,000 is invested, it may yield $1,000–$2,000 at a CD rate of 1%–2%, for a total of $101,000–$102,000 each year. Concurrently, the Consumer Price Index reports an inflation rate. If the inflation rate during the year is 2.5%, then the sum of $100,000 will have the investment buying power of only $97,500 in the next year. The choice of the most appropriate discount rate, typically >2%–3%, depends to a large extent on how inflation rates are addressed. Financial software packages and personal computers can perform these calculations. A health economist should be consulted for computation and analyses.

## STEP 5: Define Behavioral Impact or Health Outcome Rates (Output)

The implementation of the next step involves the documentation of impact or outcome rates of change (effect size range) attributable to the HP-DP program. These data are derived from two sources. An evaluation team needs to conduct a meta-evaluation (ME), or use data and results produced by a prospective RCT for the same problem and comparable population. These steps provide an estimate or document specific behavioral impact and/or health outcome rates produced by an existing versus new HP-DP program. *In examining these output data, the methodological issues related to internal validity defined in Chapters 1 through 5 must be addressed.* Valid evidence needs to be presented to confirm that the significant changes and E versus C group differences in observed impact or outcome rates are attributable to the HP-DP program. Cost analyses should not be performed unless a methodologically rigorous outcome evaluation has been conducted to produce results with high internal validity.

### Estimation of Behavioral Impact and/or Health Outcome Rates: A Meta-Evaluation

An economic evaluation needs to define what level of effect is a reasonable (defensible) estimate of significant change over time. In some cases, measurement may be complicated, for example, measurement of the quality of adjusted life years (QUALY) attributable to an intervention. However, almost all HP-DP programs, if effective, produce behavioral impact or health status outcomes over a one- to three-year period of successful implementation, for example, high blood pressure, diabetes, or asthma control, reduced high blood cholesterol levels, or behavioral effects such as changes in smoking status or weight. All of these rates can be measured in very valid and reliable ways.

An evaluation needs to conduct a meta-valuation (ME) and a meta-analysis (MA) to define the range (low-medium-high) of intervention effects. For example, as noted in Table 6.7 (Case Study 3), an ME by Windsor (2010) confirmed that the range of cessation rates reported for pregnant smokers (E Groups) exposed to a "best practice" Smoking Cessation and Reduction In Pregnancy Treatment (SCRIPT) program was 12%–27%. This level of impact can be compared to a 0%–11% rates from the usual counseling (C group) rate. The range behavior changes reported in the ME was 4.0%–15.7%: the average E minus C difference was 8.5%.

All eight SCRIPT evaluations met ME criteria for high internal validity. Each evaluation measured behavior change, smoking status, and levels of tobacco exposure at baseline and end of pregnancy by self-report and an independent biochemical test. All evaluations had sufficient sample size and confirmed exposure to treatment or control intervention procedures. Almost all evaluations were conducted among patients in Medicaid-supported prenatal care. These data and methods are essential to estimate the level of effect and costs associated with producing each percent of change for a problem and population for a CEA and CBA. An example of the potential effectiveness and CBA of dissemination derived from an ME of a "best practice" intervention, the SCRIPT methods, for the annual US cohort of pregnant smokers (N = app. 800,000) is presented in Case Study 3 of this chapter.

### Confirmation of Behavioral Impact and/or Health Outcome Rates: A Prospective Evaluation

Assume a rigorous evaluation of a worksite disease management program for employees with Type 2 (T2) diabetes was conducted among 300+ E group employees and 300+ C group employees. It measured physical activity, weight control, diabetes, and absenteeism for the last 12 months, and blood glucose levels (HbA1C) at baseline. At a 12-month follow-up, the evaluation documented that the E group intervention produced "an average weight loss of 10 pounds from baseline observations, a 12% reduction in the worker absenteeism rate, and confirmed a HbA1C (glucosylated hemoglobin) T2 diabetes control rate of 80%, and a 15% reduction in the average Hb1AC values." The C group intervention produced a "4 pound weight gain from a baseline observation, a small increase in the absenteeism rate of 4%, and an Hb1AC diabetes control rate of 65%." If a program decides to conduct a CEA of the E versus C group intervention, it needs to confirm which of the differences were statistically significant, to document the actual costs to deliver the E group intervention method #1 and C group method #2, and compare weight loss, absenteeism, HbA1C/Type 2 diabetes rates, and control effectiveness rates. These analyses should produce a cost-effective ratio (CER), and cost per unit of effect for each impact rate.

From a cost-benefit analysis (CBA) perspective, a program could also decide to document the costs of method #1 and method #2, and the associated economic benefits for each method. Did the significant reduction in workdays lost, reduced weight, improved rates of diabetes control, produce reduced use of diabetes-related healthcare services, for example, doctor visits, medications, and/hospitalizations? Were there significant cost savings and lower expenditures for diabetes-related care and services observed for intervention #2? Did the HP-DP intervention pay for itself? In a CBA evaluation of method #1 versus method #2, a cost-to-benefit ratio (CBR) would be computed, and economic benefits, a return on investment (ROI), and dollars saved per year would be reported to employing organization management and to the workers.

Excellent discussions of successful impact and cost evaluations of adult diabetes management are presented by Rothman, DeWalt, Malone, et al., "Influence of Patient Literacy on the Effectiveness of a Primary Care-Based Diabetes Management Program," *Journal of the American Medical Association* (2004) (Impact Evaluation) and by Rothman, So, Shin, et al., "Labor Characteristics and Program Costs of a Successful Diabetes Disease Management Program," *American Journal of Managed Care* (2006) (Cost Evaluation).

## STEP 6: Perform a CEA or CBA

A detailed picture of its cost-effectiveness is needed before an organization establishes a new HP-DP policy or program and commits a large amount of money to its development and routine delivery. If a statistically significant impact of an intervention is documented, these results should be examined in the context of variations of behavior and health effects (output) and costs (input) at different sites and systems, or with similar groups of program participants in other geographic locations. These sensitivity analyses and data will inform the evaluation and program leadership about how the original conclusions about cost-effectiveness and cost-benefit might change. Sensitivity analysis may produce at least four results: (1) dependence on a specific assumption of a level of impact; (2) assumption that does not significantly affect conclusion; (3) confirmation of the assumption of the minimum or maximum value that a cost must have for a program to appear worthwhile; and (4) issues and uncertainties deserving future evaluation.

### STEP 7: Sensitivity Analysis (SA)-Vary Cost and Impact Assumptions

Several sensitivity analysis (SA) options can be selected: one variable, multiple variable, and threshold analysis. An SA may vary intervention cost, and impact rates, or conduct an analysis to determine at what point cost and impact reach a "threshold." Personnel and material costs for an HP-DP program will differ by program infrastructure, type of staff, location, from state to state, and by levels of behavioral impact or health outcome rates. The cost of staff and variations in effectiveness of a program in Boston, Massachusestts, will be very different from those of a program in Columbia, South Carolina.

An organization may decide in an SA to vary staff or costs by 10% or 20% and effectiveness by 10% or 20%. By varying impact levels and cost assumptions, using low-medium-high estimates, an SA documents what changes would occur in the conclusions with each variation. In performing an SA, it is important to emphasize that variations of assumptions should be rational. The following five case studies provide examples of the application of the steps and methods used to conduct a CEA and CBA, including performing sensitivity analyses.

## Cost Analyses and CEA-CBA Case Studies

### Case Study 1: Cost Effectiveness Analysis of a Clinic-Based Disease Management Program

R. Windsor, W. Bailey, J. Richards, et al., "The Efficacy and Cost Effectiveness of Health Education Methods to Increase Medication Adherence Among Adults with Asthma," *American Journal of Public Health* (1990), 1519–1521 (see publication for references).

## Introduction

The prevalence, hospitalization, and mortality from asthma among adults in the United States is a serious national problem. This evaluation was designed to document the following three outcomes:

**Efficacy**: The level of behavioral impact produced by a tailored patient education program with optimal resources, provided by specialty staff;

**Cost:** The resources, personnel, and materials needed to routinely deliver the existing and new intervention programs to adults with asthma who were receiving routine care from pulmonary and critical care specialists; and

**Cost-effectiveness:** The cost per unit of asthma medication adherence (in percent).

## Methods

The study was conducted at the Comprehensive Pulmonary Medicine Clinic of the University of Alabama Medical Center in Birmingham. Of 280 adults > 17 years screened during a one-year period with a diagnosis of asthma, 267 (95%) agreed to participate. Following consent and baseline assessment, 135 patients were randomized to a C group and 132 to an E group. Prior to randomization, patients were stratified by level of asthma severity in each of 11 pulmonary physician practices. Using Power = 0.80, alpha = 0.05, estimated improvement in adherence of > 20% for 12 months, and a 10% attrition rate, > 120 patients were needed in each group.

### Patient Education Intervention

In addition to all 267 patients receiving regular asthma care and counseling from their MD and RN, the E Group also received a peak flow meter and a standardized, four-component counseling program from an MPH trained and Certified Health Education Specialist:

- P1 = A 30-minute one-to-one session with instruction on peak flow-meter use of inhaler use skills, and use of *A Self-Help Guide to Asthma Control*;
- P2 = A 60-minute support group session of 4–6 patients and asthma control partners; and
- P3 + P4 = Two brief telephone reinforcement calls < one month of the group session.

Four focus group sessions and pilot tests with patients were held to develop intervention Procedures (P1, 2, 3, 4). NHLBI Asthma Treatment Guidelines were discussed with all 11 MDs/RNs at the clinic by the PI (William Bailey, MD, Professor of Pulmonary Medicine).

## Measurement

All patients received a baseline (O1) and 90% completed a 12-month follow-up (O2) medical and behavioral assessment with four outcomes: correct inhaler use, inhaler adherence, medication adherence, and total adherence rating. Medication adherence (MA) and inhaler adherence (IA) were assessed using existing instruments. A Total Adherence Score was derived by combining patient medication and inhaler scales scores. Patients lost to follow-up were counted as failures.

## Behavioral Impact Results

Data in Table 6.3 confirmed E and C group baseline equivalence. A comparison of the 13 patients who refused (5% rate) versus 267 who participated confirmed no baseline differences by gender, race, age, education, and asthma severity. Thirty-four C group (25%) and 8 E group patients (6%) were lost to follow-up. Baseline analyses confirmed that the 42 dropouts were not significantly different from the 238 participants. A low potential for selection bias was documented.

A process evaluation of E group patients confirmed the use of the Asthma Guide by 124 (94%); 110 (89%) participated in the group session; and 124 (94%) received both reinforcement calls. *The Program Implementation Index (PII) for the E group was PII = 0.93.* The behavioral impact of the intervention is presented in Table 6.4. Using a 95% confidence interval (CI) to evaluate differences between rates of group

TABLE 6.3 Baseline Patient Characteristics by Study Group

| VARIABLES | C GROUP (N = 135) | E GROUP (N = 132) |
|---|---|---|
| Sex: female | 71% | 61% |
| Race: black | 28% | 32% |
| Median age | 49 | 53 |
| Median years: education | 13 | 13 |
| Current smoker | 13% | 10% |
| Asthma severity: Mild | 39% | 37% |
| Moderate | 45% | 48% |
| Severe | 17% | 16% |

TABLE 6.4 Cost Effectiveness of the Asthma Management Program

| GROUP | COST PER PATIENT | ADHERENCE SCORE IMPROVEMENT | TOTAL COST-EFFECTIVENESS* |
|---|---|---|---|
| Control Group | $ 3.61 | +02% | $244 (N = 135) |
| Experimental Group | $32.03 | +44% | $ 96 (N = 132) |

*Cost effectiveness = Total cost per group divided by adherence score increase

improvement, a consistent pattern of E group adherence was confirmed for a 12-month period. Significant improvements for the E group in inhaler skills use (CI = .29, .61), inhaler adherence (CI = .24, .50), medication adherence (CI = .31, .57), and total adherence score 100% adherence (CI = .28, .59) were observed.

### Cost Estimation and Analysis

Because an agency perspective was applied in this CEA, patient time and intervention development costs were not used to compute costs. While an MPH-Health Education Specialist provided the intervention, a nurse would be the typical provider. A salary of $25,000 plus a fringe benefit rate of 20% was used to estimate nursing cost: $30,000/year/2,080 hr. = $14.42/hr. Total personnel time cost for the E group was $24.30: Component #1 = $7.21, Component #2 = $14.42 and Component #3 = $2.40. The Asthma Guide cost $8.00 for a Total Intervention Cost = $32.03/patient. The total C group costs for a 10-minute general discussion about the importance of adherence and two brief follow-up contacts for a total of 15 minutes were $3.61/patient.

Cost analyses in Table 6.4 confirmed the cost-effectiveness of the tailored intervention. The results of this trial indicated that if an adult asthma management program wants to significantly improve patient adherence levels, it will need to allocate additional types of resources.

### Discussion

The significant increase in E group adherence exceeded rates from previous reports. Feasibility, patient and provider acceptance was very high. From an administrative and programmatic perspective, these results indicated that this type of intervention may have potential for adaptation and use by other asthma programs.

The tailored intervention provided may have been too resource-intensive and costly for other care sites. Although the methods and results reported were encouraging, future research needs to evaluate the impact of a streamlined program on health services utilization, for example, ambulatory care, emergency care, hospitalization, and clinical outcomes.

*This is a useful case study for an HP-DP evaluation class exercise, using the same levels of impact and use current, average estimates of salary and fringe benefit cost of RNs, and the Bureau of Labor Statistics (BLS) Consumer Price Index (CPI) for medical care for RN expenses to inflate and estimate to 2015 dollars.* Another excellent economic evaluation of an asthma intervention for children for considered for in-class discussion is "Easy Breathing," presented by Clouthier et al., *American Journal of Managed Care* (2009).

## Case Study 2: A Cost-Benefit Analysis of Worksite Health Promotion Programs

K. Baicker, D. Cutler, and Z. Song, "Workplace Wellness Programs Can Generate Savings," *Health Affairs* (2010) (see publication for references).

### Introduction

Because of significant annual increases in healthcare costs and spending, multiple stakeholders, especially employers, have expressed growing interest in identifying HP-DP programs that improve worker health, reduce absenteeism, and lower employee healthcare costs. Systematic reviews revealed that most EHP evaluation studies lacked an adequate comparison or control group. They were not able to account for possible unobserved variables or alternative explanations responsible for observed differences in costs between participants and non-participants. Most employee health promotion (EHP) evaluations were not able to attribute observed differences to the HP program. The primary threat to internal validity was selection bias. The healthiest employees were most likely to enroll in voluntary wellness programs.

Reviews also confirm that most methods used by employers to calculate costs and benefits of health-related investments may not reflect valid estimates of program impact. Because of multiple deficiencies, past reviews have indicated that there is limited evidence of the efficacy of EHP programs (poor internal validity) and the reported results cannot be generalized to comparable worker settings (poor external validity).

## Purposes

This study conducted a meta-analysis on effectiveness, costs, and savings associated with employer-based wellness promotion programs and policies. Eligible studies were screened for analytical rigor, and standardized estimates of ROI from those studies were calculated. This review included only evaluation studies for which there was a comparison group. Effectiveness of health program interventions and impact on healthcare costs and absenteeism were documented.

## Methods

A literature search from peer-reviewed meta-analyses of employee wellness programs produced a sample of > 100 peer-reviewed studies of employee programs spanning the past three decades. Analyses were restricted to evaluations that met the following criteria: (1) well-defined intervention; (2) well-defined E and C group, even if the comparison (C) group was not randomly assigned; and (3) presented analysis of a distinct new intervention, rather than analysis of an intervention examined in one of the other studies. Applying these criteria reduced the sample to 32 original publications. These studies are listed in the report. A uniform wage rate was used to define comparable estimates of ROI associated with reduced workdays lost.

## Results

This meta-analysis confirmed that 90% of the health promotion programs were implemented in large firms (> 1000 employees). Information in Table 6.5 identifies the typical methods provided to the employees and the primary risk factors: weight loss/fitness and smoking.

Table 6.6 presents a synthesis of the average impact on costs, average savings, and impact on absenteeism of the health promotion interventions, and average return on investment (ROI). Absenteeism was monetized using an average hourly wage for 2009 of $20.49.

## Discussion

This systematic review and meta-analysis and cost and economic analysis of the 36 evaluation studies presented strong and consistent evidence for the cost-benefit of employee health promotion (EHP)

TABLE 6.5 Characteristics of Worksite Wellness Programs Studied[+]

| METHOD OF DELIVERY | PERCENT OF FIRMS |
|---|---|
| Health risk assessment | 81% |
| Self-help education materials | 42% |
| Individual counselling | 39% |
| Classes, seminars, group activities | 36% |
| Added incentives for participation | 31% |
| Focus of intervention | |
| Weight loss and fitness | 66% |
| Smoking cessation | 50% |
| Multiple risk factors | 75% |

[+] SOURCE: Author's calculations based on studies in Appendix Table 1. Available online at http://content.healthaffairs.org/cgi/content/full/29/2/hlthaff.2009.0626/DC2
Per employee/year, costs in 2009 dollars

TABLE 6.6 Summary of Employee Wellness Studies Analyzed

| FOCUS | NUMBER OF STUDIES | AVERAGE SAMPLE | | AVERAGE DURATION | AVERAGE SAVINGS | AVERAGE COSTS | AVERAGE ROI |
|---|---|---|---|---|---|---|---|
| | | E | C | | | | |
| Healthcare Costs | 22 | 3,201 | 4,547 | 3.0 years | $358 | $144 | 2.49 |
| Absenteeism | 22 | 2,683 | 4,782 | 2.0 years | $294 | $132 | 2.23 |

programs. EHP investments produced a $3.27 reduction in healthcare savings for each $ spent, and a $2.73 savings from reduced absenteeism for each dollar spent. The authors acknowledge that the size and characteristics of the company and employee workforce and employee risk status play salient roles in the potential for impact and cost savings. This report is an excellent methodological review of how to evaluate the impact and how to conduct economic evaluations of HP-DP programs for employees and worksites.

## Case Study 3: A Cost Benefit Analysis for Dissemination of an Evidenced-Based Program

R. Windsor, "Smoking Cessation and Reduction In Pregnancy Treatment (SCRIPT) Methods: A Meta-Evaluation of the Impact of Dissemination," *American Journal of Medical Sciences* (October 2003), 216–222 (see publication for references).

## Introduction

Active and passive exposure to tobacco smoke during pregnancy and infancy are the most serious and preventable causes of adverse maternal, fetal, and infant outcomes in the United States. This meta-evaluation provided a synopsis of the state of the science in five areas of this specialized area: (1) the validity of patient reports of smoking status and trends during pregnancy: (2) a definition of "best practice" cessation methods for pregnant women; (3) a description of the cost of the SCRIPT methods (niput); (4) an estimate of the impact of dissemination of the Agency for HealthCare Research and Quality (AHRQ, 2000) recommended SCRIPT methods among the 800,000 pregnant US smokers in 2002 (output); and (5) an estimate of the evidence from a cost-benefit analysis of improved maternal and infant outcomes from cessation attributable to SCRIPT methods, including a Sensitivity Analysis (ouput).

### Defining the Problem and Population at Risk

Approximately 4 to 4.2 million women gave birth in the United States from 1990 to 2003: about 1.6 million (40%) were Medicaid patients. During this period, the smoking prevalence rate during pregnancy had been monitored annually by federal agencies. Data in Table 6.7 are based on the PRAMS (Pregnancy Related Assessment and Monitoring System) reports from the CDC National Center for Health Statistics.

All smoking rates are based on self-reports in response to a multistage, mailed survey (70% response rate) sent two to four months after babies were born. The CDC reported that the rate during pregnancy had been reduced from 18.4% in 1990 (736,000 smokers) to 12.2% in 2000 (488,000 smokers) to 10% in 2003 (410,000 smokers). Thus, the CDC

TABLE 6.7 Smoking Rates During Pregnancy and Percent Change by Group: 1990–2003

| YEARS | TOTAL | BLACK | WHITE | HISPANIC | OTHER |
|-------|-------|-------|-------|----------|-------|
| 1990 | 18.4% | | | | |
| 1993 | 15.8% | 15.9% | 21.0% | 6.7% | 8.6% |
| 1995 | 13.9% | | | | |
| 1997 | 13.2% | 10.6% | 17.1% | 4.3% | 7.5% |
| 2000 | 12.2% | 9.1% | 15.7% | 3.7% | 5.9% |
| 2003 | 10.0% | | | | |

% < 45% < 320,000 smokers = self-reported estimate Use 1 < only

reports indicated that approximately 320,000 more smokers quit during their pregnancy in 2003, compared to the 1990 data: a > 40% reduction in the annual smoking rate during pregnancy.

Data in Table 6.8 documented the average smoking rate for three-year periods among pregnant women from 1990 to 2003 based on the National Annual Household Survey on Drug Abuse by the Substance Abuse and Mental Health Services Administration (SAMHSA). These data represent a subsample of women, ages 15–44, from the annual 70,000 face-to-face interviews in the home, also with a 70% response rate. The SAMHSA data do not agree with the CDC data. The SAMSHA interviews, however, were much more likely to have elicited a valid statement of smoking status compared to a survey mailed two to four months after birth.

*Because NONE of the CDC or SAMSHA surveys used a biochemical test (e.g., a saliva or urine cotinine analysis) to corroborate patient self-reports, all national estimates of the prevalence and number are significant underestimates of the problem.* Because of the high social desirability of a nonsmoking response, high rates of patient deception/ nondisclosure about smoking status at the onset and during care have been well documented. The CDC documented a deception rate of 48% by a urine cotinine test (N = 6,000), and the Alabama Smoking Cessation/ Reduction In Pregnancy Treatment Trial II documented a deception rate 24% by a saliva cotinine test (N = 1000). If the SAMHSA rate of 17.0% is adjusted, by adding a low estimate of deception (5%), the true prevalence rate was > 20% (> 800,000 smokers) in 2003. When the CDC and SAMHSA data are considered, it is a plausible conclusion that the CDC prevalence rates are very inaccurate.

### Assessing Smoking Status and Exposure in Prenatal Care

In 1991 in the *Journal of the American Medical Association*, Fiore presented a discussion on the need to routinely assess smoking status

TABLE 6.8 Average Smoking Rates, Women 15–44: 1990–2003

| YEARS | PREGNANT | NOT PREGNANT |
|---|---|---|
| 1990–1992 | 20.0% | 30.0% |
| 1994–1996 | 20.6% | 31.8% |
| 1998–2000 | 19.4% | 30.2% |
| 2001–2003 | 17.5% | 30.0% |

and recommended its inclusion as a standard procedure in clinical practice: "a new vital sign." The Agency for Healthcare Research and Quality Clinical Practice Guideline (2000) recommended routine assessment of patients: "The first step in intervention is assessment of tobacco use status. Biochemical confirmation was recommended."

### Defining the Effectiveness of Health Education Methods for Pregnant Smokers

The PHASE 1 and 2 SCRIPT evaluations, cited by the Clinical Practice Guidelines, documented the quality, efficacy, and cost effectiveness of standardized patient education for pregnant smokers: SCRIPT internal validity. According to the Guidelines, "clinicians should offer effective smoking cessation interventions to pregnant smokers at the first prenatal visit as well as throughout the course of pregnancy." Examples of effective interventions with pregnant smokers from the meta-analysis and Guidelines (p. 94) are presented in the article.

### Defining the SCRIPT Program for Dissemination

Phase I, II, and III Trials (1982–2002) and meta-evaluation of the eight studies among 2,700 patients from four countries (US, Canada, Sweden, and Norway) comprehensively evaluated the SCRIPT Program. A synopsis of the SCRIPT program is presented below

#### SCRIPT ASSIST Component

The ASSIST component of SCRIPT, the core methods, includes a three-part patient education process at the first visit.

**Component #1:** "Commit to Quit Smoking—During and After Pregnancy," a 10-minute video, was designed to enhance motivation to quit, improve comprehension of risk information, introduce the Guide, ensure exposure to recommended cessation methods, and reduce counseling time.

**Component #2:** "A Pregnant Woman's Guide to Quit Smoking" is a 32-page tailored guide with a fifth- to sixth-grade reading level. It is introduced by the video and the clinic counselor.

**Component #3:** This is a 5–7-minute patient-centered counseling session delivered by a physician, nurse, midwife, social worker, or WIC nutritionist during regular prenatal care.

## Cost Analysis of SCRIPT Methods

The primary cost of SCRIPT methods is staff time and patient education materials. Because an agency perspective was applied, patient time, facilities, and intervention development costs were not used in the cost analysis. An RN would be a typical SCRIPT provider. *An average salary + fringe of $60,000–80,000/year can be used to estimate nursing staff costs to estimate intervention costs in 2015 for in-class discussion and computation of costs/CEA/CBA.*

An average staff cost for delivery of the 10-minute intervention was $5.00/patient. The bulk order (1,000 +) price for "A Pregnant Woman's Guide to Quit Smoking" is approximately $3.00. The commercial price of the "Commit to Quit Smoking" video is $25.00/unit. The video cost can be divided by 100 patients/year for a cost of $0.25/patient for clinical use, not for individual or commercial distribution. Because a television and DVD player are standard equipment at a clinic, they were not included in the cost estimates. Total intervention cost was $8.00/patient.

Patient flow analyses at the prenatal care sites would confirm that nurses, with reinforcement by other staff, would spend about 3–5 minutes with smokers. C group patients typically received "Ask and Advise" procedures. Nurses provided printed handouts on the risks of smoking and the benefits of quitting. *The average total new time needed would be about 6–8 minutes.* The costs associated with staff time to deliver the usual cessation advice are about $1–2 per C group patient. *Thus, the approximate NEW cost to an agency of the SCRIPT methods would be about $6.00/patient.*

## Estimated Behavioral Impact of SCRIPT Dissemination

Table 6.9 presents a synopsis of the impact of the eight SCRIPT evaluation studies.

The evaluations in Table 6.9 documented, by a self-report and biochemical measure, the effectiveness of SCRIPT methods. As noted, the overall average behavioral impact level was 7.7%, and US behavioral impact level was 8.5%. Table 6.10 presents estimates of the impact that can be used to conduct a CBA of national dissemination of SCRIPT methods. It applies three dissemination impact levels: low = 4%; moderate = 5%; high = 6%, to estimate the additional number and percentage of patients who might quit from SCRIPT methods. As indicated in Table 6.7, exposure among the 700,000 smokers (17% X 4 million +) to effective methods might produce annually an additional 4% cessation rate (low impact N = 28,000

TABLE 6.9 Behavioral Impact of SCRIPT Methods

| PI: EVALUATION STUDY | MEASURE | E GROUP | | C GROUP | | DIFFERENCE |
|---|---|---|---|---|---|---|
| | | N | % | N | % | (E–C) |
| Windsor, 2000 (US) | S-COT | 139 | 17.3% | 126 | 8.8% | 8.5% |
| Gebauer, 1998 (US) | S-COT | 84 | 15.5% | 94 | 0.0% | 15.5% |
| Hartmann, 1996 (US) | CO | 107 | 20.0% | 100 | 10.0% | 10.0% |
| Valbo, 1996 (Norway) | CO | 107 | 27.0% | 105 | 11.4% | 15.7% |
| Windsor, 1993 (US) | S-COT | 400 | 14.2% | 414 | 8.4% | 5.8% |
| O'Connor, 1992 (Canada) | U-COT | 90 | 13.3% | 84 | 6.0% | 7.3% |
| HJfrson, 1991 (Sweden) | SCN | 444 | 12.6% | 209 | 8.6% | 4.0% |
| Windsor, 1985 (US) | SCN | 102 | 13.7% | 104 | 1.9% | 11.8% |
| US Studies (N = 1,670) | Total | 15.4% | | 6.9% | | 8.5% |
| Non-US Studies (N = 1,039) | Total | 15.0% | | 8.8% | | 6.2% |
| (N = 2,709) | Total | 15.2% | | 7.5% | | 7.7% |
| | **E minus C Group difference = 4.0% to 15.7%** | | | | | |

TABLE 6.10 Estimated Smokers and Impact of AHRQ-SCRIPT Methods

| LEVEL-CPD | SMOKERS (A) | STANDARD METHODS RATE | IMPACT | AHRQ-SCRIPT METHODS RATE (B) | IMPACT | DIFFERENCE (B–A) |
|---|---|---|---|---|---|---|
| Light (10) | 400,000 | 8% | 32,000 | 16% | 64,000 | 32,000 |
| Mod (11–19) | 200,000 | 6% | 12,000 | 12% | 24,000 | 12,000 |
| Heavy (20) | 100,000 | 2% | 2,000 | 4% | 4,000 | 2,000 |
| Total | 700,000 | 6.2% | 46,000 | 12.5% | 92,000 | + 46,000 |

quitters: cohort 1), an additional 5.0% cessation rate (moderate impact N = 35,000 quitters: cohort 2), or an additional 6% cessation rate (high impact N = 42,000 quitters: cohort 3).

The estimated cost to deliver the SCRIPT methods to all pregnant smokers would be $8.00/patient in 2003. Thus, the cost for a pregnant smoker cohort would be about $5.6 million ($8.00 X 700K). The cost of SCRIPT can be varied to $10.00/patient ($7.0M) and $12.00/patient ($8.4M) to reflect regional cost variations. With these assumptions, a CBA and sensitivity analysis, describing the cost-benefit of nationwide SCRIPT dissemination, can be performed.

Using the excess smoking-attributable savings of $1,500/patient who quit in 1995 (Miller et al., 2001), and adjusting this cost for inflation by the Consumer Price Index (CPI)—US Bureau of Labor Statistics (BLS)

TABLE 6.11 Estimated Impact, Cost, and Savings of AHRQ-SCRIPT Methods

| COHORT | IMPACT | QUIT RATE | SAVINGS | SCRIPT COST | NET SAVINGS RANGE |
|--------|--------|-----------|---------|-------------|-------------------|
| #1 700K | 4% | 28,000 | $56M | $5.6M | $50M–$49M–$48M |
| #2 700K | 5% | 35,000 | $70M | $7.0M | $64M–$63M–$62M |
| #3 700K | 6% | 42,000 | $84M | $8.4M | $78M–$77M–$76M |
| M = millions | | (A) | (B) $2,000 | (C) | (B1-2-3... C1-2-3... D1-2-3) |

for increases in maternal and infant healthcare costs, in January 1, 2003, the average estimated savings for each quitter would > $2,000. When the savings from the excess smoking-attributable care costs of $2,000/patient is multiplied by each impact level (column A = $2,000 X column B), the potential benefits of dissemination is $56 million (low effect cohort 1), $70 million (moderate effect cohort 2), and $84 million (high effect cohort 3). CBA data in Table 6.11 indicate that dissemination is cost-beneficial.

When sensitivity analyses are performed, varying and subtracting low-moderate-high estimates of SCRIPT costs ($8.00 = $5.6 million, $10.00 = $7 million, and $12.00 = $8.4 million per patient (column C) from the low-moderate-high average estimates of gross savings (column B), the estimates net savings range (column D) would be $49 million, $63 million, and $77 million per year. If the lowest estimate of behavioral impact (4%/28,000) and highest estimate of intervention costs ($12/$8.4M) are applied in a CBA, the CBR = $1: $5.7 ($47.6 M/$8.4 M). If the impact from SCRIPT dissemination is set at 5% (+ 35,000 quitters), the estimate of excess smoking attributable healthcare cost is reduced 25%, $2,000 to $1,500 (35,000 X $1,500 = $52.5M), and the highest SCRIPT cost of $12/patient (700K X $12 = $8.4M) is applied in a sensitivity analysis, the estimated savings from dissemination would be $27 million ($35M/$8.4 M), and ROI = $1: $4.17.

## Summary

Cost and economic evaluations, if successfully implemented, should produce valid data and insight about the efficiency of HP-DP programs. They define program costs and what it will cost to break even, if a new intervention is introduced. CBA defines the potential or actual opportunity to save money. Efficiency of intervention methods in producing either behavioral impact–health outcome rates described in non-monetary terms, or impact or outcome rates described in dollars, should be documented using the appropriate analyses. Conducting economic evaluations of HP-DP methods should be a routine process for HP-DP programs. Many funding agencies require a cost-economic evaluation for all major HP-DP proposals.

The Congressional Office of Technology Assessment concluded in 1981 that healthcare decision-making could be significantly improved by the process of identifying relevant costs and benefits of a decision and policy. While a voluminous body of literature and evidence confirms the validity of this 30-year-old statement, past and present reports indicate that cost-economic analyses and evaluations are typically *not* part of an HP-DP program plan or its evaluation. CEA or CBA are infrequently part of an evaluation of public health or primary care services.

It is also important to emphasize from a philosophical perspective that a preoccupation with cost analyses and solely judging a program's economic value-cost is usually not justifiable. Cost-economic evaluation, for most programs, should seldom serve as the primary determinant of HP-DP program decision-making. Cost and efficiency are only one part of rational decision-making. *A broader range of issues, especially effectiveness, quality, and equity, reflecting concern for the health and welfare of a target population, should be the primary guides to decision-making.*

# REFERENCES

Allegrante, J., and Barry, M. June 2009. *Galway (Ireland) Consensus Conference on Credentialing in Health Promotion and Health Education (Conference proceedings). Health Education and Behavior.*

American Association for Health Education. 2002. CD *Cynergy: A tool for health communication planning and evaluation.*

American Public Health Association, Committee on Professional Education. 1957. Educational qualifications and functions of public health education. *American Journal of Public Health* 47: 1.

Baicker, K., Cutler, D., and Song, Z. 2010. Workplace wellness programs can generate savings. *Health Affairs* 1–8.

Bandura, A. 1977. *Social learning theory.* Englewood Cliffs, NJ: Prentice Hall.

Bandura, A. 1986. *Social foundations of thought and action: A social cognitive theory.* Englewood Cliffs, NJ: Prentice Hall.

Baranowski, T., and Stables, G. 2000. Process evaluations of the 5-a-day projects. *Health Education and Behavior* 27(2): 157–166.

Barry, D., Chaney, B., Piazza-Gardner, G., and Chavarria, A. 2013. Validity and reliability reporting practices in the field of health education and behavior: A review of seven journals. *Health Education & Behavior* 12–18.

Barry, P., and DeFriese, G. 1990. Cost-benefit and cost-effectiveness analysis for health promotion programs. *American Journal of Health Promotion* 4(6): 448–452.

Basch, C., Sliepcevich, E., Gold, R., et al. 1985. Avoiding type III errors in health education program evaluation: A case study. *Health Education Quarterly* 12(3): 315–331.

Berg, G., and Wadha, S. 2007. Health services outcomes for a diabetes disease management program for the elderly. *Disease Management* 10(4): 226–234.

Biglan, A., Ary, D., and Wagenaar, A. 2000. The value of interrupted time-series experiments for community intervention research. *Prevention Science* 1(Mar 1): 31–49.

Blackburn, H., and Leupker, R. Minnesota Heart Health Project (MHHP). 1980–1990. PMID 7719388.

Boyd, N., and Orleans, T. 1999. Intervening with older smokers. In *Helping the hard-core smoker: A clinician's guide*, ed. D. F. Seidman and L. Covey. Mahwah, NJ: Lawrence Erlbaum Associates.

Boyd, R., and Orleans, C. 2002. Smoking cessation for older adults. In *Treating alcohol and drug use in the elderly*, ed. A. Gurnack, R. Atkinson, and N. Osgood. New York: Springer.

Boyd, N., and Windsor, R. 1993. A meta-evaluation of nutrition education intervention research among pregnant women. *Health Education& Behavior* 20: 327–345.

Boyd, N., and Windsor, R. 2003. Formative evaluation in maternal and child health practice: The Partners for Life Nutrition Education Program for Pregnant Women, *Journal of Maternal & Child Health* 2: 137–143.

Campbell, D. 1969. Reforms as experiments. *American Psychology* 24(4): 409–429.

Campbell, D., and Fiske, D. 1959. Convergent and discriminant validation by the multitrait-multimethod matrix. *Psychological Bulletin* 56(2): 81–105.

Campbell, D., and Stanley, J. 1966. *Experimental and quasi-experimental designs for research*. Chicago: Rand McNally.

Carmines, E. G., & Zeller, R. A. 1979. *Reliability and validity assessment*. Issue 17, Sage Publishing, New York.

Chen, Y., Jin, G. Z., Kumar, N., and Shi, G. 2013. The promise of Beijing: Evaluating the impact of the 2008 Olympic Games on air quality. *Journal of Environmental Economics and Management*, 66(3): 424–443.

Clouthier, J., Grosse, S., and Wakefield, D. 2009. Easy breathing. *American Journal of Managed Care* 15(6): 345–351.

Cohen, J., and Cohen, P. 1975. *Applied multiple regression/correlation for the behavioral sciences*. Hillsdale, NJ: Lawrence Erlbaum Associates.

Cohen, S., Neumann, R., and Weinstein M. 2008. *New England Journal of Medicine*. PMID 18272889.

Committee for the Study of the Future of Public Health, Institute of Medicine. 1988. *The future of public health*. Washington, DC: National Academy Press.

Cook, T., and Campbell, D. 1979. *Quasi-experimentation: Design and analysis for field settings*. Boston: Houghton Mifflin.

Cook, T., and Reichardt, C., eds. 1979. *Qualitative and quantitative methods in evaluation research*. Beverly Hills, CA: Sage.

Cronbach, L. 1951. Coefficient alpha and the internal structure of a test. *Psychometrika* 16: 297–334.

Dale, E., and Chall, J. 1948. A formula for predicting readability. *Educational Research Bulletin* 1: 37–54.

DiClemente, R., Wingood, G., Harrington, K., et al. 2004. Efficacy of an HIV prevention intervention for African American Adolescent Girls: A randomized clinical trial design. *Journal of the American Medical Association* 171–179.

Driscoll, D., Appiah-Yeboah, A., PSalib, P., and Rupert, D. 2007. Merging qualitative and quantitative data in mixed methods research: How to and why not. *Ecological & Environmental Anthropology* 3(1): 19–28.

Driscoll, D., Lynch, M., Burke, M., et al. 2008. *A formative assessment of knowledge and beliefs about pandemic influenza mitigation among culturally distinct audience segments*. Report to CDC.

Driscoll, D., Rojas-Smith, S. Sotnikov, K., et al. 2006. An instrument for assessing public health system performance: Validity in rural settings. *National Rural Health Association* 22(3): 254–259.

Driscoll, D., Rupert, C., Golin, L., et al. 2008. Promoting prostate-specific antigen informed decision-making: Evaluating two community-level interventions. *American Journal of Preventive Medicine* 35(2): 87–94.

Eisenberg, M., Ringwalt, C., Driscoll, D., et al. 2004. Learning from Truth (sm): Youth participation in field marketing techniques to counter tobacco advertising. *Journal of Health Communication* 9(3): 223–231.

Farquhar, J., Fortmann, S., Flora, J., et al. 1990. Effects of communitywide education on cardiovascular disease risk factors. The Stanford Five-City project. *JAMA* 264: 359–365.

Fiore, M. C. 2000. US Public Health Service clinical practice guideline: treating tobacco use and dependence. *Respiratory Care* 45(10): 1200–1262.

Flay, B. 1986. Efficacy and effectiveness trials (and other phases of research) in the development of health promotion programmes. *Preventive Medicine* 15: 451–474.

Fleiss, J. 1990. *Statistical methods for rates and proportions*. New York: Wiley.

Flesch, R. 1948. A new readability yardstick. *Journal of Applied Psychology* 32: 221–233.

Freudenberg, N. 1989. *Preventing AIDS: A guide to effective education for the prevention of HIV infection*. Washington, DC: American Public Health Association.

Fries, J., Green, L., and Levine, S. 1989. Health promotion and the compression of morbidity. *Lancet* 481–483.

Gebauer, K., et al. 1998. A nurse-managed smoking-cessation intervention during pregnancy. *Journal of Obstetrics & Gynecology in Nursing* 21: 47–53.

Glaser, B., and Strauss, A. 1967. *The discovery of grounded theory: Strategies for qualitative research*. New York: Aldine.

Glass, G. 1976. Primary, secondary, and meta-analysis of research. *Educational Research* 5: 3–8.

Glass, G., McGaw, B., and Smith, M. L. 1981. *Meta-analysis in social research*. Beverly Hills, CA: Sage.

Green, L. 1974. Toward cost-benefit evaluations of health education: Some concepts, methods, and examples. *Health Education Monographs* 2(1): 34–64.

Green, L., and Glasgow, R. 2006. Issues in external validity and translational methodology. *Evaluation and the Health Professions*. PMID 16510882.

Green, L., and Kreuter, M. 1987. *Health promotion planning: An educational and ecological approach*. New York: McGraw-Hill.

Green, L., and Kreuter, M. 1991. *Health promotion planning: A diagnostic approach*. Mountain View, CA: Mayfield.

Green, L., and Kreuter, M. 1994. *Health promotion planning: An educational and ecological approach*. 2nd ed. Mountain View, CA: Mayfield.

Green, L., and Kreuter, M. 1999. *Health promotion planning: An educational and ecological approach*. 3rd ed. Mountain View, CA: Mayfield.

Green, L., Kreuter, M., Deeds, S., and Partridge, K. 1980. *Health education planning: A diagnostic approach*. 1st ed. Mountain View, CA: Mayfield.

Green, L., and Lewis, F. 1986. *Evaluation and measurement in health education*. Mountain View, CA: Mayfield.

Green, L., and Kreuter, M. 2004. *Health promotion planning: An educational and eco-logical approach.* 4th ed. New York: McGraw Hill.

Greenberg-Seth. J. et al., 2004. Evaluation of a community-based intervention to promote rear seating for children. *American Journal of Public Health* 1009–1013.

Greenwald, P., and Cullen, J. 1985. *NCI Journal.* PMID 3883037.

Grossman, J., and Tierney, J. P. 1993. The fallibility of comparison groups. *Evaluation Review* 17(5): 556–571.

*Handbook for certification of health education specialists.* 1990. New York: National Commission of Health Education Credentialing.

*Health inequalities.* 2009. The UK report, House of Commons Health Committee, Third Report of Session 2008–2009. Vol. 1, HC 286-I [Incorporating HC 422-I to vii, Session 2007–2008] London: The Stationery Office Limited.

Hochbaum, G. 1965. Research to improve health education. *International Journal of Health Education* 8: 141–148.

Institute of Medicine. 1988. *Future of public health.* Washington, DC: National Academy Press.

Jamison, D. T., Breman, J. G., Measham, A. R. et al. 2006. *Disease control priorities in developing countries*, 2nd ed. World Bank Publications. Chap. 2: Intervention cost-effectiveness by Laxminarayan, Chow, and Shahid-Salles.

Kenny, D., 1979. *Correlation and causation.* New York: John Wiley.

Khodyakov, D., Stockdale, S., Jones, A., et al. 2013. On measuring community participation in research. *Health Education & Behavior*, 40(3): 346–354.

Levine, R., ed. 2004. *Millions saved: Proven successes in global health.* 3(3). Peterson Institute.

Lewin, C., Lavis, A., Oxman, R., et al. 2008. Supporting the delivery of cost-effective interventions in primary health-care systems in low-income and middle income countries: An overview of systematic reviews. *Lancet.*

Manandhar, D., Orsin, D., Shrestha, B., and the MIRA Trial Team. 2004. Effect of a participatory intervention with women's groups on birth outcomes in Nepal: Cluster-randomized controlled trial. *Lancet* 364: 970–979.

Millennium Development Goals (MDG) Report. 2013. United Nations. Available at mdgs.un.org.

Minkler M., and Wallerstein.N. 2003. *Community-based participatory research for health.* San Francisco, CA: Jossey-Bass. Chapter 13, Issues in participatory evaluation, by Springett presents a succinct reflection about the differences and complementarity of conventional evaluation and participatory evaluation.

Montforton, C., and Windsor, R. 2010. An impact evaluation of federal mine safety training regulation and policies on fatality and injury rates among U.S. stone, sand and gravel workers: an interrupted time-series analysis. *American Journal of Public Health* 100(7): 1334

Morgan, G., Noll, E., Orleans, T, et al. 1996. Reaching midlife and older smokers: Tailored intervention for routine medical care. *Preventive Medicine* 25: 346–364.

Morisky, D., et al. 2008. Predictive validity of a medication adherence measure (MAS) in an outpatient setting. *Journal of Clinical Hypertension* 10(5): 348–354.

Moyo, D. 2009. Dead aid: Why aid is not working and how there is a better way for Africa. New York: Farrar, Straus, and Giroux.

Murray, D. 1998. *Design and analysis of group randomized trials*. New York: Oxford University Press.

National Cancer Institute. 2005. *Making health communications programs work*. Washington, DC: NIH.

Neumann, P., Palmer, J., Daniels, N., et al. 2008. Strategic plan for integrating cost-effectiveness analysis into the US healthcare system. *American Journal of Managed Care* 14(4): 185–188.

Orleans, C., Rimer, B., Fleisher, L., et al. 1989. *Clear Horizons: A quit smoking guide especially for those 50 and over*. Philadelphia: Fox Chase Cancer Center.

Oxman, A. D., Bjorndal, A., Becerra-Posada, F., et al. 2010. A framework for mandatory impact evaluation to ensure well informed public policy decisions. *Lancet* 375(9712): 427–431.

Parker, D., Windsor, R., Hecht, J., et al. October 2007. Feasibility, process, efficacy, and cost effectiveness evaluation of motivational interviewing by telephone for pregnant medicaid patients: The New England SCRIPT Trial. *Nicotine and Tobacco Research*.

Patton, M. 2000. *Qualitative research and evaluation methods*, 2nd ed. Thousand Oaks, CA: Sage.

Pearson, J., Windsor, R., El-Mohandes, A., and Perry, D. August 2009. A formative evaluation of the immediate impact of the Washington, D.C. smoke-free indoor air policy on bar employee ETS exposure. *Public Health Reports*.

Prochaska, J., and DiClemente, C. 1983. Stages and processes of self-change of smoking: Toward an integrative model of change. *Journal of Consulting and Clinical Psychology* 51: 390–395.

Public Affairs Institute. 1973. *Report of the President's Committee on Health Education*. New York: Public Affairs Institute.

Puska, P., Koskela, K., and McAlister, A. 1979. A comprehensive television smoking cessation program in Finland. *International Journal of Health Education* 22 (4, suppl.): 1–28.

Repace, J. 2004. Respirable particles and carcinogens in the air of Delaware hospitality venues before and after a smoking ban. *Journal of Occupational and Environmental Health* 46: 887–905.

Rogers, E. 2003. *Diffusion of innovations*, 5th ed. New York: Free Press.

Rosenstock, I. 1960. Gaps and potentials in health education research. *Health Education Monographs,* 21–27.

Rossi, P., ed. 1982. Standards for evaluation practice. *New Directions for Program Evaluation* 15 (September). San Francisco, CA: Jossey-Bass.

Rossi, P., and Freeman, H., 2004. *Evaluation: A systematic approach*, 7th ed. Newbury Park, CA: Sage.

Rossi, P., Freeman, H., and Wright, S. 1979. *Evaluation: A systematic approach*. Beverly Hills, CA: Sage.

Rothman, R. L., DeWalt, D. A., Malone, R., et al. 2004. Influence of patient literacy on the effectiveness of a primary care-based diabetes management program. *Journal of the American Medical Association*

Rothman, R. L., So, S. A., Shin, J., et al. 2006. Labor characteristics and program costs of a successful diabetes disease management program. *American Journal of Managed Care*

Russell, L. 1987. *Evaluating preventive care: Report on a workshop*. Washington, DC: Brookings Institution.

Savedoff, S., Levine, S., and Birdsall, N. (2006). *When will we ever learn: Improving lives through impact evaluation by the Evaluation Gap Working Group in Washington, D.C*. Center for Global Development (CGD).

Scriven, M. 1972. Pros and cons about goal-free evaluation. *Evaluation Comment* 3(4): 1–4.

Society for Public Health Education, Ad Hoc Committee. 1968. Statement of functions of community health educators and minimum requirements for their professional preparation with recommendations for implementation. Professional preparation of community health educators, National Commission on Accrediting. Washington, DC: DHEW, Public Health Service, CDC.

Society for Public Health Education, Committee on Professional Preparation and Practice of Health Education. 1977a. Guidelines for the preparation and practice of Community Health Educators at the Baccalaureate Level. 1997b. Criteria and guidelines for baccalaureate programs in community health education. *Health Education Monographs* 5(1): 90–98.

Society for Research on Nicotine and Tobacco (SRNT), Sub-Committee on Biochemical Verification of Tobacco Use and Cessation. 2002. *Nicotine and Tobacco Research* 4: 149–59.

Steckler, A., and Goodman, R. 1998. How to institutionalize health promotion programs. *American Journal of Health Promotion* 3(4): 34–44.

Steckler, A., and Linnan, L. 2002. *Process evaluation in public health interventions*. San Francisco, CA: Jossey

Steckler, A., and McLeroy, K. 2008. The importance of external validity. *American Journal of Public Health*.

Stone, E. 1994. Process evaluation in the multicenter child and adolescent trial for cardiovascular health (CATCH). *Health Education Quarterly* (suppl. 2): S1–S143.

Suchman, E. 1967. *Evaluative research: Principles and practice in public service and social action programs*. New York: Russell Sage Foundation.

Sudman, E. 1967. *Applied sampling*. New York: Academic Press.

Suhrcke, G., Nugent, T., Stuckler, R., and Rocco, T. 2006. *Chronic disease: An economic perspective*, oxa.org.

Thompson, M., and Fortress, E. 1980. Cost-effectiveness analysis in health program evaluation. *Evaluation Review* 4(4): 549–568.

Tengs, T., Adams, M., Pliskin, J., Safran D, et al. 1995. Five hundred life-saving interventions and their cost effectiveness. *Risk Analysis* 15: 369–390.

The Evaluation GAP, Working Group Report. 2006. www.cgdev.org/publication/when-will-we-ever-learn-improving-lives-through-impact-evaluation,CDG, Washington, DC.

*Treating tobacco use and dependence*. 2000. Agency for Healthcare Research and Quality. Clinical Practice Guideline. US Department of Health and Human Services, Public Health Service.

US Centers for Disease Control. 2008. Framing an economic evaluation: A self-study guide, and (2) Applying cost analysis to public health programs: A self-study course. Health Economics Research Group, US Centers for Disease Control, epopeb@cdc.gov.

US Congress Office of Technology Assessment & United States of America. 1988. *How effective is AIDS education?* Washington, DC: GPO.

US Department of Health, Education and Welfare. 1971. *Findings and recommendations: National activities in support of health education.* Report of the President's Committee on Health Education. Washington, DC: GPO.

US Department of Health and Human Services. 1990b. *Healthy people 2000: National health promotion and disease prevention objectives.* Washington, DC: GPO.

US Department of Health and Human Services. November 2000. *Healthy People 2010.* Washington D.C.: GPO.

Vaughen, R. 2004. Editorial, Associate Editor for Statistics and Evaluation. *American Journal of Public Health.* American Public Health Association.

Waage, J., Banerji, R, Campbell, O. et al. 2010. The Millenial Development Goals: A cross-sectional analysis and principles for goal setting after 2015. *Lancet* (September 13): 1–33.

Ward, K., Windsor, R., and Atkinson, J. 2012. A process evaluation of the friendships and dating program for adults with developmental disabilities: Measuring the fidelity of program delivery. *Research and Practice for Persons with Disabilities.*

Warner, K., and Luce, B., 1982. *Cost benefit and cost-effectiveness analysis in health care.* Ann Arbor, MI: Health Administration Press.

Weatherly, H., Drummond, M., and Claxton, K. 2009. Methods for assessing the cost-effectiveness of public health interventions. *Health Policy* 93(2–3): 85–92.

Webb, D., Boyd, R., Messina, T., and Windsor, R. 2003. The discrepancy between self-reported smoking status and urine cotinine levels among women enrolled in pre-natal care at four publicly funded clinical sites. *Journal of Public Health Management Practice* 9(4): 322–325.

Weiss, C. 1972. *Evaluation research: Methods for assessing program effectiveness.* Englewood Cliffs, NJ: Prentice Hall.

Weiss, R. 1994. *Learning from strangers: The art and method of qualitative interview studies.* New York: Free Press.

Williams, J., Belle, G., Houston, C., et al. 2001. Process evaluation methods of a peer-delivered health promotion program for African American women. *Health Promotion Practice* 2(2): 135–142.

Windsor, R., 1981. Improving patient education assessment skills of hospital staff: A case study in diabetes. *Patient Counseling and Health Education* 3(1): 26–29.

Windsor, R. 2010. Behavioral treatment methods for pregnant smokers: The evidence base for prenatal care practice. Invited Chapter in Arden Handler, Joan Kennelly, and Nadine Peacock, Editors. "Reducing Racial/Ethnic Disparities in Reproductive and Perinatal Outcomes: The Evidence From Population-Based Interventions", Springer Publishing, New York.

Windsor, R. 2003. Smoking Cessation and Reduction In Pregnancy Treatment (SCRIPT) Methods: A meta-evaluation of the impact of dissemination. *American Journal of Medical Sciences* 216–222.

Windsor, R., et al. 2005. *A pregnant woman's guide to quit smoking.* Washington, DC: SOPHE.

Windsor, R., Bailey, W., Richards, J., et al, 1990. Evaluation of the efficacy and cost-effectiveness of health education methods to increase medication adherence among adults with asthma. *American Journal of Public Health* 80(12): 1519–1521.

Windsor, R., Baranowski, T., Clark, N., and Cutter, G. 1984. *Evaluation of health promotion and education programs*. Mountain View, CA: Mayfield.

Windsor, R., Baranowski, T., Cutter, G., and Clark, N. 1994. *Evaluation of health promotion, and disease prevention programs*. Mountain View, CA: Mayfield.

Windsor, R., Boyd, N., and Orleans, T. 1998. A meta-evaluation of smoking cessation intervention research among pregnant women: Improving the science and art. *Health Education Research* 13: 419–438.

Windsor, R., Clark, N., Boyd, R., and Goodman, R. 2004. *Evaluation of health promotion, health education, and disease prevention programs*, 3rd ed. New York: McGraw-Hill.

Windsor, R. Clark, J. Cleary S, et al. 2013. Evaluation of the effectiveness of AHRQ Recommended Practice Guidelines and the Smoking Cessation and Reduction In Pregnancy Treatment (SCRIPT) Program: A science to primary care practice partnership. *Maternal and Child Health Journal* 18: 180–190.

Windsor, R., Cleary, S., Ramiah, K., et al. 2013. Development and Evaluation of the Smoking Cessation and Reduction In Pregnancy Treatment (SCRIPT) Adoption Scale (SAS) for prenatal care programs and providers. *Journal of Health Communication* 6: 1–20.

Windsor, R., Cutter, G., and Kronenfeld, J. 1981. Communication methods and evaluation design for a rural cancer screening program. *American Journal of Rural Health* 7(3): 37–45.

Windsor, G. Cutter, J. Kronenfeld, et al. 1981. Increasing utilization of rural cervical cancer detection program. *American Journal of Public Health* 71(6): 641–643.

Windsor, R., Cutter, G., Morris, J., et al. 1985. Effectiveness of self-help smoking cessation intervention research among pregnant women: A randomized trial. *American Journal of Public Health* 76(12): 1389–1392.

Windsor, R., Kronenfeld, J., Ory, M., and Kilgo, J. 1980. Method and design issues in evaluation of community health education programs: A case study in breast and cervical cancer. *Health Education Quarterly* 7(3): 203–218.

Windsor, R., Lowe, J., Perkins, L., et al, 1993. Health education for pregnant smokers: Behavioral impact and cost benefit. *American Journal of Pubic Health* 83(2): 201–206.

Windsor, R., Middlestadt, S., and Radosh, A. 1997. *Evaluation of secondary school HIV/STD prevention education programs: Methodological and design issues to improve the science base*. Project Report: Academy for Educational Development & CDC, Division of Adolescent and School Health (DASH).

Windsor, R., Whiteside, H., Jr., Solomon, L., et al. 2000. A process evaluation model for patient education programs for pregnant smokers. *Tobacco Control* 9(suppl. 3): ii29–ii35.

Windsor, R., Woodby, L., Miller, T., et al, 2000. Effectiveness of agency for health care policy and research clinical practice guidelines and patient education methods for pregnant smokers in Medicaid maternity care. *American Journal of Obstetrics and Gynecology* 182: 68–75.

Windsor, R., Warner, K., and Cutter, G., 1988. A cost-effectiveness analysis of self-health smoking cessation methods for pregnant women. *Public Health Reports* 103(1): 83–87.

Windsor, R., Woodby, L., Miller, T., et al. 2000. Effectiveness of AHCPR clinical practice guideline and patient education methods for pregnant smokers in Medicaid maternity care. *American Journal of Obstetrics and Gynecology* 182: 68–75.

Woolf, S. H. (2009). A closer look at the economic argument for disease prevention. *JAMA* 301(5): 536–38.

World Health Organization. 1986. The Ottawa Charter for Health Promotion. Geneva: WHO.

World Health Organization. 1991. The Sundsvall Statement on Supportive Environments. Geneva: WHO.

World Health Organization. 1997. Jakarta Declaration on Leading Health Promotion into the 21st Century. Geneva: WHO.

World Health Organization. 2000. The Mexico Charter. Geneva: WHO.

World Health Organization. 2005. The Bangkok Charter. Geneva: WHO.

# INDEX

Note: Page numbers followed by an f or t indicate a figure or table respectively.

alpha level
  for environmental tobacco smoke
    reduction program, 136
  in HIV/STD Prevention Intervention, 159
  measure of internal consistency, 202
  in Nepal birth outcomes program, 134
American Heart Association, 38
American Legacy Foundation, 276
American Lung Association, 38
Analysis of Covariance, 112, 260
analysis of validity, 185–190
Appiah-Yeboah, A., 282–284
"Applying Cost Analysis to Public Health
  Programs" (CDC), 289
appropriateness of program, 79
Ary, D., 117
Ask-Advise-Assess-Arrange- Assist
  Procedures, 164
Procedures, 164
assessment, 15t. *See also* evaluation designs;
  evaluation of HP-DP programs
assurance, 15t
asthma patients
  behavioral adherence to intervention,
    181, 301
  cost effectiveness analysis of treatments,
    294, 303–307, 305t, 306t
  designing a program for, 80–81
  health cost in 2015, 307
  physical consequences of intervention, 75
  published consensus reports of, 29
Atkinson, J., 266–276, 271t
attitude variables, 182
attrition bias, 103t, 105–106
attrition rate, 105, 106
audiotaping, 219, 239, 255, 281
availability of programs, 79

background data, 85
Baicker, K., 307–309, 309t
Bailey, William, 303–307, 305t, 306t
Bandura, A., 92, 174
Bangkok Charter for Health Promotion, 45
Baranowski, T., 38, 39
Barnett, S., 170
Barry, D., 179–180
Basch, C., 39, 229
Beccera-Posada, F., 47

behavior impact analysis for HIV/STD
  prevention, 160–161, 161t
behavior science theory, 174
behavioral assessment
  criteria and standards for, 67, 68–69
  for quit-smoking program for older
    adults, 88
behavioral data, 219
behavioral impact
  for asthma education program,
    305–306, 306t
  confirmation of, 301–302
  as core objective of HP-DP programs, 6
  defined, 22
  defining for economic evaluation, 300
  estimation of, 300–301, 310t
  estimation of for SCRIPT program, 313
Behavioral Impact Aims, 147, 148
behavioral intervention program, 174
behavioral risk factors, 21–22
behavioral science research, 174–175
behavioral variables, 182
behaviors
  factors influencing, 74
  interventions designed for
    modification of, 78
  measurement of, 208
  rating by importance and changeability,
    68, 69, 69t
belief variables, 182
Belle, G., 254–258, 256t, 257t
Berg, G., 263–265, 265t
Best Practice Guidelines, 101
biases
  of abstracted medical records, 223–224
  defined, 184
  evaluation designs and, 107–109
  expressed in town hall group
    interviews, 280
  group randomized community trial
    control of, 125–126
  for health-clinical-physiological
    measures, 222
  identification of, 100
  of individual interviews, 277
  to internal validity, categories of, 103t, 104t
  to internal validity, synthesis of, 103–104
  in interviews, 216

discriminant validity, 186t, 192

discussion groups, 62–63, 76

*Disease Control Priorities in Developing Countries* (Jamison, et al.), 289

Dissemination-Translational Evaluation, 8, 21t. *See also* PHASE 4 Dissemination-Translational Evaluations

divergent validity, 194

domains of planning and evaluation, 31–36

downstream indicators, 2

Driscoll, D.

"Formative Assessment of Knowledge and Beliefs Regarding Pandemic Influenza Mitigation Among Culturally Distinct Audience Segments, A," 280–281

"Learning from Truth (sm)," 276–279

"Merging Qualitative and Quantitative Data in Mixed Methods Research," 282–284

"Promoting Prostate-Specific Antigen Informed Decision-Making," 279–280

Drummond, M., 287–288

duration of program, 79

"Easy Breathing" (Clouthier, et al.), 307

ecological assessment, 74–77

ecological variables, 183

economic evaluation

cost-utility analysis, 291, 292–293

defined, 22

development of for HP-DP programs, 286–288

experimental design and, 107–108

purposes of, 315–316

reasons for poor quality, 99

STEP 1: define economic evaluation question-population-problem, 294–295, 294t

STEP 2: define program-intervention-methods-setting, 294t, 295–296

STEP 3: define cost perspective, 294t, 296–297

STEP 4: define program costs and cost analysis methods, 294t, 297–300

STEP 5: define behavioral impact or health outcome, 294t, 300–302

STEP 6: perform a CEA or CBA, 294t, 302–303

STEP 7: perform sensitivity analysis varying plausible cost and impact assumptions, 294t, 303 *See also* cost-benefit analysis (CBA); cost-effectiveness analysis (CEA)

economic recession (2007-2009), 44

education

academic programs for HP-DP specialists, 53

of providers, 231–232

educational assessment, 74–77, 89

"Effect of a Participatory Intervention With Women's Group" (Tripathy, et al.), 170

"Effect of a Participatory Intervention With Women's Groups on Birth Outcomes in Nepal" (Manandhar, et al), 166–170, 168t, 169t

effect size (ES)

as criteria for meta-evaluations, 7

defined, 33, 72

documentation for economic evaluation, 300

effect on sample size, 25

effects of errors, 197

for environmental tobacco smoke reduction program, 136

estimates for HIV/STD Prevention Intervention, 159

estimation of, 131, 171

of media campaigns with/without enforcement message, 73

meta-evaluation estimation of, 7, 18, 22, 70, 71

specification of in meta-analysis, 72

variability by problem, 24

effectiveness, 227, 229

Effectiveness Evaluations, 8, 21t. *See also* PHASE 3 Effectiveness Evaluations

"Effectiveness of AHCPR Clinical Practice Guideline and Patient Education Methods for Pregnant Smokers in Medicaid Maternity Care" (Windsor, et al), 162–166, 165t, 166t

efficacy, 227, 229, 304

"Efficacy and Cost Effectiveness of Health Education Methods to Increase Medication Adherence Among Adults with Asthma, The" (Windsor, et al. 1990), 303–307, 305t, 306t

internal consistency (*Cont.*)
   evaluation of instruments, 214
   of Health Belief Scale and Social Support
      Scale, 202–205, 204t
   methods of analysis, 202
   of SCRIPT Adoption Scale,
      194–196, 196t
internal consistency and item analysis
   case study
   factor and psychometric analysis of SSS
      and HBS, 203–204
   item analysis: item difficulty and
      discrimination for knowledge-skills
      tests, 204
   methods, 201–202, 203t, 204t
   test-retest or stability reliability, 205
internal historical events (Hi), 107
internal peer review, 231
internal program review, 100, 234
internal validity (IV)
   for AHCPR Clinical Practice Guideline
      evaluation, 165–166
   barrier to use, 120
   categories of biases to, 103–107,
      103t, 104t
   of cervical cancer screening program,
      152–153
   controlling for biases, 125–126
   defined, 8, 101
   design of evaluation of, 26
   design selection and, 109
   documentation of, 22
   of environmental tobacco smoke
      reduction program, 138–141
   evaluations of, 23–27
   factors affecting, 20, 101–102
   of federal mine safety training regulation,
      157–158
   generation of current statement of, 30
   of HIV/STD Prevention Intervention,
      161–162
   meta-evaluation of, 71
   of Nepal birth outcomes evaluation,
      169–170
   in non-randomized comparison (C) group
      design, 119
   of quasi-experimental design, 144
   for RFTS-SCRIPT Dissemination Project,
      147–148

   for SCRIPT program, 312
   of worksite health promotion program,
      307–308
International Classification of Disease
   (ICD), 224
international consensus reports on specific
   diseases, 29
*International Initiative for Impact
   Evaluation*, 19
International Union Against Tuberculosis
   and Lung Disease (IUATLD) Bronchial
   Symptoms Questionnaire, 137, 139
inter-observer reliability. *See*
   inter-rater reliability
interpersonal violence interview (IVI),
   268, 269
inter-rater reliability
   defined, 197–198
   internal consistency and item analysis,
      202–205, 203t
   methods establishing, 198–199, 198t
   of observations, 219
   of Partners for Life Program, 260
   reproducibility-consistency, 200–201
   results, 199–200, 200t
   split-half reliability, 201
Inter-Rater Reliability Coefficient, 200t
intervention ( *Xn*), 20
intervention procedures
   definition of, 248–249
   process variables and program tasks,
      248–249, 248t
interventions
   criteria for, 79
   development of, 77–79, 174–175
      *See also* Health Promotion and
         Disease Prevention Program (HP-
         DP); PRECEDE-PROCEED
         Planning Model
interviewer effect, 207
interviewer training, 216–218
interviews
   biases in, 216, 277
   computer assisted telephone
      interviews, 218
   in-depth interviews, 276–277, 284
   as education and ecological assessment
      method, 76
   face-to-face interviews, 215–216, 217

in cervical cancer screening program, 149
  criteria for number in a program, 79
  degree of representation of target
    population, 110
  determining sample size, 129–132, 132t
  in environmental tobacco smoke
    reduction program, 136, 137, 139–140
  in Friendships and Dating Program, 266,
    268, 271t
  in HIV/STD Prevention Intervention, 159
  inclusion and exclusion criteria, 105–106
  interviews with, 276–278
  involvement in planning, implementation,
    evaluation, 59–60, 62
  in Nepal birth outcomes evaluation,
    168, 168t
  randomization of, 122–123
  ratings of *Clear Horizons* program, 95t
  recruitment and retention in Smoke Free
    Family Program, 252, 253
  recruitment for *Clear Horizons* program,
    92–93, 97
  recruitment for environmental tobacco
    smoke reduction program, 136
  recruitment of, 80
  representativeness, 210–211
  in RFTS-SCRIPT Dissemination
    Project, 144 *See also* target population
participation monitoring, 235–237
participatory learning techniques, 167
Partners for Life Program (PFLP)
  conclusion, 263
  formative evaluation design and sample
    size estimation, 260–261
  instrument and measurement, 260
  introduction and background, 258–259
  location and methods, 259–260
  measurement and analysis methods, 261
  peer educator recruitment and
    training, 260
  process evaluation, 261–262, 261t
  results and discussion, 262–263
Partridge, K., 60
patient adherence, 253
patient competence, 222
patient education programs, 176
patient knowledge and self-care skill
    program, 191–193, 191t

Patton, M., 37, 51
Pawtucket Heart Health Project, 38
PBPR-CBPR (Practice-Based and
    Community-Based Participatory
    Research and Program
    Evaluation), 27–28
Pearson, J., 135–141, 138t, 139t
Pearson correlation, 197, 201
peer educators, 255, 260
peer reviews, 12, 50, 53
peer support groups, 56
peer-delivered health promotion program
  introduction, 254–255
  peer training, 255
  process evaluation, 255
  results, 255–256, 256t, 257t, 258
PEM (Process Evaluation Model). *See*
    Process Evaluation Model (PEM)
perceived health, 62
Performance Standard (D)
  for Friendships and Dating Program,
    270, 271t
  for Partners for Life Program, 262
  for Smoke Free Families Program,
    250–251
performance standard/metric (Ps)
  defined, 229
  for health education specialists, 233t
  of peer-delivered nutrition program items,
    256t, 257t
permanently disabling injury (PDI) rates,
    156–157
Perry, D., 135–141, 138t, 139t
personnel costs, 81, 84, 298
personnel services, 85
personnel training, 80–81
PFA (practice flow analysis), 249
PFLP (Partners for Life Program). *See*
    Partners for Life Program (PFLP)
PHASE 1 Formative Evaluations
  for AHCPR Clinical Practice Guideline
    evaluation, 162, 163
  application of factorial designs, 108
  conceptual framework for, 174
  conducting theory-based evaluations,
    174–175
  defined, 7–9
  definition of internal validity, 101

for PHASE 3 and 4 evaluations, 24–25
sampling
  convenience strategy, 273–274
  defined, 65
  methods of, 210–211
  purposive strategy, 273
  random strategy, 273
  representativeness of, 210–211
Sanchez, V., 272
Santayana, George, 173
school-based evaluation of HIV/STD
    prevention program. *See* Healthy &
    Alive (HA) curriculum evaluation
science domain
  description of, 33–34
  as foundational domain, 36
  stakeholders of, 31–32
science-policy-practice gap, 3–4, 46–50, 148
science-policy-practice partnerships,
    3, 35–36
scientific horizon, 30
SCRIPT Adoption Scale (SAS)
  administration of, 194
  construct validity, 193–194
  development of, 179, 193
  factor and convergent validity analysis,
    194, 194t, 195t
  internal consistency and stability,
    194–196, 196t
  reliability evaluation, 196t
  validity evaluation, 187–188, 193–194,
    195–196t
SCRIPT ASSIST components, 312–313
SCRIPT Dissemination Project, 142–143
SCRIPT Policy and Management Committee
    (PMC), 163
SCRIPT procedures, 162, 163, 164
SCRIPT Program
  cessation rates, 301, 310t
  components of, 312
  cost analysis of methods, 313
  cost-benefit analysis of, 309–315, 310t,
    311t, 314t, 315t
  definition of, 312
  dissemination project, 142
  estimation of behavioral impact, 313–314
  evaluation of, 312–315
  factor analysis for scale development
    and construct validity, 193–194,

195–196t *See also* pregnant smokers;
    RFTS-SCRIPT Dissemination Project;
    Smoking Cessation and Reduction
    In Pregnancy Treatment (SCRIPT)
    Adoption Scale (SAS)
Scriven, M., 37
SCT (social cognitive theory). *See*
    social cognitive theory (SCT)
secondary data analysis, 66
secretarial-clerical staff, 81
secretary, 85
selection bias (S)
  in AHCPR Clinical Practice Guideline
    evaluation, 166
  in cervical cancer screening program, 152
  control of, 111
  defined, 103t, 104, 104t, 105–106
  demographic variables revealing, 180–181
  determining effects in environmental
    tobacco smoke reduction program,
    138–140
  in federal mine safety training
    regulation, 157
  for HIV/STD Prevention Intervention,
    161–162
  of Nepal birth outcomes evaluation, 170
  non-randomized comparison group
    control of, 117, 144–145
  one group pre-post test control of,
    112, 113
  in quasi-experimental design, 120, 144
  randomization of sample minimizing, 210
  in randomized pre-test and post-test
    design, 123
  in RFTS-SCRIPT Dissemination Project,
    146, 147
  in school-based evaluation studies,
    125–126, 127, 128
  time series control of, 118–119
  in worksite health promotion
    program, 307
selection-treatment interaction bias, 110–111
self-completion questionnaires, 214–215
self-efficacy
  as core construct of SCT, 175
  measurement in HP-DP programs using
    SCT, 174
  as predictor of impact or outcome rates,
    176, 177